DATE

Psychotherapy with Women

Psychotherapy with Women
EXPLORING DIVERSE CONTEXTS AND IDENTITIES

EDITED BY
Marsha Pravder Mirkin
Karen L. Suyemoto
Barbara F. Okun

FOREWORD BY
Monica McGoldrick

THE GUILFORD PRESS
New York   London

© 2005 The Guilford Press
A Division of Guilford Publications, Inc.
72 Spring Street, New York, NY 10012
www.guilford.com

Printed in the United States of America

This book is printed on acid-free paper.

Last digit is print number: 9 8 7 6 5 4 3 2 1

Library of Congress Cataloging-in-Publication Data

Psychotherapy with women : exploring diverse contexts and identities /
  edited by Marsha Pravder Mirkin, Karen L. Suyemoto,
  Barbara F. Okun.
    p. cm.
  Includes bibliographical references and index.
  ISBN 1-59385-189-8
  1. Women—Mental health—Social aspects. 2. Women—
Psychology—Mental aspects. 3. Psychotherapy—Social
aspects. 4. Women—Social conditions. I. Mirkin, Marsha Pravder,
1953– II. Suyemoto, Karen L. III. Okun, Barbara F.
RC451.4.W6P796 2005
616.89′0082—dc22

                                                    2005005951

*In memory of Ann Goldman Pravder,
Sadie Sunshine Goldman,
and Annie Olarnik Prafder,
my mother and grandmothers, for their courage in
starting all over again in this country and for
allowing me to stand on their shoulders and reach
for the stars*

—M. P. M.

*For Jim (James Meyer, Jr.),
my friend and mentor, who taught me the meaning
of good therapy and helped me develop strategies to
resist oppression*

—K. L. S.

*In memory of Henry G. Altman,
who empowered me to grow as a woman in my
personal and professional lives*

—B. F. O.

About the Editors

Marsha Pravder Mirkin, PhD, is a clinical psychologist and resident scholar at the Brandeis University Women's Studies Research Center. She is on the faculty at Lasell College. Dr. Mirkin's interest in unheard voices and alternatives to the dominant discourse led her to edit *Women in Context: Toward a Feminist Reconstruction of Psychotherapy* (1994, Guilford Press) and write her recently released book *The Women Who Danced by the Sea: Finding Ourselves in the Stories of Our Biblical Foremothers* (2004, Monkfish). She has served on the faculties of the Cambridge Hospital Couples and Family Training Program, Harvard Medical School, and the Jean Baker Miller Institute of the Stone Center at Wellesley College.

Karen L. Suyemoto, PhD, is Assistant Professor in Psychology and Asian American Studies at the University of Massachusetts–Boston, where she teaches classes related to race, culture, and gender. She has published and presented primarily on topics related to racial and cultural identity, particularly in multiracial and Asian American people. Dr. Suyemoto's current research projects explore how interventions of education and community programs may affect racial and ethnic identities and empowerment in Asian American youth and college students.

Barbara F. Okun, PhD, is Professor and Training Director of the combined school and counseling psychology doctoral program at Northeastern University. She served for 10 years on the faculty of the Cambridge Hospital Couples and Family Therapy Training Program, Harvard Medical School. Dr. Okun maintains a diverse clinical practice in individual, couple, and family therapy. Her books include *Effective Helping: Interviewing and Counseling Techniques* (6th ed., 2002, Brooks/Cole), *Understanding Diversity: A Learning-as-Practice Primer* (with J. Fried and M. L. Okun; 1999, Brooks/Cole), and *Understanding Diverse Families: What Practitioners Need to Know* (1996, Guilford Press).

Contributors

Mizuho Arai, PhD, is a full-time faculty member at the University of Massachusetts–Boston, where she teaches courses in sociology, psychology, and women's studies. She has focused her research on the professional development of women and issues of family violence from a cross-cultural perspective. Her greatest satisfaction comes from seeing her students realize their potential as they succeed in life.

Marilyn Braithwaite-Hall, EdM, is a doctoral student in counseling psychology at Northeastern University. She is personally and professionally curious about the ways that African American spirituality informs and guides the individual and the collective. She maneuvers through her multiple identities of mother, wife, student, and human being with a sense of gratitude and determination.

Vanessa Jackson, LCSW, is a therapist in private practice in Atlanta, Georgia. She is the author of *In Our Own Voice: African-American Stories of Oppression, Survival and Recovery in Mental Health Systems* and *Separate and Unequal: The Legacy of Racially Segregated Psychiatric Hospitals,* two monographs on the history of African American psychiatric experiences; she also contributed the chapter "Surviving My Sister's Suicide: A Journey through Grief" to the book *Living Beyond Loss: Death in the Family.* She is a nationally recognized speaker on mental health issues

Sandra J. Jones, PhD, is a developmental psychologist and resident scholar at the Brandeis University Women's Studies Research Center. She was a visiting scholar at the Wellesley College Center for Research on Women for 2 years, as well as an adjunct faculty member at Lesley University and the University of Massachusetts–Boston. Her work in narrative analysis, women's subjectivities, upward mobility, and working-class consciousness has been published in journal articles and book chapters.

Judith V. Jordan, PhD, is the codirector of the Jean Baker Miller Training Institute of the Stone Center, Wellesley College, where she is also director of training and a founding scholar. She is an attending psychologist at McLean Hospital and an assistant professor of psychology at Harvard Medical School. She founded the Women's Studies Program and Women's Treatment Network at McLean Hospital, and served as its first director. Dr. Jordan works as a psychotherapist, supervisor, teacher, and consultant. She is coauthor of *Women's Growth in Connection,* editor of *Women's Growth in Diversity,* and coeditor of *The Complexity of Connection.*

Grace S. Kim, MA, is a PhD candidate in clinical psychology at the University of Massachusetts–Boston. Her research and clinical interests focus on how experiences of belonging and exclusion relate to racial and ethnic identity development. She has conducted research on Korean transracial adoptees and Asian American high school students.

Jodie Kliman, PhD, is a psychologist and family therapist on the faculty of the Massachusetts School of Professional Psychology, where she teaches family therapy and narrative therapy and trains doctoral students placed at a local high school. She is on the board of directors of the American Family Therapy Academy, and is a member of the Network for Multicultural Training in Psychology and the Council on Contemporary Families. Dr. Kliman offers training in culturally respectful family therapy, systems work on the collective trauma of war and terror, and network therapy. Her private practice is in Brookline, Massachusetts. She is also the editor of *Touched by War Zones: Oscillations of Despair and Hope.*

Roxana Llerena-Quinn, PhD, is a psychologist in the Latino Program at Children's Hospital in Boston. She is eternally indebted to the many Latino/Latina families from whom she has learned the wisdom that is born out of living in the shadows. She facilitates with others a cultural self-awareness course for faculty and medical students at Harvard Medical School.

Sukie Magraw, PhD, is the director of the doctoral psychology program at John F. Kennedy University in Pleasant Hill, California, the mission of which is to train students to work with culturally diverse and underserved populations. She also maintains a small private practice. She lives with her partner and their daughter in Oakland, California.

Marsha Pravder Mirkin, PhD (see "About the Editors").

Lise Motherwell, PhD, PsyD, is a faculty member in the Center for Psychoanalytic Studies and an associate in psychology at Massachusetts General Hospital, an instructor at Harvard Medical School, and the president of the Northeastern Society for Group Psychotherapy. She recently published *Complex Dilemmas in Group Therapy: Pathways to Resolution* with coeditor Joseph Shay. Dr. Motherwell maintains a private practice in Brookline, Massachusetts, where she treats children, adolescents, and adults in individual and group therapies.

Barbara F. Okun, PhD (see "About the Editors").

Tracy L. Robinson-Wood, EdD, is a professor in the Department of Counseling and Applied Educational Psychology at Northeastern University. She teaches master's- and doctoral-level courses in research, research design, multicultural psychology, and diversity. She is the author of the textbook *The Convergence of Race, Ethnicity, and Gender: Multiple Identities in Counseling*. Dr. Robinson-Wood's research interests focus on the intersections of race, gender, class, and culture in psychosocial identity development. She has developed an instrument called the Robinson Resistance Modality Inventory (RRMI), and is conducting empirical research on African American women, resistance, stress, and racial identity development.

Patricia Romney, PhD, is a psychologist who consults with individuals and organizations throughout the United States. Using her finely honed assessment skills as a starting point for change efforts, she has assisted organizations in the areas of diversity, community building, conflict resolution, and leadership development.

Maria P. P. Root, PhD, is a psychologist in private practice in Seattle, Washington. She has published several books dealing with the topics of interracial couples, families, and their children, including the award-winning *Racially Mixed People in America* (1992), *Love's Revolution* (2001), and *The Multiracial Child Resource Book* (2003). She is also known for her published work on trauma, disordered eating, and Asian American mental health.

Eileen Santa, MA, is a doctoral student in the clinical psychology program at the University of Massachusetts–Boston. She is interested in the contribution of cultural protective factors to Latino/Latina maternal and child health. Currently, she is in the Washington, D.C., area, pursuing her interest in applying psychological research to public policy issues related to ethnic minorities and women.

Gretchen Schmelzer, PhD, is a senior consultant with Teleos Leadership Institute, an international consulting firm serving leaders of Fortune 100 businesses and major not-for-profit organizations such as the United Nations. Her expertise includes extensive work in psychological and cognitive assessment, family and organizational systems, and interventions for treating traumatic stress in children and adults. Dr. Schmelzer is also a lecturer in the Department of Counseling and Applied Educational Psychology at Northeastern University.

Ester R. Shapiro, PhD, is an associate professor of psychology at the University of Massachusetts–Boston, and a research associate at the Mauricio Gaston Institute for Latino Public Policy and Community Development. She helped found a clinical training program dedicated to delivering urban services from cultural, developmental, interdisciplinary, and health promotion perspectives. Dr. Shapiro is the author of *Grief as a Family Process: A Developmental Approach to Clinical Practice* (1994), as well as numerous articles on family development, culture and grief, resilience among urban immigrant adolescents and families, and multimethod program evaluation based on a sociocultural developmental model.

Barbara A. Stewart, MD, is an internist on the staffs of both Beth Israel Hospital and Brigham and Women's Hospital in Boston. She is also a nationally ranked runner. In 2002, she founded Strategies for Health, a company that allows her to focus her medical practice on prevention, women's issues, and strategies to optimize medical (and other) outcomes.

Karen L. Suyemoto, PhD (see "About the Editors").

Nadine Tafoya, MSW, has spent over 20 years addressing issues of cultural diversity and the behavioral health needs of Native Americans locally and nationally. She was a recipient of the 19th Annual Governor's Award for Outstanding New Mexico Women.

Hugh Vasquez, MSW, is the founder of the Todos Institute and a partner with the Center for Diversity Leadership in the San Francisco Bay Area. Now a private consultant, Mr. Vasquez conducts trainings, provides consultation, and delivers presentations on equity, social justice, and diversity-related topics to organizations throughout the United States.

Lauren Gallo Ziady, MA, is a doctoral student in counseling psychology at Northeastern University in Boston, Massachusetts. Her interest in the career development of women with disabilities developed during a doctoral seminar in lifespan development. She is currently working on her doctoral dissertation studying the neuropsychological implications of disorganized attachment.

Foreword

Psychotherapy with Women: Exploring Diverse Contexts and Identities reflects another decade of the leavening of the multidimensional perspective presented in *Women in Context* (Mirkin, 1994). The book is a remarkable accomplishment by a group of brilliant, creative women about the multidimensional process of therapy with women.

Psychotherapy with Women is an extraordinary resource for clinicians on women's issues, as well as a timely rethinking of many of the issues we have been taught about until now primarily from a white, male, privileged perspective, in spite of feminist efforts and lip service that now gets paid to multiculturalism in psychology. In its multidimensional approach, the book offers a complete re-visioning of traditional psychological thinking. Its perspective transforms even the developing literature on women and psychotherapy by considering culture, race, class, and gender as basic to any discussion of women, their problems, the life cycle, and clinical practice. As the editors note in their introduction, to understand women in context "necessitates looking beyond the now and addressing multiple historical contexts of individual women and the social systems to which they belong." Marsha Pravder Mirkin, Karen L. Suyemoto, and Barbara F. Okun have taken a major leap forward in helping us to think in more inclusive ways—they are lighting the way for this crucial paradigm shift. This contemporary update to *Women in Context* has brought in two additional editors and many new authors. Each chapter is full of theoretical, clinical, and cultural insights and expands our understanding of women's lives as reflected in the clinical work of these amazing writers. The authors and editors have followed through on their promise to examine each issue from multiple cultural perspectives and to include the therapist's own cultural experience as part of their focus (Chapter 16). There are wonderful insights: about the gender and generational dilemmas of immigrant women (Ester R. Shapiro and Eileen Santa, Chapter 6), women's particular dilemmas regarding class differences within a family because of their socialization to be responsible for maintaining family relationships (Sandra J. Jones, Chapter 7), and women in the workplace transforming hierarchical gender and racial structures (Judith V. Jordan & Patricia Romney, Chapter 9). Hugh Vasquez and Sukie Magraw (Chapter 3) challenge us to become active agents for understanding how privilege and oppression operate in our therapy work and to make our efforts at cultural competence a lifetime effort involving ongoing social action in and out of the therapy room. Roxana Llerena-Quinn and Marsha Pravder Mirkin (Chapter 4) provide many insights about working with immigrant mothers and the specific problems for transnational mothers who work as caregivers for U.S. children, while their own children remain in their country of origin. Maria P. P. Root and Karen L. Suyemoto (Chapter 5) raise some crucial clinical questions about love across class, race, and accepted gender lines. Barbara F. Okun and Lauren Gallo Ziady (Chapter 10) help us consider the many problems women have balancing family responsibilities in a context that provides inadequate child care support and work systems that still largely discriminate against women.

This book offers a creative weaving together of the theoretical perspectives on the multiple dimensions of our identities (Chapters 2 and 16)—gender, race, ethnicity, class, sexual orientation, and religion—with very readable case examples. It presents a nuanced analysis of the ways our multiple identities in therapy are co-constructed (Chapter 1), elucidating how much more useful we are the clearer we are about these dimensions and the interface of our multiple identities with those of our clients. Having read this book, no one can go back to the standard texts without a profound awareness of their glaring inadequacy. Every chapter addresses women in their multifaceted complexity. Each author has done her or his homework in reviewing the subject at hand from the standpoint of diversity. What a boon to our field to read so many articulate, well-informed authors who are able to steer our thinking in the new and important direction of overcoming our racism, sexism, classism, and heterosexism.

The examples in the book offer a sophisticated and well-written analysis of the multiple layers of women's cultural identities through the lifespan and how these are reflected in clinical situations. The writing draws you in—no dry treatises that preach a new vision, but human and practical discussion, with all the lumps and difficulties of real life that do not fit well together. The authors move comfortably from theory to the complexities of our sociopolitical world to real women in their everyday lives. The theoretical discussion is tied brilliantly to case implications, and the chapters range over the life cycle and through a broad array of issues central to women's lives. Gretchen Schmelzer and Lise Motherwell (Chapter 12) explore the importance of play in working with women, who so often do not feel entitled to create the space in their lives of caring for others to play themselves. Issues of women's health and mental health, which have until now been largely ignored, are covered (Barbara A. Stewart and Barbara F. Okun, Chapter 15), as are women in relation to therapy (Jodie Kliman, Chapter 2). Most important, this discussion of psychological issues includes all kinds of women. Nadine Tafoya (Chapter 14) discusses culturally congruent interventions with Native Americans and ways of incorporating native healing customs in work with women emerging from adolescence. Mizuho Arai (Chapter 8) explores the differences among Asian cultures in basic gender attitudes and values and in adaptation of Asian immigrant women to the United States, and the implications of these differences for clinical practice. Tracy L. Robinson-Wood and Marilyn Braithwaite-Hall (Chapter 13) discuss how one encourages dialogue about religion and spirituality within clinical contexts, such as working with a Christian lesbian African American. They emphasize the importance of understanding how the structural issues of therapy may differ from other relationships in that therapy has a beginning and an end, the client shares more information than the therapist, and the therapist, but not the client, is required to maintain confidentiality. Within these constraints the authors explore the importance of considering the intersections of culture, religion, spirituality, gender, and sexual orientation in our clinical work.

This book shows how we can develop and share a collective consciousness with other women about the patriarchal, hierarchical context of all our behavior. Vanessa Jackson (Chapter 11) raises pivotal issues about the concept of poverty as trauma, discussing the themes of survivor guilt and of being a class traitor for those who are upwardly mobile, and the extent to which poverty keeps people invisible in this society. She places the issue of poverty squarely in its historical context.

We must radically change our training to encourage our field to have the courage to acknowledge and deal with the complexity made apparent in this book. Bravo and good luck to all who will read this book for the new paths it suggests for our work and our lives!

MONICA MCGOLDRICK, LCSW, PHD (h.c.)

Reference

Mirkin, M. P. (Ed.). (1994). *Women in context: Toward a feminist reconstruction of psychotherapy.* New York: Guilford Press.

Acknowledgments

We are very fortunate to have worked with a supportive, professional team at The Guilford Press. We would like to thank Jim Nageotte, Senior Editor, who helped nurture this project from the start; Judith Grauman, Managing Editor, for always having such helpful answers to our questions; and Laura Patchkofsky, Senior Production Editor, whose attention to the process allowed us to complete this book in a timely way.

A special thank you to our clients who have taught us and challenged us and helped us to better understand both them and ourselves.

We are deeply appreciative of the thoughtfulness, responsiveness, and dedication of our chapter authors who have shared so much of their expertise here. The three of us are also grateful that we had the chance to work with each other—that we could challenge and support each other through the sometimes murky waters of our own multiple identities that incorporate our own privilege and marginalization.

We would like to add that we contributed equally to the text and the order of editorship does not reflect any difference in level of contribution.

I (M. P. M.) would like to acknowledge the women and men in my life who have inspired me, challenged me, and helped me develop my commitment to psychological explorations of social justice. A thank you to Dr. Shulamit Reinharz, Director of the Women's Studies Research Center (WSRC) at Brandeis University, for providing me a "home" where I could edit this volume. I am grateful to my colleagues at the WSRC for energizing my writing through exposure to their inspirational work and ideas.

I would also like to thank my dear friends and colleagues at the American Family Therapy Academy for giving me a circle of people with whom to honestly explore the issues represented in this book. While I know this is only a partial listing, I'd like to thank Nancy Boyd-Franklin, Rachel Dash,

Donna DeMuth, Mona Fishbane, Nydia Garcia-Preto, Ann Hartman, Jaime Inclan, Hugo Kamya, Jodie Kliman, Joan Laird, Judy Libow, Roxana Llerena-Quinn, Don-David Lusterman, Monica McGoldrick, Elaine Pinderhughes, Pat Romney, CharlesEtta Sutton, David Trimble, and Marianne Walters.

I want to thank my students at Lasell College. It is a true privilege to learn from you.

And to my dear husband, Mitch, and our daughters, Allison and Jessica: I couldn't have done this without you—your love inspires me all the time to learn more, do more, and change more about myself and our society.

I (K. L. S.) would like to thank the colleagues, mentors, and friends who have opened my eyes, validated my perspectives, worked with (and through) difficult moments of oppression and privilege, and helped me develop the abilities to build bridges and map terrains. An incomplete list includes: Julie Ahn, Mary Ballou, Chris Bobel, Stephanie Day, Juanita Dimas, Peter Kiang, Grace Kim, Terrell Lasane, Joan Liem, Nancy Lin, Phuong Nguyen, Maria Felix Ortiz, Lizabeth Roemer, Carin Rosenberg, Willie Sanchez, Rajini Srikanth, John Tawa, Claudia Fox Tree, and Jennifer Wolfrum.

My deep gratitude to the many students in the classes I have taught (about race, culture, and gender particularly) who have pushed me to think more, feel more, and challenge my own assumptions. You have taught me so much through sharing your lives and perspectives, through taking the risk to expose your fears and vulnerabilities, and through daring to show me my own areas of bias and blindness.

I (B. F. O.) would like to acknowledge the significant female influences in my life: Donna Raymer, devoted friend and mentor; Goldie Okun, inspirational mother-in-law; Marcia Okun, daughter and coauthor; and Jane Fried, coauthor and colleague.

In addition, I want to acknowledge my appreciation to my students, trainees, and colleagues (both at Northeastern University and at the national and international sites where I have been privileged to work) who continuously stimulate my learning and growth by sharing their own perspectives and thinking.

Contents

Psychotherapy with Women

Introduction

Marsha Pravder Mirkin
Karen L. Suyemoto
Barbara F. Okun

This second edition of *Women in Context* emerges from the impact of dramatically changing sociocultural systems on women's lives. Over 10 years ago, when the first edition of *Women in Context* was published, we lived in a different world. Our demographics have shifted so that the dominant white population is no longer the majority in this country (Hacker, 2003). Our understandings have become more complex and less compartmentalized to reflect our greater comprehension of the diversity of women in the United States as well as the many social changes experienced by these diverse women. For example, although women working outside the home has become an expected and unremarkable phenomenon in the last few decades, most of the scholarship on women in the workforce has investigated white, middle-class, married women or college students. However, the factors of class, sexual orientation, race, culture, disability, and so on, significantly impact the ways that women create balance between family and work and the meanings of the choices involved for each woman and her family. Lesbian marriages were only a dream 10 years ago, whereas now legal lesbian weddings take place in Massachusetts. Lesbian couples with adoptive or biological children (in contrast to those with children from previous heterosexual marriages) were practically unheard of 10 years ago, but now becoming more the norm. There are more interracial marriages, international adoptions, and upward and downward social mobility than ever before (Hacker, 2003). These shifts revise and revamp our understanding of the intersections of privilege and marginalization. Given the changing world, how women create balance in their lives and take care of themselves need to be re-visioned. Our understandings of and scholarship related to work, relationships (such as marriages and mothering), and self-care need to encompass these changes.

Before we continue our discussion of changes in the past decade, let us focus on what we mean by the term "context." Actually, "context" has several meanings for us. Our primary meaning addresses context as the macrosystem(s) that impacts a person. Here, when we use the word *context* we are specifically referring to social categorizations and systems, such as gender, race, culture, class, ethnicity, sexual orientation, etc. We understand these social systems as related to hierarchies of power and privilege because (1) one's opportunities and resources are shaped by one's status/categorization within these systems; (2) one's status/categorization within these systems is not necessarily individually chosen, but may be assigned or ascribed by others with more power (although this labeling can, of course, be resisted); and (3) the meanings in these systems related to "acceptable" or "healthy" living are defined by the dominant group within a society (e.g., in the United States by white, European American, heterosexual, Christian, middle/upper-class men). Exploring the contexts in which women live means exploring their lives, experiences, and challenges in interaction with these social systems.

"Context" has two additional meanings that emerge in this text. One is temporal: Several chapters (particularly the three chapters in Part I) refer explicitly to a *sociohistorical* context, and most chapters rest implicitly on an understanding that the context can be understood as the social systems that have shaped the meanings attached to people and groups over time. Although women of color may have greater opportunities now than ever before, the legacies of slavery, wars, and/or colonization within communities are internalized within families and individuals and affect their current experiences. Similarly, although women from working-class backgrounds may develop financial status related to being middle class, their own personal histories as working-class women continue to affect their experiences. To understand women in context necessitates looking beyond the now and addressing historical contexts of individual women and the social systems to which they belong.

Finally, there is a situational meaning of "context" that is reflected in the structure of this book: relationships, work, and self-care are all different types of situational contexts. Situational contexts vary in their relationships, their goals, their importance to women, etc. The meanings of a social systemic context for a particular woman will vary according to the situational context which she is addressing at a given moment. For example, the meaning, rewards, and challenges of being an African American woman who is economically disadvantaged will be very different in relation to her context as a partner to an Asian American lesbian, in relation to her context as a mother, in relation to her working context, her religion/spirituality, her need to develop a healthy lifestyle that minimizes her risk of disease, and so on. To work successfully and sensitively with women in context necessitates understanding that women's meanings vary in relation to different people and life demands. Therapists must explore the different situational contexts within which a woman moves to fully understand her social systemic context and its effects on her functioning, whether healthy or problematic.

Although considerable social changes have opened doors to new experiences for women, at the same time women's rights and choices are being chipped away. Constitutional rights are being challenged and the role of the Supreme Court is in transformation. Since 9/11, the privileged, for the first time in the United States, now feel unsafe; the nonprivileged never felt safe. The Patriot Act curtails the rights and choices of women as well as men. The anti-immigrant and anti-Arab response to 9/11 and the current conservative administration affect women as well as men. The results of the 2004 presidential election challenge women's choices regarding abortion, economic and emotional security, access to health and social services, lesbian civil unions or marriage, immigration, bilingualism, and so on. In the United States, the rich are getting richer and the poor are getting poorer; the middle class is disappearing. Poor health benefits, unemployment, and homelessness are impacting groups that heretofore enjoyed privilege. It is certainly likely that the national efforts to support wars such as the one in Iraq will affect women's lives, not only because every soldier has or is a mother, sister, or friend, and every death is mourned, but also because the national discourse will have to address conscription of women. At the intersection of contexts, we see that it is the financially disadvantaged and people of color who are often the targets of military recruiters, and an increasing number of women are volunteering to join the armed forces.

In the international arena, we have noticed an alarming increase in the polarization of liberal/progressive groups pitted against fundamentalist/conservative groups. This polarization leads to heightened conflicts over civil rights and cultural sensitivity. The political ramifications are enormous. Relationships are changing, the international community has changed, and mistrust and fear of terrorism have made everyone feel vulnerable.

The climates of our professional disciplines have also changed, in that they now actively support, and even mandate, multicultural training. There is a major expectation from professional and training institutions that all clinicians work in a culturally sensitive manner. However, there is variation in the definitions and implementation of "cultural sensitivity." Clinical practice has become more subsumed into a managed care mentality, in which services are regulated more by cost-effectiveness than by clinical judgment. Community mental health services have been reduced in scope and are time limited; symptom reduction therapy has become the norm. Brief, empirically validated practices are encouraged along with the increased use of medication. These changes result in a fixed formula: "One short-term/medication therapy type for all."

These changes are among the many that have influenced our focus in this volume. The interaction of social justice and psychotherapy receives short shrift during these times. Whereas basic multicultural considerations and studies were cutting edge 10 years ago, today we are more aware of the dilemmas created from the complexities and interactions in our social contexts. As we live in a more multicultural society, we look at race, sexuality, gender, ethnicity, religion, and sexual orientation in multidimensional, interdependent contexts. We are more cognizant of the intragroup diversity and, hopefully, more sensitive to the impact of privilege on individuals as well as on groups. We feel it is necessary, but no longer sufficient, to consider single aspects of diversity as if they affect women's lives in one single way. Rather, we need to explore the *intersections* of social systemic contexts such as race, gender, class, and ethnicity within particular lived contexts, such as women's intimate relationships, their work environments, and their self-care habits. We believe that the contributions of our diverse authors share our commitment to understand women in their changing multiple contexts, and we believe that the material in this volume must be integrated into current psychotherapy theory and practice.

We aim to provide a clinical understanding of, and suggestions for, interventions with diverse women as we address issues related to identity, roles, rules, functions, and strengths and weaknesses in love, work, and play. Our major focus is on psychotherapy issues of gender, race, culture, sexual orientation, and class, as they are experienced in lived contexts. We seek to make connections between larger contexts and systems of oppression and the lived experiences of women, particularly related to relationships, work, and self-care. The topics and approaches chosen for inclusion in each section represent areas that have not been widely explored from this perspective. The contributing authors embody diversity in race, ethnicity, sexual orientation, class, age, religion, and spirituality. Each writes from her or his unique perspectives and also from a broad systemic/ecological perspective. We believe that this broad systemic/ecological context enables clinicians and their clients to transcend conventional/traditional notions of development and difficulties as well as to achieve balance in the three major life areas (love, work, and self-care) and a fuller appreciation of the interactions between strengths and difficulties.

This volume is divided into four parts. Part I, which formulates the conceptual framework for the book, consists of three chapters that explore the systemic/ecological and social justice perspectives generally and in relation to individual and family therapy and the role of the therapist. Each chapter addresses the interaction between therapist and client within this ecological framework. The section provides a foundation for the chapters in each of the remaining sections that focus on relationships, work, and self-care. Chapters 1 and 2 emphasize the multiple models of intersection—individual, family, and larger systems, along with the individual and systemic variables of gender, class, religion, race, ethnicity, sexual orientation, and so forth—that shape all aspects of human development and behavior. Chapter 3 focuses on the therapeutic relationship, stressing the collaborative, activist position of therapist as ally.

Part II focuses on women's interpersonal relationships, particularly the differences within those relationships. Much has already been written about relationships generally, so in this book we focus on how intersecting contexts and statuses affect different types of relationships: intimate relationships (among lesbians as well as heterosexuals), sibling relationships, and parent–child relationships across cultural, geographical, and generational divides. Chapter 4 discusses the issues that affect immigrant mothers and their children. Chapter 5 studies interracial and intercultural intimate relationships, and Chapter 6 focuses specifically on the intersection of gender and generation within Latina immigrant families. Part II concludes with Chapter 7, which discusses research on the impact of upward class mobility within family systems, with particular attention to sibling relationships.

Part III covers areas of women's work that have not received much attention in the literature. Today, work outside of the home is so prevalent that clinicians must consider how women balance their lives and how work status affects women's identity, strengths, and limitations. The influence of Asian American women's cultures on their work choices and behaviors is explored in Chapter 8. The focus on organizational consulting from a psychological model in Chapter 9 raises questions about how work done individually with middle management impacts the larger system. Chapter 10 addresses the organizational contexts of work and career development as well as the work issues of lesbians and women with disabilities. Chapter 11 attends to the intersection of work and class; most of the literature about women's work has focused on professional and educated women's issues.

There is not much talk among therapists and in the literature about self-nurturance, which is therefore the focus of Part IV. Chapter 12 discusses the importance and experience of play in women's lives throughout the lifespan, and the importance of play as a component of the therapy experience. Focusing on African American women, Chapter 13 explores the significance of addressing spirituality in psychotherapy. Chapter 14 focuses on the importance of community in fostering Native American women's resiliency, healthy living, and ability to deal with sociopolitical oppression. Chapter 15 highlights relevant information about women's salient health issues and mind–body connections, with the goal of preventing disease or at least achieving early diagnosis and intervention. These writers suggest strongly that an essential part of any psychotherapy includes attention to lifestyle, the cultivation of healthy living habits, and collaboration with clients' health care providers.

In Part V, the final chapter elucidates the editors' reflections about their learning and collaboration processes and their ideas for future directions of study.

We three editors are of different generations, classes, races, ethnicities, religions, and sexual orientations (although we are all in heterosexual relationships). We came together gradually over 1½ years after our editor at The Guilford Press, Jim Nageotte, queried Marsha about revising the first edition of *Women in Context*. Marsha asked Barbara if she would be interested in collaborating on this project, and they began to think about how they could update the topics covered in the first volume. After discussing her thoughts with Karen and reading some of Karen's work on multiple identities, Barbara suggested that Karen join us, and Marsha was open to that possibility. As we began to discuss this project, our thoughts veered from a revision of previously covered topics to extending the theme of the last volume to look not only at diversity but also at the intersections among contexts. Jim suggested we look at the three aspects of women's lives: relationships, work, and self-care.

Over time, as we began to share our visions of this book and as we listened to each other and to our editor, we developed trust and our excitement mounted. We learned that, despite our differences, we share a passion for lifelong learning and for understanding diverse women in multiple contexts, as well as a commitment to challenging traditional assumptions and paradigms. We have learned so much from our work with each other and with our chapter authors. Our personal and professional relationships have deepened and we have become, despite Marsha's original concerns and uncertainties about how much energy and time she could commit to yet another project, a truly egalitarian, collaborative team.

We believe that our authors, who represent diversity in terms of their levels of experience, professional training, and fields of interest (in addition to the cultural diversities previously mentioned), will excite your appetite for learning and diverse thinking.

Reference

Hacker, A. (2003). *Mismatch*. New York: Scribner's.

PART I

Foundational Contexts

CHAPTER 1

Journeys through Diverse Terrains

MULTIPLE IDENTITIES AND SOCIAL CONTEXTS
IN INDIVIDUAL THERAPY

Karen L. Suyemoto
Grace S. Kim

Maria was a single, second-generation Mexican American woman in her late 20s from the southwest United States. She was referred by her primary care physician and came to see me (KLS) during the winter with symptoms of severe depression that included dysphoria, loss of appetite, sleep disturbance, fatigue, anhedonia, difficulty concentrating, feelings of worthlessness, and excessive guilt. These symptoms had begun approximately 1 month after she had entered graduate school. As a result, she dropped out of graduate school and returned to her older brother's family home to live. Maria stated that she thought she was not good enough because she was not doing what she should do: living up to her family's expectations and ideals.

Maria's emotional difficulties first occurred in her early teens, when she felt despondent, lethargic, and had difficulty concentrating. During the fall and winter of each of her college years, Maria experienced depressive episodes that were treated primarily with medication and short-term psychotherapy through her college mental health services. Maria experienced no depressive episode in the 2 years after college when she lived with her older brother's family and worked, prior to returning to graduate school.

Maria's parents were devout Catholics. Her father was a blue-collar worker and her mother worked part time as a domestic. When Maria first came to therapy, she was involved in a relationship with a Latino

man, whom she had been seeing for approximately 1 year; she identified herself as heterosexual.

Jenny was a third grader who was referred to therapy with me (GSK)
by her school guidance counselor because of her behavioral problems
and hyperactivity. According to the school guidance counselor, Jenny
had been "bullying" several other girls at school. Jenny and her
mother explained that in the previous year, Jenny had been bullied by
the same girls; they had pushed her and called her names. This year she
started to retaliate against them. Jenny was involved in a few fights
with these girls, which included verbal arguments and kicking (by
Jenny). Following a recent argument with one of the girls, Jenny was
placed on in-school suspension status, which prompted her mother to
seek therapy for her. Jenny also exhibited concentration difficulties,
general impulsivity, and hyperactivity.
     Jenny was a multiracial child who lived with her white European
American mother and her white European American stepfather. She
had not had contact with her African American father since very early
childhood. Jenny had a close relationship with her mother, obtained
average to high-average grades at school, and maintained a few close
friendships at school. A high school graduate, Jenny's mother worked
as a bank teller, and Jenny's family lived in subsidized housing in an
affluent suburb. Jenny's stepfather, who had only recently married
Jenny's mother, worked as a mechanic. Although Jenny had limited
contact with her biological father's and stepfather's families, she was
very close to her maternal grandparents, aunts, and uncles, and frequently visited her cousins.

As is the case with most clients, there are myriad ways to understand
Maria and Jenny, multiple areas to explore, and many places from which to
begin asking questions. To use a metaphor, there are an infinite number of
pathways to the central goal of understanding and helping. Therapeutic
orientation as well as general values will have a great impact on which
pathway is chosen. Some may be narrow pathways, paved and constrained
by walls and relatively disconnected from the environmental contexts
through which they pass. Others may travel across uncharted open fields or
wind through forests, with guidance only visible to those trained to see.
Many of these paths will stay within one terrain at a given time or explore
each in sequence (moving from forest to savanna to desert to ocean). We
believe that the challenge for multicultural feminist therapists committed to
social justice is not only to understand how these environments affect the
individual (and vice versa), but also to understand how these environments
interact within, and depend upon, each other to create meaning and sustain
health. In this chapter we have two primary aims: (1) to provide basic
understandings of definitions, contexts, and the complexity of interactions

and thereby create a foundation for the later chapters; and (2) to share our attempts to create a map that connects the multiple pathways and assists us as therapists to see their interdependence. In less metaphorical language, we will share our attempts to conceptualize the multiple contributions of individual, group, and systemic contexts and meanings as they are integrated and enacted in individuals, so that we as therapists can provide a therapy that embraces the holistic person within her multiple contexts. We will return to Maria and Jenny repeatedly throughout the chapter.

Multiple Identities:
Social and Individual Meanings

Western philosophy and social sciences, including psychology, have conceptualized identity as an endeavor that is primarily individually formed or decided upon, although influenced by social relationships. For instance, various ego identity theories (e.g., Blasi, 1988; Erikson, 1968; Marcia, 1994) suggest that individuals contemplate their identities internally and individually, while referencing different social groups. Social discrepancies create internal conflicts that the individual works through in order to maintain a continuous and authentic self-identity. This individualistic idea of identity works well with an individualistic orientation to therapy, in which the focus is helping the individual change internal affects and understandings to create a sense of self that fits well within his or her social environment. However, this individualistic orientation has been criticized by many feminist and multicultural therapists as overpathologizing, potentially oppressive to minorities and women, and depoliticized (see, e.g., Sue & Sue, 2002): We see this view as the narrow, walled, paved pathway mentioned above.

In contrast, we (and others) conceptualize identity as a more interactive co-constructive process embedded in multiple contexts, systems, and meanings (Huo, 1998; Kim, 2003; Shotter, 1993; Suyemoto, 2002a). "Context" includes all of the social systems (e.g., family, community, larger social systems of gender, race, class, ethnicity) that contribute to and shape one's multiple identities. "Identity" is an ongoing process in which people consider, co-create, and organize meanings about themselves in interrelation with social meanings from others in their particular sociocultural, political, and historical contexts (Gergen, 1991; Shotter, 1993). As such, "identity" as used here is one way to conceptualize how an individual might internalize and individually organize social meanings related to group experiences and references (e.g., *social systemic contexts* such as gender, race, culture, class). Exploring identity may also be a way to consider how an individual's internalizations related to group referencing may change in relation to different life experiences and demands (e.g., *situational contexts* such as different kinds of relationships, in the experience of work, in relation to play or self-care). Thus, for an individual woman in therapy, exploring identity can be a way to explore the lived social meanings, enabling therapist and client to map the complex terrain as it is negotiated by the client.

Although individuals appear to have choices in how they create identities, these identities are actually claimed in light of how others perceive, understand, and presume them to be and how the individuals understand the others' perceptions. For instance, individuals' identities are usually influenced by how their families understand who they are (e.g., as members of certain races, ethnic groups, nationalities, or religious communities) and transmit these perceptions of shared memberships and associations to the individuals (Rigazio-DiGilio, 1997). Individuals' identities are also influenced by relationships with significant groups of people, such as close friends, colleagues, or members of a particular community or geographical region. These groups of people may actively accept or reject individuals as belonging within their group membership and identity. This influence constitutes the social contexts for considering the meanings of identities in relation to others (Kim, 2003; Suyemoto, 2002b). Thus, the *meaning* of an identity is created through an interactive process that includes the identity meanings created by other individuals and groups and the shared meanings created by individuals and groups together (Cox & Lyddon, 1997; Gergen, 1991, 1999; Suyemoto, 2002a).

For example, the meanings of our identities as Asian Americans are continually recreated from our unique experiences, our experiences with other individuals (such as our family members and our relationships with each other), and our experiences with different groups. For example, the Asian American group has its own meaning of Asian American identity that is agreed upon and co-constructed by Asian Americans within the group (Sodowsky, Kwan, & Pannu, 1995). This group identity inevitably influences our identity meanings, even if we do not fully agree with the parameters of it. Although the Asian American group's meaning of Asian American in a given time and location may be monoracial and heterosexual, I (KLS) claim an Asian American identity although I am multiracial and bisexual. Similarly, the Asian American group's meaning of Asian American may include being American born, but I (GSK) claim an Asian American identity although I am an immigrant. We both create a meaning of Asian American identity that includes multiracial; lesbian, gay, and bisexual (LGB); and immigrant people. However, the process of claiming and meaning creation is different for us than for someone who agrees with the group meaning of Asian American as monoracial, heterosexual, or

American born. Simultaneously, an individual's meaning of a group-referenced identity may affect the groups' identity meaning, although the extent of these effects will vary according to the power that the individual has or creates within the group (Suyemoto, 2002b). When we speak to Asian American people about including multiracial, GLB, or immigrant people, we are attempting to change the group's meaning to be more inclusive. The points of agreement and disagreement between groups and individuals can have implications for group interactions, individuals' identity development, and mental health.

How others impact identity is developmentally related (Rigazio-DiGilio, 1997). The importance of different relationships (parents, peer groups, significant others, children) varies in different personal and family developmental contexts. One's ability to differentiate what is positive, what is negative, what is personal, and what is social depends upon cognitive abilities that are also developmentally related. One reason to discuss Jenny (as a fourth grader) along with Maria (as an adult woman) is to consider some of these developmental processes and meanings and how different social influences may have different impacts at different developmental ages.

Power issues are crucial to include when thinking about individual identities. Sociohistorical and systemic contexts are embedded in intergroup power dynamics and discourses (see Kliman, Chapter 2; Vasquez & Magraw, Chapter 3), and they affect individuals' identities in significant ways. Identities are shaped not only by groups with which one actively identifies but also by groups with which one does not identify, particularly groups that are dominant in relation to privilege and power (Suyemoto, 2002b). Racial identity is a good example of how groups and individuals with more power have more influence over inclusion criteria for their own group as well as more power to affect the identity meanings of groups and individuals who have less power.

In relation to racial identity, white Americans influence the socially agreed-upon meanings and the inclusion criteria of racial minority groups more than racial minority groups influence the socially agreed-upon meaning of the white American identity. The dominant white American group has the power to create group-identity criteria for their own group (socially, institutionally, and legally) that makes it more difficult for marginalized racial groups to claim identities associated with that group that would create access to rights or privileges. This process is evident, for example, in historical legal challenges to the denial of rights based on racial categorization, such as the 1922 case of *Ozawa v. United States* and the 1923 case of *United States v. Thind* (described in Ancheta, 1998). Ozawa argued that he should be eligible for naturalization because he (and other Japanese people) were white on the basis of skin color. His argument was rejected by the

Supreme Court, who said that the intended meaning was Caucasian. A year later, in *United States v. Thind*, the Supreme Court ruled that Asian Indians were barred as well, in spite of their classification as Caucasian, due to the popular (racial) equality of white and Caucasian (Ancheta, 1998). The rulings, made by white judges, defined and redefined Asian Americans in ways that maintained their exclusion from privilege; the meaning of *white* was never articulated and was not affected by the attempts of the Asian Americans to influence it.

White European American groups also influence racial minority groups' own meanings of their group identities. For example, many Asian Americans accept and support the model minority myth, although the creation and maintenance of this stereotype is not primarily located within the Asian American community.[1] Although groups and individuals do not have to take on these dominant meanings and may create and claim their own identities, their identity journeys tend to become more complex when those with more power do not accept the identities or meanings they have chosen or created. For example, despite the fact that Japanese Americans identified themselves as loyal Americans during World War II, they were incarcerated as traitors and foreigners and the social and identity development of multiple generations of (Japanese) American citizens was affected (Mass, 1991; Nagata, 1993).

Groups with more power may also actively shape how groups with less power see each other. The dominance of the black–white paradigm and the race "hierarchy" are largely due to the historical constructions of race by the dominant white European American group in the United States (Omi & Winant, 1994; Perea, 2000). These dominant understandings of race and race relations affect the ways in which racial minority groups interact and are maintained today by the dominant group because of the benefits to them of the "divide-and-conquer" strategy.

Furthermore, the choice and meanings of identities are interactively enacted and created within a specific sociohistorical and political context. It is not only current relationships that affect identity meanings and interactions but also (1) the social meanings that have arisen and become dominant, given the specific histories within a particular context; and (2) historical and current power relations between different types of individuals and groups. My identity (GSK) as a Korean American has been informed by both historical and current experiences. Historically, I grapple with being perceived by others as a "perpetual foreigner" and through the lens of the legacies of the Korean War (1950–1953) and the role of the United States in the war. At the same time, my identity as a Korean American is affected by the current administration's (George W. Bush's) discourse on North Korea as part of an "Axis of Evil." As a Korean American immigrant from South Korea, the current discourse makes me ponder the relationship between

North and South Korea, and the U.S. relationship with these two countries. The current discourse simultaneously makes me wonder about how Koreans are viewed in the United States (i.e., Is there a differentiation between North and South Koreans? How do Korean Americans fit into this view? What about Korean Americans who are immigrants?). These current experiences remind me of the historical experiences of Korean Americans, in particular, and Asian Americans, in general, and affect the way I think about my own identity as a Korean American. My identity as a Korean American is thus co-constructed in the process of thinking about, reflecting on, and negotiating how I see myself and how I, or people like me, have been perceived historically and currently by others in the United States.

Conceptualizing identity in this co-constructed manner is one way to connect our understanding of the individual—with her or his own internal and interpersonal experiences, reflexive awareness, and agency—with our analysis of the social systemic *contexts* that influence group formation and reflect the current and historical social system of power and privilege. Conceptualizing therapy as a means of exploring and changing the meanings of these co-constructed identities in order to improve mental health and functioning enables us to bring our critical social justice analysis into the treatment. This conceptualization sees therapy as aiming to change individuals' understandings of themselves in relation to, and as shaped by, social experiences (Neimeyer, 1995). Therapy is, itself, a co-constructive process in which the therapist and the client reconstruct identities, partially through exploring and explaining the construction process itself. Many identity theorists discuss how identity formation is a process of moving between the *experiencing I* and the *explaining me*, whereby we consider our experience and explain it (see, e.g., Ashmore & Jussim, 1997; James, 1890/1989). Therapy, too, is conceptualized as contributing to the creation of a balance between experiencing and explaining (or observing, integrating, actively shaping, etc.; Guidano, 1995), whereby clients move between experiencing (relating their experience, feeling in the moment with the therapist) and explaining (reflecting on their experience, considering its connection to other experiences, exploring alternative meanings, practicing new ways of reacting).

The conceptualization of *co-constructed* identity provides us, as therapists, with a framework that integrates our social, systemic, and political understandings. The view of identity as an interactive, multilayered, political process can be used by therapists to consider the ways in which individuals interact with, are influenced by, and influence, their social environments. Indeed, this perspective can be used as the foundation from which to develop new knowledge that can increase both the types and the meanings of possible identities. Understanding identity as a complex interactive process can thus build conceptual bridges across contextual "terrains." By *ter-*

rains we mean both various group affiliated identities, such as gender, race, or class, and also various life contexts, such as social/intimate relationships, work, and self-care.

Mapping the Terrains

Frequently, the social contextual terrains and the associated identities of an individual's experience are understood as relatively separate. By "contextual terrains" (or, in less metaphorical language, "social contexts") we mean socially salient categories that are frequently related to dynamics of power and privilege, both currently and historically. *Identities* are created by the individual to negotiate and personalize these terrains, and are therefore associated with them and created in interaction with them. Within individuals' lives (in contrast to abstract discussions), the identities are not really separable, although individuals may be able to separate the abstract terrains: For example, a working-class lesbian of color will never be able to completely separate her own lived lesbian identity from her lived identity as a woman of color, although she may be able to discuss how the specific concepts of sexual orientation and race affect her. In conceptualizing client difficulties and strengths and in planning therapeutic interventions, separating the concepts may be necessary initially in order to define each concept (as we do here), create shared meanings, and attempt to understand the environmental demands of each terrain. Such a separation is also important in that it makes explicit what may be implicitly imposed. For example, racial meanings and power relations are frequently hidden behind the language of ethnicity (Omi & Winant, 1994), and class or racial differences between women may be obscured by focusing on their common gender oppression (Williams, McCandies, & Dunlap, 2002). However, defining what something *is* also inherently describes what it *is not*. Defining a concept or an identity frequently results in a decontextualization of what is being defined. Thus we found that although we could abstractly define each of these concepts as distinct from the others, when applying them to our understanding of Maria and Jenny, we were compelled to discuss the ways in which multiple identities interacted.

In this section we seek not only to provide basic understandings of definitions and contexts that create a foundation for the later chapters in this book,[2] but also, through discussion of Maria and Jenny, to explore (1) how each of these areas of identities are socially as well as individually constructed, and (2) how actively considering the interaction of identities and bridging the terrains contributes to a better understanding of the individual in therapy. We focus on those statuses and identities that the editors of this book have chosen to make their relative focus—gender, race, ethnicity, socioeconomic status and class, religion and spirituality, and sexual orientation—in order to provide definitions and identify complexities, with particular attention to the first four variables, which are especially salient to Maria and Jenny.

Each of the concepts discussed here is socially constructed and socially contested as to its meaning and implications. Therefore, there is no agreement on the meanings and boundaries of gender, race, ethnicity, socioeconomic class, religion, and sexual orientation. This disagreement means that each individual and each group must work out for herself or itself where she or it fits, where she or it does not fit, and what it means to claim that identity given the multiple meanings offered by different individuals and groups in the particular sociohistorical context. Wehrly (1995), citing Das and Littrell, notes the distinction between the *modal construct* of a culture, which reflects those practices/beliefs/values that are held by most people in the group that are also used to define the group itself, and the *individual manifestation* of a culture, which reflects how a single individual might choose from, and enact the meanings within, the culture. Each individual manifestation will be slightly different from another. This distinction is important when working with socially interactive identities in therapy, because there may be disagreement between the individual's understanding of the modal construct and her own individual manifestation or meaning construction.

Each of the concepts we discuss not only reflects individual differences but also social systemic differences in power, which are associated with socially constructed and maintained hierarchies of privilege. Thus the meanings created by individuals, groups, and therapists have implications for social justice and personal empowerment because of the value-laden nature of the constructed identities.

Gender

"Gender" is defined as beliefs about what each sex means in the culture. Although frequently confounded with sex, gender is more about the social meanings associated with categorization, whereas sex is the categorization between male and female based on physical and biological determinants such as hormones, gonads, external genitalia, and secondary sex characteristics (e.g., facial hair; Calhoun, 2002b; Colman, 2001).[3] The meanings and social norms related to gender vary across culture and certainly across historical context. State licensing boards and the American Psychological Association policies make it clear that therapists are expected to have a minimal understanding of the personal and social implications of gender, the ways in which the system of gender has contributed to inequities between men and women, and the ways in which therapy needs to resist contributing to these inequities. The feminist movement has contributed to our field's great progress in holding us as therapists accountable for the effects of our own gender socialization on the services we provide to our clients. Nevertheless, not only does gender continue to be an important aspect of identity, it continues to be an area that involves great discrepancy in power and privilege.

As the basic influence of the social meanings of gender differences becomes widely accepted, we also begin to understand the many other statuses and systems with which gender interacts. One of the primary criticisms of the feminist movement continues to be its relative inattention to intersecting identities and statuses, for example, attention to the ways that gender intersects with race, ethnicity, religion, sexual orientation, social class, and other variables at the individual and systemic levels (e.g., Williams et al., 2002). Being a woman of color is not the same as being a white woman; being a working-class woman is different from being an upper-class woman, being a Jewish woman is different from being a Hindu woman, and being a black, lesbian, Muslim, middle-class woman is different from being a Latina, heterosexual, Christian woman living in poverty. Although some experiences may be shared, gender cannot stand alone as the primary source of influence or oppression.

Although Maria never stated an explicit identification as a woman or a feminist, it was clear that the individual and social meanings of her gender were contributing to her presenting difficulties. In many areas, Maria felt trapped by meanings and identities that she simultaneously valued and perceived as conflicting with her own desires. For example, the meaning of "woman" for Maria affected her experiences in relationships, at school/work, and in relation to herself and her self-care. Maria felt that "woman" essentially meant being subservient to men and sacrificing herself to the needs and desires of others. This meaning was created in interaction with her family's meanings, as well as those of her peers and her cultural communities. Maria's first model of woman was her mother, whom Maria described as "like a slave" to her husband and family. Maria's mother created her identity primarily in relation to her family relationships; even at work, she was particularly polite to the male members of the families for whom she worked. She taught Maria to be deferential to her father and brothers. She tolerated her husband's alcoholism and gave Maria the message that husbands and fathers should be indulged and accommodated, even if abusive or intoxicated, and even if it meant denying or suppressing one's own emotions. When Maria was a child and her father was intoxicated, he wanted most to be with her and hear her say how much she loved him. Although Maria made it clear to her mother that these moments were hurtful to her, and she frequently hid to avoid them, her mother would bring Maria to her father and encourage her to tell him that she loved him, regardless of what she was feeling at the moment (fear, anger, hatred) in order to avoid angering her father. As an adult, Maria resisted expressing her love to her partners, because she felt that to say "I love you" would be to lose herself.

Maria's friends were similarly deferential to their boyfriends. Furthermore, the majority of role models in Maria's cultural and religious communities supported the subservient meaning of "woman." Maria's understanding of herself as a woman affected her perception of herself in school and at work. She was the only woman in her social group to continue on to graduate school and one of only a few who had graduated from college.

In therapy, Maria came to realize that, as a woman, she did not expect her needs to be met and attempted to suppress her own recognition of the existence of her needs and feelings in order to avoid being disappointed. As we explored the pattern of her depressive episodes (occurring in the fall of years she attended college or graduate school), Maria expressed a strong feeling of being an imposter, as if she did not really belong in school and as if her achievements were somehow a mistake or a fraud that would soon be discovered by others.

Clearly, Maria's identity as a woman had been, and continued to be, shaped by her family and by the social groups with which she identified. If we were to understand Maria's struggles using gender as an individualistic and relatively isolated aspect in relation to her other identities, we might approach treatment of Maria by (1) helping her understand the relational orientation associated with the gender socialization of women, (2) creating insight about the effects of her childhood experiences on her current relationship attitudes, and (3) recommending assertiveness training or a woman's group that would help Maria feel empowered to reclaim her own experience and redefine the meaning of woman. However, although Maria's understanding of the meaning of "woman" may be similar to women from different racial and ethnic groups, for Maria it was strongly associated with her particular ethnicity. Maria rarely spoke about the meaning of being a woman but frequently discussed what it meant to her to be a *Mexican American woman.* Thus, for Maria, to change the meaning of being a woman had implications for her identities and feelings of belonging in relation to her ethnicity and her religion (among other aspects). Because some of these identities, social meanings, and group criteria were cherished by Maria, it was important to explore with her how these groups defined their own identities (e.g., Mexican American) and how they defined these identities in interaction with the meaning of "woman." In essence, as a therapist, it was necessary for me to help Maria see how her identity as a woman was embedded in a network of social and individual meanings connected to her ethnicity, her race (Maria's complexion was quite dark), her sexual orientation, and her religion, and to find a path to alternative meanings that respected the social meanings that maintained the social connections that supported her.

Race

"Race" is a categorization system that creates groups of people who are distinguished (by themselves or others) in social relationships and interactions by their physical characteristics (Pinderhughes, 1989; Root, 1998; Spickard, 1992; Suyemoto, 2002b). Although frequently assumed to be biological, race is actually a social construction rather than a biological "reality" (American Psychological Association, 2003; Helms & Cook, 1999). Race is frequently confounded with ethnicity. However, whereas certain ethnic cultures may be related to certain racial categorizations, there are clear distinctions between the two concepts in multiple areas, including compass (e.g., there are many ethnic groups within a single race and potentially many races within an ethnic group), criteria (physical characteristics vs. cultural knowledge), and sociohistorical intent (e.g., the purpose of race is to create social categorizations and power hierarchies [Omi & Winant, 1994], whereas the purpose of ethnicity is to create and maintain shared cultural experiences).

The boundaries of racial groups are unclear and highly contextual, depending on historical period, geographical region (e.g., in the United States vs. in Cuba), and politics. Different people have developed between 3 and 200 categories of race (Schaefer, 1988, as cited in Atkinson, Morton, & Sue, 1998). Criteria for membership in different racial groups also vary according to the person or group judging. As described above, the ways in which various groups define a particular racial identity affects an individual's identity meaning and choices. However, because the meanings of race are so uncertain, discrepancies between individuals' and groups' identities are even more frequent and magnified. For example, multiracial individuals judged as Asian by white people may not be judged as Asian by Asian people, which may create challenges in the construction of racial identity for these individuals. Another example is that the criteria for Native American identity or tribal affiliation varies among nations, between the criteria set by the nation and that set by the U.S. government, and/or among different groups or individuals about the same person (Garroutte, 2001; Nagel, 1997), again creating problems for those individuals who claim the identity but are not accepted by the group. Although we colloquially discuss race as if anyone with certain racial or ethnic heritages were clearly within a given racial group, the boundaries and lived meanings are much less clear in actuality. A multiracial individual who "looks white" will have a significantly different daily experience from one who is easily categorized as black, Asian, Latino, or Native American, based on unchangeable physical characteristics such as skin color or shape of features (rather than changeable cultural or ethnic displays such as clothes). The ambiguity of the meaning of race is strongly evident within the Latino population. Although the census distinguishes white Hispanics from nonwhite Hispanics, it is unclear what the "nonwhite Hispanics" are if they are not black, Native American, or Asian.

Groups and individuals with less power due to historical or current social systems may also have less access to knowledge or experiences that would increase the number of identity options open to them. It may therefore be significantly more difficult for them to create and claim adaptive empowering identities. For example, the social "scripts" associated with being a black woman may cover a narrower range than those possibilities open to white women (see Stephens & Phillips, 2003) as reflected in the types and number of media images of white women and black women. The "procedural knowledge" (i.e., the information and resources) needed to create an identity may also be limited by a group's access to a systemic power (see, e.g., Yowell, 2002): If one has never seen a black intellectual, for example, then the ability to imagine oneself with that identity is significantly constrained.[5]

Given that identities are socially constructed, it is imperative to understand social meanings and uncertainties of race when treating girls and women of color.

> For Jenny, what it meant to be a multiracial white and black girl became salient in her relationships with others, at school, and in her self-attitude. Jenny had a very close relationship with her immediate family, feeling close to her white European American mother and building a positive relationship with her stepfather. She spent a lot of time with her maternal white European American cousins and extended family. Although her white maternal family accepted her and loved her dearly, the family members did not speak much about the effects that race might have had in her relationships with others. Initially, Jenny seemed not to have contemplated her own multiracial identity much but accepted the identity offered by her family (e.g., that she was just a girl who was loved by her family, and that racial differences did not matter), which seemed developmentally appropriate for a latency-age child.
>
> At school, however, issues related to race and racial differences had become extremely salient. The girls who had bullied Jenny the previous year and whom Jenny was currently bullying were all African American girls who were bused from the inner city to Jenny's suburban school. Other than these girls, there were few African American girls in Jenny's grade. It became apparent that the teasing and name calling from these girls toward Jenny was race related. Jenny thought of herself as an African American and, prior to her interaction with these girls, seemed to have made little distinction between African American and black. But Jenny had quickly been told by these girls

that she was different; she was not really black because she had only one African American parent. Jenny reacted to the other girls' labeling by trying out various behavioral options, which included ignoring, walking away, arguing, and/or kicking and fighting ("bullying them back").

The distinction at the core of this conflict involved not only the individually chosen identities and meanings of the girls, who considered themselves "monoracial" or true "blacks," but was also heavily embedded in social meanings about what it meant to be black. The girls' understanding of black identity reflected an internalization of the inconsistencies that exist in our society about the meanings of race, and how the boundaries around who gets to claim being black depend heavily on the social contexts and politics at a given time, ignoring the "reality" that most blacks are actually multiracial (Atkinson et al., 1998).

The urban girls' black identity also reflected the intersections of their racial identities with ethnic and class identities. The urban African American girls told Jenny that she was not tough (and black) like them because she had a white mother. In this case, black racial identity seems to have been connected with being tough and may have also been related to the way some girls linked being urban with being black. Being tough and knowing how to be assertive may be adaptive for some girls of minority backgrounds, helping them to navigate social systems that historically have been racist and classist. Constructing collective identities around the racial identity and the attribute of assertiveness can serve as a strong, inner holding space in which young girls develop positive identities and a sense of community. However, in Jenny's context, the preadolescent girls connected toughness, black racial identity, and class differences in a way that differentiated Jenny from them and from a black racial identity. By framing black as being tough, the girls not only restricted the black identity to their own immediate experiences, but also demonstrated their internalization of the limited "scripts" available for African American girls. They may also have judged Jenny as less black because they perceived her as less ethnically/culturally African American, based on Jenny's primary ethnic socialization in her European American family. Furthermore, the preadolescent girls seemed to have related the perceived differences in class between Jenny and others, based on where they lived (in a surburb vs. city), even though Jenny's family lived in a subsidized housing in a suburb.

Jenny's responses toward these girls were complicated by her ADHD, particularly impulsivity, which often led her to spring into action when provoked (she would often respond to others by arguing or kicking) and to get involved in disruptive behaviors in the classroom (e.g., participating in side conversations during class time). It is possible that having ADHD and being perceived as one of the girls who bullies others or gets into fights might have led to a quicker referral for therapy than if Jenny had presented with more internalizing problems. Given social perceptions of black children, it is also possible that Jenny's behavioral problems might have seen as being related to the "script" of being a tough black girl at school—which is ironic, given the other girls' accusations about Jenny not being tough or black enough.

In therapy, Jenny did not want to discuss her racial identity in depth, but she made a point of saying that she considered herself African American but not black. She explained her logic by saying that if one had two black parents, then one was black, but if one had one black parent and one white parent, then one was African American. Jenny's logic might have described her understanding of the intersection between race and ethnicity and reflected her attempts to negotiate the multiple meanings of being a black girl from multiple sources (e.g., from her own thinking about her experiences, from her family, from her white peers, and from these African American peers). Jenny's attempts to grapple with the multiple meanings of race were also subtly played out in her relationship with her family. When her African American paternal grandparents wanted to spend more time with her, Jenny responded by telling her mother that she would be willing but that she was not thrilled by the prospect. Jenny also said that she did not care much about seeing her father, who had been absent in her life, but later expressed curiosity about him and her grandparents, at one point even writing a letter to her father.

Developmental aspects are clearly relevant to understanding Jenny. As a preadolescent, she was trying to struggle with the pull toward trying to be the same with everyone else while simultaneously exploring the similarities and differences between herself and others—and noticing her uniqueness. She did not talk in depth about her identity, because it was not her primary concern at this developmental phase, but instead focused on social interactions at school. At the same time, she was willing to explore how issues related to race, as illustrated by her social relationships with the other girls, affected her peer relationships and the behavioral choices she made. Jenny experienced some tension between her identities formed within her family and her identities that were being challenged by her peers. Balancing these identity tensions might be a general developmental task for any latent-age child (i.e., noticing differences between what one has learned/been taught at home vs. what one notices/hears at school). Jenny's situation, however, was complicated by a very challenging set of factors: how racial identities and their meanings are socially constructed and embedded in sociopolitical history, the intergroup dynamics between black and white groups, and associated issues of power and privilege.

Culture

"Culture" refers to meanings that are shared by an identifiable group of people and passed on to others within that group (Tomlinson-Clarke, 1999; Triandis, 1995, 2001). "Meanings" are broadly defined to include cognitive, affective, and behavioral aspects of individual and group functioning, such as values, beliefs, customs, norms, gender roles, affective styles, social behavior, language, and ways of self-understanding. Although we most frequently discuss ethnic culture (and, specifically, ethnic-minority culture), there are many types of culture associated with many types of identifiable groups. Most of the other identities and statuses discussed here have cultures associated with them, such as women's culture, ethnic cultures, lesbian culture, cultures associated with religion or spirituality (e.g., Jewish culture,[6] Muslim culture, Wiccan culture). There are cultures associated with other oppressed or marginalized groups, such as with differentially abled groups (e.g., deaf culture or a more general culture of disability); with privileged groups, such as American culture; or with other identities such as Democrats or Republicans. Culture is also constantly changing, both in the modal construct and in the individual manifestation (American Psychological Association, 2003).

Ethnicity

"Ethnicity" refers to cultural patterns usually related to a shared national or geographical origin (Pinderhughes, 1989; Suyemoto, 2002b). Ethnicity is not determined by physical characteristics and is much less frequently an imposed identity compared to race. Within the five major racial groups in the United States (white, black, Latino, Asian, Native American), there are hundreds of ethnicities. The ways in which race and ethnicity are confounded are affected by the differential salience of ethnicity and ethnic differences and the presence or absence of a dominant ethnicity within a given racial group. Both the white and black racial groups have a largely dominant ethnic identity and culture within them (European American for the white group and African American—meaning, descended from the legacy of slavery in the United States—for the black group). For these groups, the confounding of ethnicity with race, such that ethnic differences are discussed in relation to race (e.g., black culture), is extremely common, as demonstrated by the discussion of Jenny. Within these groups the confounding of race and ethnicity may be less problematic for those within the dominant in-group space (i.e., black African Americans who are the children of two black African American parents descended from slaves; white European Americans descended from early colonists). However, for those within these racial groups who do not belong to the dominant in-group space (e.g., Caribbean or African immigrants,

Bosnian refugees), the erasing of distinct ethnicity in the service of "racialization" may be significantly more problematic (see, e.g., Bailey, 2000; Thompson & Bauer, 2003).

The confounding of race and ethnicity is similarly problematic for Latinos, Asian Americans, and Native Americans who do not have a dominant ethnic identity within the racial group that the majority of members would reference and could therefore be used interchangeably with a racial label (see, e.g., Ancheta, 1998; Espiritu, 1992). For example, there is such great heterogeneity within Asian American ethnic groups that to speak of an "Asian American" culture may be a disservice to many individuals' identity meanings (e.g., compare Pakistanis with Thais, Hmong with Japanese, Indonesians with Filipinos). Individuals within these racial groups may identify primarily with their specific ethnic or sociolinguistic group rather than a pan-ethnic or racial grouping or identity; for example, a Mexican American woman such as Maria may identify primarily as Mexican American rather than Latina and may not feel racial or cultural affinity with a Cuban American woman, even though both are labeled Latina. Or a Vietnamese American may make strong distinctions between Vietnamese Americans and Chinese Americans (perhaps influenced by histories of discrimination in Asian home countries) and may therefore struggle with imposed racialization (Bailey, 2000; Suyemoto, 2002b).

The modal construct of any given ethnic culture is constantly changing in relation to the composition of the group and the groups' interactions with other groups, cultures, and subcultures. Ethnic minority groups in the United States that are characterized by ongoing immigration (such as most Latino groups, most Asian American groups, and some black groups such as Haitians and Cape Verdeans) are constantly renegotiating the meanings of their ethnic identities in response to the infusion of cultural patterns brought from the homelands. Thus there can be widely discrepant meanings of ethnic identity within a particular group, and especially across immigration generational status (e.g., immigrant generation, first U.S.-born generation) and across family generational status as it intersects with immigrant generational status (e.g., between immigrant parents and their U.S. born children).

> Maria strongly identified as Mexican American and saw this identity as created by and reflected in her daily life, including her bilingual ability, her values, her family structure and expectations, and her traditions (holidays, foods, etc.). Maria's parents had met and married in Mexico and immigrated to the United States for better economic opportunities for themselves and their children. Throughout Maria's life her family had lived with many members of the extended family, including many recent immigrants. Maria's parents and her married

older brother's family lived in largely Mexican American communities, and her parents' friends were of similar backgrounds. Maria and her three siblings (her older and younger brothers and her younger sister) were all born in the United States, although her oldest brother had been raised by his grandparents in Mexico for many years. Like her siblings, Maria attended Catholic school prior to college, with many other Mexican American children from her neighborhood. Her closest friends were Mexican American girls who were also U.S. born children of immigrants. Maria lived with her older brother and his family while attending a large state college with a diverse student body. Maria's first language was Spanish, and she spoke Spanish exclusively with her parents at home. However, in contrast to her parents, Maria spoke English fluently and at college she found that she felt comfortable in social situations with individuals and groups from varied backgrounds.

Maria's identity as a Mexican American woman affected her relationships, her school and work experiences, and her ability to enjoy her experiences and feel entitled to self-care. Her understanding of women (and daughters) as subservient was shaped not only by the dominant social meanings but particularly by the meaning of women within the Mexican American community with which she identified and by the experiences and meanings of her parents' immigrant generation. In therapy, Maria discussed her perceptions of her mother's attitudes toward her father, her sister-in-law's attitudes toward her brother, and their relationships as related to her Mexican American heritage and the gender mores with which her parents had grown up in Mexico. Maria struggled with feeling that if she expected more egalitarian and intimate relationships, she would somehow be less traditional or less Mexican American. Although she initially framed this fear in relation to disappointing her parents, it soon became clear that maintaining a strong Mexican American identity was inherently important to Maria herself as well.

In some ways, Maria's parents were less traditional in their gender expectations than the stereotypical first-generation Mexican American parents that Maria expected them to be. Specifically, Maria's parents had always supported and encouraged her pursuit of education and a career. Similarly, they had encouraged her brother to marry an educated woman who had a career. Although this was a rather untraditional attitude toward Mexican American daughters, Maria did not see this divergence as a challenge to the stereotype and a means to consider multiple possible meanings of being a Mexican American woman. Instead, Maria framed her parents' acceptance of her educational and career goals in a way that reflected her identity meaning: Mexican American woman as subservient and trapped. Maria felt that her parents' support of her own educational and career goals was actually a burdensome obligation and that she must do well in school to please them (particularly her father), fulfill expectations, and be obedient. Furthermore, Maria associated her need for academic success with her ethnic identity: She believed that because so few Mexican Americans had the opportunity to get a doctorate, she must therefore fulfill her *obligation* to her community by doing so, even if she did not personally want to do so. Maria's feeling that her success was an indication of her subservience and her experience of obligation as burdensome and dystonic contributed to her feeling like an imposter and made it difficult for her to feel connected to her own achievements and to her ethnicity. Although her Mexican American identity engendered a genuine desire to contribute to the Mexican American community (a more positive view of "obligation"), she could not conceive of genuine and positive ways to make this contribution because being a Mexican American woman meant being a woman who was subservient and who erased her own needs. Thus Maria's achievements and relationships gave her little joy.

Maria set an initial goal in therapy of increasing her self-esteem. To meet this goal, it was important to "map the terrain" together. We needed to explore the individual and social meanings that were contributing to her beliefs and emotions and try to create alternative meanings of her chosen and cherished identities that felt positive and enabling, rather than being constrained by social meanings that felt foreign or imposed upon her. For example, although Maria acknowledged that her father's views toward education were less than traditional, this acknowledgment had never been connected to a possibility that perhaps her father's views about being a good Mexican American daughter were not limited to simple obedience and subservience. In therapy, we explored the multiple possible meanings of being a good daughter, being a woman, being an intimate partner, being Mexican American, and the multiple ways these identities could interact.

Therapy also enabled Maria to differentiate these social meanings of her identities from her own meanings, noting when meanings were positive and when she would like to change some to be more flexible or growth promoting. For example, exploring how "obligation" and "desire to serve her community" were related areas helped Maria feel positively about achieving both for herself and for others. Therapy also helped Maria understand how these meanings had developed and how they may need to change in response to new contexts and demands. This understanding applied to the social meanings (e.g., the ways in which her parents' meanings developed within their Mexican context and how some flexibility within these in response to the new context of the United States might be helpful) and her own meanings (e.g., the ways in which her own understandings had developed in response to childhood views and developmental experiences that were no longer seen or experienced in the same way).

As Maria began to see new possible meanings and identities, she sought out different experiences and considered behaving in ways with her family that affirmed her connection to them and to her role as a Mexican American daughter, but did not feel subservient or self-sacrificing to her. Maria began to more actively explore relationships that supported her new identities. For example, she sought out discussions with her sister-in-law regarding her immigrant experiences, her view of being Mexican American, and her seeming subservience to Maria's brother. Through these conversations, Maria learned more about how her brother actively supported his wife and her career and how her sister-in-law made active choices about balancing caretaking of others with her own needs and desires to achieve and be connected to the Mexican American community. Maria's view changed from seeing this relationship as forcing her sister-in-law into submission to seeing how her sister-in-law was a strongly identified Mexican American woman in a mutually supportive heterosexual relationship, who was doing work that she loved and that also contributed to the Mexican American community. Although Maria had known her for years, she had never perceived her sister-in-law in this way or identified with her so strongly.

We also explored the pattern of her depression in relation to her feelings about her field and discipline. Although it took some time to work through her feelings that to not get a doctorate was to renege on her obligation to the Mexican American community, Maria eventually decided to return to school to pursue a master's degree in a human-service-related field, where she would be working directly with Latino/a children and families. She returned to school and completed the academic year without any depressive episode.

Class

Although social class in psychological studies is frequently operationalized as income and education, authors writing about the effects of social class make it clear that there are multiple meanings potentially unrelated to current income or individual educational achievement. "Class" is a complex social system that groups families and individuals in relation to power, privilege, and resources, including economic capital (assets of all sorts), symbolic capital (resources from fame or recognition; Calhoun, 2002c), cultural capital (resources from education, knowledge, or cultural learning; Calhoun, 2002a), and social capital (resources from relationships and social networks; Burchardt, 2003). The inclusion of symbolic, cultural, and social capital recognizes that class position is affected not only by one's current economic assets, but also by one's family's historical position and the ongoing ramifications of that position. Furthermore, these types of capital emphasize the cultural aspects of class; class background is associated with cultural experiences, including values, behavioral knowledge, and norms. One may or may not be aware of one's class culture, but changing contexts that involves crossing class boundaries can frequently make class culture salient and recognizable.

Given the current and historical racial discrimination, class is strongly associated with race and, in some racial groups, with specific ethnicities. Blacks, Latinos, Native Americans, and some Asian Americans (such as Cambodian and Vietnamese refugees) are overrepresented within the lower class (Sue & Sue, 2002; U.S. Department of Health and Human Services, 2001). For these groups, class and ethnic cultures may become linked, so that to be accepted by some groups as Vietnamese or African American may mean enacting cultures associated with class-specific experiences of race or culture.

In Jenny's case, issues related to class intersected with gender and race issues.

Jenny was one of the few black children at her school who lived in an affluent suburb; the other black girls were being bused in from economically challenged areas of the inner city. Jenny's family lived in subsidized housing in the suburb, and they received some support from her maternal extended family, particularly around child care. To me (GSK) it was unclear how Jenny was seen in the socioeconomic status hierarchy at school, in relation to the girls from the inner city as well as the other children who were residents of the suburb. To these girls, living in a suburb related to being white and affluent—and therefore not black. The range of choices relating to race, culture, and class was limited; they could not conceive of a rich, suburban black girl, or even a poor, suburban black girl. Jenny did not fit into the group of black girls who strongly identified with being black, urban, and from a lower socioeconomic class. Although most of the categorizations the girls were making were dualistic and based on their perception of class differences (especially given Jenny's actual socioeconomic status), they were no less real in the girls' lives.

Before her social interactions with the group of black girls, Jenny's racial identity seemed to be relatively unrelated to her class identity or status. But for the urban black girls, race seemed to be linked to class culture, and class culture was linked to ethnic culture. The city girls linked the idea of being less black with living in the affluent white suburb. Thus class, race, and ethnic culture criteria all needed to be met in these girls' meaning of black. For the urban girls, being tough in this school situation was important, if not necessary, for survival. As black girls from the inner city, they may not have been readily accepted by other children at the affluent, predominantly white and Asian school; they may have found a way to support each other by forming an exclusive group that linked their racial minority status with being tough and acting in ways that associated urban class culture with race. To maintain the group identity, it was necessary to define race in particular ways and to draw a very specific boundary that excluded Jenny. Yet on another level, Jenny and these girls might have encountered differences because of living in different geographical regions—which often involves being familiar with, and socializing in, different racial and ethnic communities as well as different cultures. Thus Jenny might have had different cultural associations with being black as compared to the urban black girls whose "color" may be similar but whose ethnic cultural and class cultural experiences may be very different. This is particularly possible given that Jenny was being raised by a white mother without much contact with her black extended family, in a suburban context primarily dominated by European American culture.

Jenny's experiences provide a glimpse into how a preadolescent girl is beginning to consider her identity in complex ways. Whereas her initial problems seemed to be confined to ADHD and behavioral issues, identity emerged as a major underlying theme in therapy. The way Jenny understood herself was very much in the light of, and was influenced by, her relations with other people and the meanings of race, class, and ethnicity that they communicated to her. Looking ahead to Jenny's development into the teenage years and adulthood, we could imagine that she might continue to encounter some of the issues she has faced in the fourth grade, and that her journey might be complicated if her identity as an African American continued to be rejected by others. Therapy served not only as a setting in which to engage problem-solving skills regarding her current relational problems, but also as a space in which she could play out various ways of seeing herself and her situations. It created and modeled multiple possibilities and meanings for Jenny's identities (e.g., expanding the meanings of what it meant to be "African American" and a suburban girl), and may have contributed to preventing difficulties that could have emerged, given continuous social rejections based on the current social meanings.

Religion and Spirituality

Therapists have been interested in religion from very early on, whether to vilify it (e.g., Freud 1953/1964) or to laud it (e.g., Fromm, 1950; Jung, 1938). Like all of the issues discussed here, religion is a complicated concept with multiple meanings. Meanings of "religion" include personal beliefs about, relationship with, and actions in relation to a spiritual being (God/god/Goddess/goddess/higher power) or spirituality more generally, as well as acceptance of, or adherence to, shared doctrine or institutions (Brown & Forgas, 1980; Fromm, 1950; Jung, 1938). Religious and spiritual frameworks/groups/communities seem to actively support the mental health of many women, especially those who are part of ethnic minorities, and to function as primary models/arenas for self-care and social support (see, e.g., Dudley-Grant, 2003).

Most of the major religious institutions also have, to a greater or lesser extent, associated cultures that not only organize or prescribe one's relationship with a higher power or spiritual understanding but also organize one's relationships with other people, oneself, and one's values, beliefs, behaviors, etc. These cultures can, and frequently do, provide important and positive sources of identity (contributing to feelings of positive self-care and nurturance). Furthermore, many religions interact strongly with ethnic cultures in the meanings they carry, the ways they are enacted, and the identities that are constructed in relation to them (e.g., a Mexican American Catholic identity may be quite different from an Irish American Catholic identity). Religious or spiritual identities also interact strongly with meanings of gender, race, sexual orientation, class, etc.

Like all of the concepts discussed here, those of religions and spiritual systems have sociohistorical meanings and hierarchies that reflect a continuum from privilege to oppression. For example, Jews have a long history of oppression, and Chesler (2003) argues that there is a new and intensifying rise in anti-Semitism in current times. Religious beliefs have also been used to oppress others, particularly those who are different in relation to other variables discussed here, such as gender (e.g., the oppression of strong women through witch hunts), race (e.g., the justification of slavery on the basis of paganism), or sexual orientation (e.g., the vilification of gay and lesbian marriages by some current religious leaders). The identities created in relation to, or in interaction with, religion reflect these complicated and dynamic aspects of power and privilege. For example, Maria's Catholicism supported her through a belief in a positive God and by contributing to the positive meaning of her Mexican American identity; but her Catholicism was also problematic for her as she tried to make sense of the church's dictates about sex and birth control, and the ways in which Mexican American women are framed within Catholicism (e.g., the meaning of the Virgin Mary as a role model of self-sacrifice). For many women, religious and spiritual identities are both salient and central, and the socially co-constructed nature of them, in interaction with other identities described here, will be important aspects of therapy.

Sexual Orientation

Identity in relation to sexual orientation(s) includes one's gender in relation to the gender of people (1) for whom one feels intimate affection or sexual desire, (2) with whom one has had sexual or intimate affectional relationships, and (3) about whom one fantasizes or dreams in sexual, intimate, or affectionate terms. These various referents may or may not be congruent with each other or with one's claimed identity (Garnets, 2002). For example, a woman may identify as a heterosexual but have sexual fantasies about other women, or a woman may feel most comfortable in intimate, long-term relationships with other women but also feel sexual desire toward men. Identity in relation to sexual orientation may also relate to one's politics or ideologies; for example, a radical separatist feminist may identify as lesbian first as a political identity, rather than because of strong feelings of desire for women. Because gender is itself a contested concept, so is sexual orientation, which is strongly confounded with gender meanings within dominant social understandings (e.g., lesbian women are expected to be masculine in their gender roles and behaviors). Furthermore, just as gender norms and meanings vary with ethnic culture, meanings of sexual orientation and the intersections between sexual orientation and gender also vary with culture (Garnets, 2002); for example, Asian lesbians may experience less flexibility in gender roles and less access to a "butch" experience (Lee, 1996) than European American lesbians.

Like religion or class, different sexual orientations as social systems and meanings have associated cultures (e.g., lesbian culture, gay culture; Pope, 1995) with cultural language, traditions/holidays (e.g., gay pride day), mannerisms, gender/social norms, etc. And like all of the variables discussed here, there is a history and current context of sociocultural power that privileges some (heterosexuals) while oppressing others (Garnets, 2002; Weber, 1998). However, unlike all of the other major social systems discussed here, discrimination on the basis of sexual orientation is not illegal. In fact, it is legally endorsed in the arena of relationships (e.g., anti-sodomy laws, laws prohibiting lesbian and gay marriage, laws related to lesbian and gay parenting), work/career (e.g., "don't ask/don't tell" in the military), and in areas and organizations related to self-care (e.g., some religions' rejection of gays, lesbians, and bisexuals). Even when a person, group, organization, or social environment is not actively homophobic, it is very frequently heterosexist, meaning that it assumes heterosexuality and imposes this assumption on all people within the context.

Similar to the other identities discussed, sexual orientation and its meanings affect one's overall identity and the process of therapy, whether or not they are explicitly stated and discussed. For instance, Maria *identified* as heterosexual. I (KLS) know this because I asked her as a standard part of the initial interview, not because it was a particularly salient identity for her that she specifically discussed. Because sexual orientation is not visible, like race, we frequently see it as less salient (unless one belongs to the minority space) and may assume heterosexual identity (particularly if the client is in a heterosexual relationship). Although Maria's sexual identity was not explicitly (for her) connected to her presenting difficulties, it certainly affected her identities and the ways in which she constructed meanings. Imagining Maria as a Mexican-American Catholic lesbian would lead to a different expectation and conceptualization of the issues with which she was struggling. This possibility points to the need to attend not only to explicitly claimed identities but also to social meanings of identities that are implicit because they are more privileged. These identities and meanings may also interact in important ways with actively claimed identities and may have positive or negative effects, even if they are not currently in clients' awareness.

Journeying Together

We'd like to comment briefly here on the impact of the therapist's identities and self-awareness on the journey (explored more fully in Vasquez & Magraw, Chapter 3). Because therapy is a co-constructed process, the therapist's own identities actively affect the conduct of therapy and the identities that are co-constructed for the client within therapy. If the therapist is a guide through the terrain of multiple socially co-constructed statuses and identities, then the therapist's own knowledge of that terrain (including the terrain that has not been personally salient in the therapist's own life) becomes of great importance. The identities of the therapist will have an impact on the therapy regardless of whether they are actively brought into the therapy or whether the client (or the therapist) is consciously aware of the impact. The conceptualizations of Maria and Jenny and the therapeutic decisions arising out of those conceptualizations may (or may not) have been very different if we had had other primary identities, but they were certainly affected by our own identities and our understandings of the identities of our clients. Our therapies with Maria and Jenny were affected by all of our identities because those identities have shaped who we are and, therefore, how we see and understand our clients. The effects of our identities occurred not only in how they shaped our understandings of Maria and Jenny, but also in relation to what they meant to Maria and Jenny and how these clients experienced us. Some of these effects are illustrated in the discussion and interpretations above. But here we would like to explicitly discuss our ethnicity, language, immigrant status, and race as examples of interacting client–therapist identities.

In therapy, Maria and I (KLS) explicitly discussed the importance to her of my being an ethnic-minority woman, an identity that we shared and that was important to both of us. This shared identity affected what she was willing to share with me, the affective tone of our interactions, and the ways that she saw me as a role model that was an alternative to her mother.

But those identities (and aspects of identities) of the therapist that are not personally salient or well explored may also have strong impacts on therapy, such as my monolingualism. Not only did I not speak Spanish, I had no experience with being bilingual in any language, and my ethnic identity was not connected to a bilingual language experience. I had not fully considered the meaning to me or to Maria of my being monolingual, because it was not personally salient to me. This lack of salience was partly *because* I was privileged in relation to language; if I were monolingual in a minority language, I might have had very different feelings, and I could not have been comfortable in my unexamined assumption that it was fine to be monolingual. My monolingualism constrained our therapy in several ways. There were times when Maria wanted/needed to speak in Spanish to express herself, and not only could I not understand her language, but also I could not fully sympathize with the cultural and personal meanings of the dilemma itself. My awareness of the impact of her bilingualism and my monolingualism led me to invite Maria to speak Spanish, even if I could not understand, so that she could access the emotional impact and experience embedded in the language. And we struggled together with this area of differential privilege between us, where it was imperative that I recognize my privilege and Maria's different experience.

My (GSK) therapy with Jenny was also shaped and influenced by my own identities, the way I thought about race, culture, and their meanings, and the way I understood Jenny. Working with Jenny was remarkable in relation to my own identity journey, as my identities intersected with her identities. While I focused on helping Jenny find creative ways to face her peers, I was very conscious of my identity as an Asian American and a woman of color. As a first-generation immigrant from Korea who is aware of the intergroup dynamics between various generations (e.g., immigrants as compared to second- or third-generation Asian Americans) within Asian American groups, and as someone who experienced discrimination based on my race, I could empathize with Jenny's situation in personal ways, and was conscious that my role was not only to be a therapist but also a role model to Jenny as a woman of color. My own awareness of, and attention to, the racial and cultural similarities and differences affected the intervention choices, such as choosing to invite Jenny to talk explicitly about the racial and cultural dimensions within her peer relationships, which had not been done before either at school or at home.

At the same time, I was quickly made aware of my lack of knowledge about black and African American identities (e.g., the group dynamics of the collective identities within African American groups, and how different they were from Asian American identity). In acknowledging my own ignorance, I was also faced with considering how emphasizing the shared similarities between myself as an Asian American woman and Jenny as an African American child, as people of color, did not always capture our lived experiences. Because the two groups have been pitted against each other by the dominant society (i.e., particularly between Korean Americans and African Americans), at times differences between Jenny and myself were highlighted more than our similarities. I also realized some of the privileges I had as a monoracial person whose identity is less contested within my own racial group, and as an Asian American who is often considered a member of the "model minority" and therefore not expected to get into fights or to have behavioral problems. As was developmentally appropriate for a latent-age girl, Jenny did not explicitly discuss race and culture and how they affected her identities; however, my perception of Jenny and the many possibilities for her future identity development interacted in my thinking about how to help her consider multiple possible meanings of being a black girl. These included thinking about the possibility that Jenny's identities as a black girl did not have to consist of being aggressive, having two black parents, getting involved in fights, and living in the city. Also, thinking about the multiple meanings of being black influenced, and was influenced by, some of my own thinking about multiple meanings of being a woman of color and Asian American.

Therapists also need to be aware that the effects of their identities are not only determined individually, but are influenced by the social systemic issues described above. Clients may project certain understandings on therapists, and therapists may project certain understandings on clients—even if they actively desire not to do so—because of social meanings that are internalized. Conscious and continuous attention is necessary to address these potential factors. The framework of constructed identities that we describe here is one way to focus that attention.

Expanding Our Horizons

In this chapter we have argued that identities are socially co-constructed and internalized negotiations of social contexts and categorizations (e.g., race, gender). Identity is not simply an "individual" claiming that resists imposition by others. Rather, one's identity—and all the social meanings that are embedded within that identity—are socially constructed in interaction with groups that have their own meanings that may change in different situational contexts. We also delineated the ways in which social contexts interact to produce a constant re-creation process among and within individuals and groups in a given sociohistorical context. This interaction includes, and is affected by, economics, politics, history, and issues of power and privilege. Not only are identities interactively created, but *multiple* identities are interactively created, and the social meanings of their interactions may be more than the sum of the parts. Multiple identities (e.g., as a woman, a member of a certain race, ethnicity/cultural background, sexual orientation, spiritual/religious community, and socioeconomic status) intersect and influence women's mental health in such a way that highlighting only one aspect of their identities could run the danger of pathologizing through overgeneralizing and ignoring the vast diversity *within* various groups of women. In particular, the separation of identities, statuses, or "terrains" can be particularly challenging for people who occupy what Anzaldúa (1999) has called "the borderlands": those of us who exist in multiple contexts of oppression within interacting social meanings.

Although therapy is not often considered as a space in which identities are co-constructed, we believe that an emphasis on social co-construction of identities can be a useful way to conceptualize therapy with individuals. To begin with, therapy provides a space in which clients can explore, examine, understand, and "imagine about" their lived experiences. These explorations take place not only in regard to a presenting problem, but also in relation to how the client understands her situations in light of the way she organizes her self-understanding, the various social relationships she maintains, and the social meanings to which she was exposed and has internalized. Using the relationship between the therapist and the client, therapy becomes a space in which the client's views of herself, her possibilities, and her relationships with others are revamped and expanded. It is a space that can facilitate identity shift, which is also a socially co-constructed process in therapy, because the therapist brings to the sessions her own perspectives, lived experiences, and identities.

Although we are clearly rooted in an ecological perspective (even our metaphors!), we have focused this chapter on conceptualizing and treating individuals. In the next chapter Kliman considers the intersections of multiple contexts and social meanings for understanding family systems and treating families. In the final chapter of this foundational section, Vasquez and Magraw focus expansively on the role of the therapist as ally. The remaining sections of the book build on these foundations and offer "maps" with which to consider more fully the particular terrains and journeys of diverse women within the life contexts of relationships, work, and self-care.

Notes

1. An additional example of this is the legacy of the one-drop rule. Legal definitions aimed at excluding blacks from accessing privileges and civil rights defined blacks as any person with "one drop" of black heritage, regardless of

appearance; thus the meaning of the black identity is less related to racial purity than for some other racial minority groups, such as Asians, although still relevant (as evident in Jenny's experience). Another example is the use of "blood quantum" in Native American nations. Although a given nation may not have originally used blood quantum to define membership, many nations now use blood quantum to determine tribal membership and identity (although many reject blood quantum requirements [Garroutte, 2001]), because of the imposition of race theories and ideology by European colonists and the U.S. government.

2. We want to note that there are multiple ways to define these concepts, and not all the authors will use the exact definitions presented here.

3. Although sex is not the focus for us here, we want to briefly note that sex itself is not unproblematic from a more constructivist, interactive view. Although it is usually assumed that there are two sexes and that all biological determinants are "in accordance," the seemingly clear binary categorization between male and female becomes problematized by individuals whose physical determinants are not all in "agreement" and by transsexuals who actively change some of those determinants (see, e.g., review in Crawford & Unger, 2003). The binary distinction itself is a social construction, and sex and gender activists are questioning why sex and sex identity must be categorical rather than continuous or fluid with multiple meanings and experiences (e.g., Kate Bornstein; see Bornstein, 1995).

4. The language for race and ethnicity are also confounded, although have at times been less so. White and black are commonly used and accepted as race terms, in contrast to European American and African American. However, there are no polite and nonoffensive race terms for Asian American, Native American, or Latino, although "yellow," "red," and "brown" have been used at different times and in different contexts. In this section on race (and throughout the chapter), we consciously use "black" rather than "African American" and "white" rather than "European American" in order to call attention to the differentiation.

5. We are indebted to Celeste Gutierriez and Jesse Tauriac and to the other members of the spring 2004 Social Construction of Self and Identities class (Sue Adams, Stephanie Day, Gillian Green, Jennifer Hamilton, Jennifer Kuhn, Nancy Lin, Liz Mongillo, Phuong Nguyen, and Michael Rollock) for these last two points.

6. And some cultures may have multiple boundaries and determinants: For example, Judaism is both a religion with a religious culture (Reform, Orthodox, Conservative, Reconstructionist, etc.) and an ethnic culture associated with ethnic designations (Sephardic, Ashkenazi, Yemenite, etc.).

References

American Psychological Association. (2003). Guidelines on multicultural education, training, research, practice, and organizational change for psychologists. *American Psychologist, 58,* 377–402.

Ancheta, A. N. (1998). *Race, rights, and the Asian American experience.* New Brunswick, NJ: Rutgers University Press.

Anzaldúa, G. (1999). *Borderlands/La Frontera: The new mestiza* (2nd ed.). San Francisco: Aunt Lute Books.

Ashmore, R. D., & Jussim, L. (Eds.). (1997). *Self and identity: Fundamental issues.* New York: Oxford University Press.

Atkinson, D. R., Morten, G., & Sue, D. W. (Eds.). (1998). *Counseling American minorities* (5th ed.). Boston: McGraw-Hill.

Bailey, B. (2000). Language and negotiation of ethnic/racial identity among Dominican Americans. *Language in Society, 29,* 555–582.

Blasi, A. (1988). Identity and the development of the self. In D. K. Lapsley & F. C. Power (Eds.), *Self, ego, and identity: Integrative approaches* (pp. 226–242). New York: Springer-Verlag.

Bornstein, K. (1995). *Gender outlaw: On men, women, and the rest of us.* New York: Routledge.

Brown, L. B., & Forgas, J. P. (1980). The structure of religion: A multi-dimensional scaling of informal elements. *Journal for the Scientific Study of Religion, 19,* 423–431.

Burchardt, T. (2003). Social capital. In I. McLean & A. McMillan (Eds.), *The concise Oxford dictionary of politics.* Oxford, UK: Oxford University Press. Retrieved May 3, 2004, from http://www.oxfordreference. com/views/ ENTRY.html?subview=Main&entry=t86.e1257

Calhoun, C. (Ed.). (2002a). Cultural capital. In *Dictionary of the social sciences.* Oxford, UK: Oxford University Press. Retrieved May 3, 2004, from www.oxfordreference.com/views/ENTRY.html?subview=Main&entry= t104.e401

Calhoun, C. (Ed.). (2002b). Sex. In *Dictionary of the social sciences.* Oxford, UK: Oxford University Press. Retrieved May 21, 2004, from http:// www.oxfordreference.com/views/ENTRY.html?subview=Main&entry= t104.e1516

Calhoun, C. (Ed.). (2002c). Symbolic capital. In *Dictionary of the social sciences.* Oxford, UK: Oxford University Press. Retrieved May 3, 2004, from http:// www.oxfordreference.com/views/ENTRY.html?subview= Main&entry=t104.e1648

Chesler, P. (2003). *The new anti-Semitism: The current crisis and what we must do about it.* San Francisco: Jossey-Bass.

Colman, A. M. (2001). Gender. In *Dictionary of psychology.* Oxford, UK: Oxford University Press. Retrieved May 21, 2004, from http://www. oxfordreference.com/views/ENTRY.html?subview=Main&entry=t87.e3412

Cox, L. M., & Lyddon, W. J. (1997). Constructivist conceptions of self: A discussion of emerging identity constructs. *Journal of Constructivist Psychology, 10,* 201–219.

Crawford, M., & Unger, R. (2003). *Women and gender* (4th ed.). New York: McGraw-Hill.

Dudley-Grant, G. R. (2003). Perspectives on spirituality and psychology in ethnic populations. In J. S. Mio & G. Y. Iwamasa (Eds.), *Culturally diverse mental health: The challenges of research and resistance* (pp. 341–359). New York: Brunner/Routledge.

Erikson, E. (1968). *Identity: Youth and crisis.* New York: Norton.

Espiritu, Y. L. (1992). *Asian American panethnicity: Bridging institutions and identities.* Philadelphia: Temple University Press.

Freud, S. (1964). *The future of an illusion* (J. Strachey, Ed. & W. D. Robson, Trans.) (revised ed.). New York: Anchor. (Original work published 1953.)

Fromm, E. (1950). *Psychoanalysis and religion.* New Haven, CT: Yale University Press.

Garnets, L. D. (2002). Sexual orientations in perspective. *Cultural Diversity and Ethnic Minority Psychology, 8,* 115–129.

Garroutte, E. M. (2001). The racial formation of American Indians: Negotiating legitimate identities within tribal and federal law. *American Indian Quarterly, 25,* 224–239.

Gergen, K. J. (1991). *The saturated self: Dilemmas of identity in contemporary life.* New York: Basic Books.

Gergen, K. J. (1999). *The place of the psyche in a constructed world.* Retrieved January 2, 2001, at http://www.swarthmore.edu/SocSci/kgergen1/manu.html

Guidano, V. F. (1995). Constructivist psychotherapy: A theoretical framework. In R. A. Neimeyer & M. J. Mahoney (Eds.), *Constructivism in psychotherapy* (pp. pp. 93–108). Washington, DC: American Psychological Association.

Helms, J. E., & Cook, D. A. (1999). *Using race and culture in counseling and psychotherapy.* Boston: Allyn & Bacon.

Huo, Y. J. (1998). *Who belongs in our community and who doesn't?: The influence of collective concerns on judgments of inclusion and exclusion.* Unpublished doctoral dissertation, University of California, Berkeley.

James, W. (1989). *Principles of psychology.* New York: Holt. (Original work published 1890)

Jung, C. (1938). *Psychology and religion.* New Haven, CT: Yale University Press.

Kim, G. S. (2003). *Belonging, exclusion, and construction of racial and ethnic identities among adult Korean transracial adopteees.* Unpublished master's thesis, University of Massachusetts–Boston.

Lee, J. (1996). Why Suzie Wong is not a lesbian: Asian and Asian American lesbian and bisexual women and femme/butch/gender identities. In B. Beemyn & M. Eliason (Eds.), *Queer studies: A lesbian, gay, bisexual, and transgender anthology* (pp. 115–131). New York: New York University Press.

Marcia, J. E. (1994). The empirical study of ego identity. In H. A. Bosma, T. L. G. Graffsma, H. D. Grotevant, & D. J. D. Levita (Eds.), *Identity and development: An interdisciplinary approach* (pp. 67–80). Thousand Oaks, CA: Sage.

Mass, A. I. (1991). Psychological effects of the camps on Japanese Americans. In R. Daniels, S. C. Taylor, & H. H. L. Kitano (Eds.), *Japanese Americans: From relocation to redress* (pp. 159–162). Seattle: University of Washington Press.

Nagata, D. K. (1993). *Legacy of Injustice: Exploring the cross-generational impact of the Japanese American internment* (M. J. Lerner & R. Vermunt, Eds.). New York: Plenum Press.

Nagel, J. (1997). *American Indian ethnic renewal: Red power and the resurgence of identity and culture.* New York: Oxford University Press.

Neimeyer, R. A. (1995). Constructivist psychotherapies: Features, foundations, and future directions. In R. A. Neimeyer & M. J. Mahoney (Eds.), *Constructivism in psychotherapy* (pp. 11–38). Washington, DC: American Psychological Association.

Omi, M., & Winant, H. (1994). *Racial formation in the United States: From the 1960s to the 1990s*. New York: Routledge.

Perea, J. F. (2000). The black/white binary paradigm of race. In R. Delgado & J. Stefancic (Eds.), *Critical race theory: The cutting edge* (2nd ed., pp. 344–353). Philadelphia: Temple University Press.

Pinderhughes, E. (1989). *Understanding race, ethnicity, and power: The key to efficacy in clinical practice*. New York: Free press.

Pope, M. (1995). The "salad bowl" is big enough for us all: An argument for the inclusion of lesbians and gay men in any definition of multiculturalism. *Journal of Counseling and Development, 73*, 301–304.

Rigazio-DiGilio, S. A. (1997). From microscopes to holographs: Client development within a constructivist paradigm. In T. L. Sexton & B. L. Griffin (Eds.), *Constructivist thinking in counseling practice, research, and training* (pp. 74–97). New York: Teachers College Press.

Root, M. P. P. (1998). Reconstructing race, rethinking ethnicity. In M. Hersen (Ed.), *Comprehensive clinical psychology* (pp. 141–160). New York: Pergamon Press.

Shotter, J. (1993). Becoming someone: Identity and belonging. In J. F. Nussbaum (Ed.), *Discourse and lifespan identity* (pp. 5–27). Newbury Park, CA: Sage.

Sodowsky, G. R., Kwan, K. K., & Pannu, R. (1995). Ethnic identity of Asians in the United States. In C. M. Alexander (Ed.), *Handbook of multicultural counseling* (pp. 123–154). Thousand Oaks, CA: Sage.

Spickard, P. R. (1992). The illogic of American racial categories. In M. P. P. Root (Ed.), *Racially mixed people in America* (pp. 12–22). Newbury Park, CA: Sage.

Stephens, D. P., & Phillips, L. D. (2003). Freaks, gold diggers, divas, and dykes: The sociohistorical development of adolescent African American women's sexual scripts. *Sexuality and Culture, 7*, 3–49.

Sue, D. W., & Sue, D. (2002). *Counseling the culturally diverse: Theory and practice* (4th ed.). New York: Wiley.

Suyemoto, K. L. (2002a). Constructing identities: A feminist, culturally contextualized alternative to "personality." In M. Ballow & L. S. Brown (Eds.), *Rethinking mental health and disorder: Feminist perspectives* (pp. 71–98). New York: Guilford Press.

Suyemoto, K. L. (2002b). Redefining "Asian American" identity: Reflections on differentiating ethnic and racial identities for Asian American individuals and communities. In L. Zhan (Ed.), *Asian voices: Vulnerable populations, model interventions, and emerging agendas* (pp. 195–231). Boston: Jones & Bartlett.

Thompson, P., & Bauer, E. (2003). Evolving Jamaican migrant identities: Contrasts between Britain, Canada and the USA. *Community, Work, and Family, 6*, 89–102.

Tomlinson-Clarke, S. (1999). Culture. In D. Sue (Ed.), *Key words in multicultural interventions: A dictionary* (pp. 82–83). Westport, CT: Greenwood Press.

Triandis, H. C. (1995). *Individualism and collectivism*. Boulder, CO: Westview Press.

Triandis, H. C. (2001). Individualism–collectivism and personality. *Journal of Personality, 69*(6), 907–924.

U.S. Department of Health and Human Services. (2001). *Mental health: Culture, race, and ethnicity—A supplement to mental health: A report of the Surgeon General.* Rockville, MD: U.S. Department of Health and Human Services, Public Health Service, Office of the Surgeon General.

Weber, L. (1998). A ceonceptual framework for understanding race, class, gender, and sexuality. *Psychology of Women Quarterly, 22*, 13–32.

Wehrly, B. (1995). *Pathways to multicultural counseling competency.* Pacific Grove, CA: Brooks/Cole.

Williams, M. K., McCandies, T., & Dunlap, M. R. (2002). Women of color and feminist psychology: Moving from criticism and critique to integration and application. In L. H. Collins & M. R. Dunlap (Eds.), *Charting a new course for feminist psychology* (pp. 65–89). Westport, CT: Praeger.

Yowell, C. M. (2002). Dreams of the future: The pursuit of education and career possible selves among ninth grade Latino youth. *Applied Developmental Science, 6*, 62–73.

CHAPTER 2

Many Differences, Many Voices

TOWARD SOCIAL JUSTICE IN FAMILY THERAPY

Jodie Kliman

My husband, David, woke up one morning chilled, feverish, and confused. His doctor diagnosed a galloping staph infection perilously close to his brain and ordered him to the hospital for IV antibiotics. Waiting in the ER, his face swelled and his nose turned black. He became belligerent. My urgent pleas turned loud and demanding until the IV was started, barely in time to save his life.

Frantic, I used class and other kinds of social privilege. I demanded immediate intervention. Did he survive at the expense of patients whose loved ones didn't share my entitlement, or of the overworked medical staff I pressed into action? We had health insurance. A doctor's daughter who has worked in hospitals, I am medically knowledgeable and unintimidated by doctors. Would David have survived otherwise? David was disabled for weeks, and I cancelled classes and clients to care for him. Our finances suffered, but we paid our bills. Without the flexible jobs and a financial cushion, would we have lost our jobs? Would college tuition, mortgage, or heat have gone unpaid?

Race protected David, who is 6′ 4″ and visibly strong. Toxic with infection, he was angry, confused, and probably frightening to others. I was aggressive on his behalf. What if we had been black or Latino, unprotected by our whiteness? Would antibiotics, sedation, or a call to security have come first? I later told a black colleague that without our class and racial privilege, I might be a widow. He replied, "If you'd been black, you also could be a convicted felon!" He reminded me that a black woman acting as I did could end up mothering bereaved children from prison.

My questions multiplied: How would David have fared if I didn't speak English, or only he, the incoherent one, did? What if we were undocumented aliens? Dominant gender narratives call for feminine acquiescence to male-dominated medical knowledge, so gender might have diminished another woman's class and racial privilege, but our gendering occurs in social contexts. My politically progressive and Jewish comfort with questioning authority and speaking out against wrongs shaped my responses. Had the dominant gender narratives of these contexts called for silent acceptance, I might have behaved differently. If the roles were reversed and he, a large man, were threatening staff on my behalf, how might things have turned out? Would I have had enough access to demand faster care for my partner if we were a lesbian couple, our relationship unrecognized by the state? What if we lived an hour from a rural clinic, not 10 minutes from a teaching hospital? Or if I'd been too infirm or mentally ill to get him to medical care?

My story and its hypothetical alternatives reflect the layered and intersecting ways in which privilege shapes life experience. Many forms of privilege and power, or lack thereof, contribute to our interactions and beliefs. They define what is possible, informing the webs of meaning that families, therapists, and their multiple communities use to understand, respond to, and predict life experience. They permeate what we say, what and whom is silenced, what we notice or overlook. They operate for those with privilege, and those without.

Psychological Experience in a Matrix of Intersecting Memberships and Group Narratives

An individual woman's streams of belonging converge at a single point that defines her place in a multidimensional social matrix. These converging memberships include, among others, gender, class position and history, race, ethnicity, immigration history, sexual orientation, religion, political affiliation, and mental and physical health and ability. Each membership generates its own systems of meaning, which operate together in shaping all relationships (Almeida, 1998; Falicov, 1995; Hardy & Laszloffy, 2002; Kliman, 1994; Laird, 1998; Laird & Green, 1996; McGoldrick, 1998; Pinderhughes, 2002).

This matrix can be conceived as a multidimensional layering of systems, like the transparent 3-D models of the body in which any organ system can be illuminated and placed in relationship to other visible but unlit systems, or like transparent organ system overlays in anatomy texts. Any anatomical system can be presented alone, but we fully grasp how, for example, the skeletal system operates by layering it onto the muscular and nervous systems that allow bones to move and the circulatory, respiratory, and digestive systems that nourish. Layers of meaning and belonging ramify out from individual to family, and on to the increasingly complex systems in which family is embedded: social network (Kliman & Trimble, 1983), neighborhood, community, nation, and global community.

Discourses—that is, the scaffolding we use to build our worldviews—provide the language we have available for thought, speech, and cultural practices (Hare-Mustin, 1994). Narratives—that is, the stories we use to identify ourselves and others and to guide us through life—are the key building blocks of discourse. Power and privilege operate through social discourse. Some discourses uphold existing institutions and power arrangements, and, like the groups who benefit from them, attain dominance. Subjugated groups often develop their own alternative discourses to reflect and illuminate their lived experience. These alternative discourses liberate by challenging existing power structures and the discourses that uphold them, or they are self-defeating and acquiesce to the oppressive dominant discourses. Alternative discourses are relegated to the margins, wielding less power to define self and others. Without access to language reflecting one's experience, one is silenced, blocked from articulating one's personal experience and having it acknowledged.

Because our many memberships generate both dominant and marginalized narratives to make sense of "us" and "others," family and personal worldviews are often shaped by contradictory narratives. For instance, Mei-Ling is a businesswoman and lesbian mother who emigrated from Taiwan. She holds class privilege as a businessperson in one sphere of her life. In others, American narratives about how to be a "generic" (i.e., white, middle-class, heterosexual) mother on the one hand and a "generic" (i.e., white, male) businessperson on the other marginalize her. She lives in relation to clashing group-specific narratives about how to be a mother, a daughter, Chinese, lesbian, and in business. Each of her memberships is salient (or not) in different contexts. Thus, aspects of her contextualized, embodied self are invisible to others, and even to herself, at any given time.

Social institutions such as schools, justice departments, child welfare authorities, and the media generate and are influenced by dominant beliefs. They respond one way to Mei-Ling, whose daughter is abusing drugs, and differently to other women whose children abuse drugs: undocumented Guatemalans; heterosexual working-class Irish Americans; professional African Americans; wealthy British Americans; and working-class Puerto Rican lesbians. Each woman's behaviors, in turn, reflect her own social circumstances and related cultural, class, and gender narratives about mothering children who have substance abuse problems.

All groups have internal heterogeneities and construct group-specific dominant and alternative discourses about their own group and about others. Differences are most often presented as hierarchies from *best* to *worst*. Hierarchical views of difference thrive at cultural borderlands (Rosaldo, 1989), where people encounter cultural differences and often define the subjugated "other" as "less than" (Llerena-Quinn, 2001; Root, 1996). Narratives clash when people from different backgrounds form or interact within a family: when the daughter of immigrant peasants goes to college against her father's wishes; when a secularly raised daughter becomes a fundamentalist Christian, Muslim, or Jew, or leaves those traditions for secular life or a lesbian partnership. Some subordinated group members operate "biculturally," shifting between cultures, partaking of dominant discourses as well as their own groups' range of discourses (Bacigalupe, 1998). Others internalize dominant narratives, see themselves as deficient, and either embody group stereotypes or strive to resemble dominant groups.

Llerena-Quinn (2001) suggests that we can most productively view difference not as about some "other" or about any particular people of color, but as about *all* of us, understanding that social diversity, like biological eco-diversity, is essential to our collective survival and well-being. Culture is a multidimensional, multicontextual domain of collective history, beliefs, and practices. It evolves, performed collectively but interpreted variously at the intersections of individuals' and families' group memberships (Falicov, 1995). Culture is imbued with differentials of power and privilege. People's location in the social matrix influences their degree of privilege and power, or lack thereof, which, in turn, supports their beliefs and practices. Each aspect of a family's plural memberships carries its own degree of relative privilege or subjugation, which is augmented or mitigated by members' degree of power and privilege in other domains. People and relationships are often harmed as each person performs his or her intersecting domains of privilege and marginalization. Despite her class privilege, Mei-Ling is marginalized by race, sexual orientation, gender, and immigrant status. Her white partner, Alix, has racial and native-born privilege. She hurts Mei-Ling by complaining about immigrants taking American jobs or insisting that Mei-Ling speak English with her daughter in public. Mei-Ling hurts Alix, a nurse, with her class/career privilege when she belittles nurses as not smart or ambitious enough to be doctors.

The discourses that dominant groups develop prevail but do not stand alone. Each group constructs its own cultural narratives recursively in relation to itself, others, and all intersecting memberships. White families' experience varies with ethnicity, as well with social class, religion, and health. Working-class experiences vary with race, ethnicity, immigration status and history, geography, and health. The experience of being Asian, lesbian, or deaf similarly varies. Changing just one domain of identity can shift an individual or family's entire experience.

Some domains, such as race, are usually stable, although interracial coupling can change racial identity. Others can shift, as when siblings' class trajectories vary when one moves "up" through education or "down" through drug abuse, teen pregnancy, or disability (Kliman & Madsen, 1999). Relatives' networks may barely overlap after immigration, intermarriage, divorce, illness, religious conversion, or coming out. The locations of the relatives in this web of meaning differ, in part, because their respective, overlapping social networks, neighborhoods, and work communities differ. Neighbors in an affluent community define a teacher's aide with college-bound children as working poor, but those in a poor community define her as middle class, even if her children drop out of school.

All our domains of identity shape us, even though we may not notice most of them. We most easily notice our domains of marginalization and overlook our domains of privilege; Mei-Ling and Alix feel unilaterally injured by the other, each oblivious to her power to hurt a differently marginalized loved one. Some domains of identity go unnoticed for a lifetime when everyone we know is (or seems) like us. Some aspects of identity become salient as memberships change, as when a family member shifts class position, forms an interracial or interfaith family, comes out, immigrates, or becomes chronically ill.

Our gender-based expectations about how to be in our families and communities reflect divergent class-bound realities (Kliman, 1998; Kliman & Forsberg, 1998). Social class is a *relationship*, not a neutral status. It is not equivalent to socioeconomic status, which is a formula that combines income, occupation, and educational attainments to place one along a "value-neutral" continuum of upper, middle, and lower socioeconomic status. Whereas social class highlights how the privileged classes live well at others' expense, socioeconomic status obscures that relationship (Ehrenreich, 1989). Members of one class live well at the expense of other classes (Ehrenreich, 1989). Women who challenge the glass ceiling and inequitable domestic relationships can do so in part because other, poorer, women face grueling labor and poverty tending the kitchens, nurseries, and office bathrooms of these more privileged women. Beth's attorney parents paid for her college, wedding, and down payment, setting her up for success. Now age 60, she easily finances family vacations and subsidizes her grandchildren and elderly parents' care. Janet, a widowed housekeeper's daughter, expected a bleak future, got pregnant, dropped out of school, married and then divorced a school dropout. At 60, diabetes and heart disease have ended her home health care job, and she lives on disability. Despite her ailments, she watches her great-grandchildren 6 days a week so that her granddaughter can care for Beth's mother and other elderly patients. Class affects and connects both women's life expectancies, family life cycles, expectations, and options (Kliman & Madsen, 1999).

Race shapes gendering as well. Each domain of privilege—or lack thereof—intensifies or counters the other's effects. Its combination with capitalism, colonialism, and sexism leaves families of color disproportionately poor and/or vulnerable to becoming poor (Boyd-Franklin, 2003; U.S. Bureau of the Census, 2000). Unemployment and related rates of addiction, incarceration, and violent death "disappear" many young black and Latino men, and more than a few poor young black women (U.S. Bureau of the Census, 2000). Slavery's residual effects are reflected in these phenomena and in lower expectations for even middle-class black boys than for white boys or girls of any race (Boyd-Franklin & Franklin, 2001). Black women therefore generally have higher educational and employment levels than black men. Because African Americans do not share other races' history of women's financial dependence on men, they have less marriage and more gender role flexibility than all other racial groups (Boyd-Franklin, 2003; Pinderhughes, 2002). In a country where whites once enslaved blacks, *race* often means "black and white" only, ignoring other races and expressions of racism. Race is socially constructed and context sensitive, defined quite differently in different countries and regions. Many Latinos/as who self-define as white or by their nationality in their original countries "become" black or brown on immigration. Multiracial identity has gained conceptual currency in recent years (Root, 1996; Suyemoto & Dimas, 2003).

Ethnicity and immigration relate recursively with gender. Cultural transitions from an original culture to bi- or multiculturalism or assimilation often occur at different rates within and between generations and genders. Some immigrants hold "old country" ideas that younger generations (and therapists) reject; some U.S.-born children of Americanized parents yearn for an idealized ancestral life. Race and skin color are factors as well. Light-skinned immigrants, especially those with class privilege in the "old country," tend to advance economically before their darker and poorer counterparts and thus more quickly adopt social narratives compatible with dominant American discourses. Most American descendants of European Jews, who, like Irish Americans, were mostly poor in their original countries, "became" white[1] after generations of biculturalism and economic mobility in the United States (Brodkin, 1998). Similarly, light-skinned Asian and Latino immigrant families tend to fare better than their darker compatriots. Language is also a salient aspect of ethnic cultural identity, most obviously for immigrants. Language influences how people think and what is accessible. Language barriers systematically marginalize non-English speakers.

Gender and ethnicity discourses intersect in complex ways with those of class, race, and religion. Women in culturally marginalized groups encounter U.S. forms of sexism, racism, and classism *and* culture-specific gender discourses. For instance, in many Latino cultures, the gender narrative of *marianismo* spiritually elevates women who, emulating the Virgin Mary, endure suffering and sacrifice in their relational lives (Hines, García Preto, McGoldrick, Almeida, & Weltman, 1999), and so renders their subjugation acceptable. This acceptance of subjugation comingles with the harsh realities of Latinas' cultural marginalization and their economic vulnerability in the United States. Similarly, stereotypes of Jewish mothers as intrusive and domineering or of middle-age black women as all nurturing "mammies" invalidate the complexity of their experiences. Young women in culturally marginalized groups often face within-group and dominant-group sexism *and* dominant cultural narratives that eroticize and subjugate them as the "exotic other" (Comas Díaz & Greene, 1994). At the same time, women in both dominant and subjugated cultural groups have developed countervailing narratives of resistance to such marginalization. For example, rather than perceiving themselves as intrusive and domineering, many feminist Jewish mothers celebrate their ability to use their voices to protect family and reject the dominant cultural norm of women as passively silencing their own needs.

Sexual orientation is a powerful, if often invisible, aspect of family and community life. Its effects are layered onto previously discussed factors. Gays, lesbians, and heterosexuals share all class positions and histories, races, ethnicities, religions, political beliefs, and mental and physical health statuses (Greene, 1994; Laird & Greene, 1996). Homosexuality, bisexuality, and heterosexuality play out differently in different cultures (Greene, 1994). In the United States, dominant culture narratives linking heterosexuality alone to the right to marry are only recently being publicly questioned and defended (Council on Contemporary Families, 2004). Many racial and ethnic groups call homosexuality a "white problem," and lesbians of color may face rejection or exclusion in their racial communities for engaging in a "white" form of sexuality (Greene, 1994). However, a lesbian couple of color may not see themselves as participating in a "white" form of sexuality and might feel that they have more in common with their heterosexual neighbors of color than with a white lesbian couple with a different class background living in a different neighborhood.

Gender narratives vary with physical and mental health and ability as well. Greenspan (1998) challenges the pathologizing as "enmeshed" of those mothers whose children's special needs require prolonged protection and care. Gender narratives guiding women to put others' needs first break down when illness requires them to care first for themselves (Weingarten, 1997). When both parent and children are sick with asthma, obesity-related diseases, HIV/AIDS, or other chronic illnesses that occur most among the poor and working class and that can be impoverishing, things are harder still. Many therapists see not hardship but "resistance" when poor asthmatic mothers and children are not able to take two buses to therapy in bad weather. A single mother with multiple sclerosis surviving on government disability does not share the illness and disability experiences of the similarly stricken married mother who can afford help.

Adding Layers: How Multiple Social Positions Shape Therapeutic Relationships

Jon, the grandson of Rumanian Jews, and Marla, the granddaughter of Russian Orthodox immigrants, are artists who couldn't decide whether to move in together or separate. Her parents were working class; his were professionals. Jon's vehement anger scared Marla; her fear baffled him. When Jon got "worked up" over political disagreements, Marla saw only a "dominating man." He retorted that he wanted her to argue back. My noting that I shared Marla's concern about men dominating women, but was at home with Jon's spirited, argumentative style piqued their interest. Marla was surprised that, like Jon, I saw philosophical arguments as opportunities to learn together, not as exercises in domination. Jon's and my family both enjoyed impassioned political debates—secular versions of traditional Jewish arguments over the meanings of sacred texts. Adding ethnicity and class to gender offered Marla new meanings for Jon's intensity during disagreement, and helped Jon understand her anxiety over open conflict. They began to connect Marla's parents' silence about their beliefs to job vulnerability as semiskilled workers raised by pre-Soviet immigrants. Contextualizing each other's positions fostered mutual empathy. We could then explore how Jon's impulsivity might also be related to attention-deficit/hyperactivity disorder (ADHD) and offer tools for better self-control, without relieving him of accountability or his subjective experience.

The layered exploration of experiences and assumptions helped us understand the contradictions of cultural narratives influencing these two individuals' shared lives, expanding the possibilities and context-rich meanings of therapeutic conversation. This exploration facilitated nonblaming, creative approaches that allowed us to reflect on their cultural, class, and neurobiological differences, as well as the combination of ways in which each had experienced marginalization and privilege. I could not have predicted which differences would be most significant; they emerged through collaborative conversation. Marla's gender subjugation intersected with her parents' class and cultural experiences of placating and assenting to the powerful in the interest of survival, and with her Christianity. Jon's marginalization as a Jew, whose argumentativeness is rejected by dominant culture, combined with gender and class privilege to endow him with confidence to the point of domination in an argument. Add to the mix Marla's "standard issue" neurobiological wiring and Jon's ADHD, and their interaction becomes yet more complex.

Therapists and clients participate in the discourses available to them. I resonated with Jon's Jewish background and Marla's feminism. I was comfortable with Marla's family's working-class experience, which some of my relatives share, yet I grew up with Jon's class privilege. I knew little about Orthodox Russian culture, about which I held uneasy prejudices; my grandmother's relatives in Russia were massacred in *pogroms*, the periodic mass murders of Jews throughout Europe. I had to connect across that chasm with Marla, just as I connected across gender with Jon. As therapists, like everyone, we easily see relationships through the lenses of our marginalization, but we must work harder to perceive the effects of our lenses of privilege on our assumptions about personal and professional relationships. I did not grasp how my family's racial and class privilege shaped my clinical assumptions until I became stepmother to children whose mother was from a poor, black/Native American family. Years after my brother came out as gay—and I married, but he could not— I saw how my heterosexual privilege, unacknowledged, silences lesbian, gay, bisexual, or transgendered clients in therapy. Even if we recognize our subjugation, we still must work to see its effects on ourselves or on others. Years into chronic health problems, I still struggle with internalized narratives that shame the physically afflicted.

Clinical training usually reflects dominant discourses and crowds out culture-specific narratives of therapists from marginalized groups. Hence, a Latina, lesbian, or originally working-class therapist guided by professional discourses can lose sight of the psychological effects of marginalization on her own family or on clients who experience subjugation. Therapists can also lose sight of the effects of power and subjugation when we have privilege in some areas and not in others. Don, a professional-class African American supervisee, felt anxious about a working-class, white gay male client, Jack, who, Don realized, acted as if Don were more powerful than he. Jack's stance confused Don, who said he had never seen a white client respond to him in this way. Exploring his heterosexual privilege in a homophobic society helped Don better empathize with Jack, whose subjugation as gay but privilege as white mirrored Don's racial subjugation but sexual orientation privilege.

Dominant discourse—and much of therapy—neglects social factors and guides families (and therapists) toward seeing the effects of differences in power and privilege as reflecting individual problems.

Sarah Hunt, a white realtor and single parent, and her son, Michael, an adopted, biracial preteen, consulted me about his angry struggles with teachers over minor infractions and with Sarah over slipping grades. Sarah, who had lived only in white communities, suspected that racism played into the disparate treatment of Mike and his white classmates, but she hesitated to excuse his behavior. Neither family nor school could turn to black elders to pass on discourses that resist the effects of racism. They could only draw on dominant racial narratives—for instance, the argument that the only way to be antiracist is to be color blind, or the popular adolescent "gangsta" narratives that depict young black men either as not too bright or as bright troublemakers. My questions, designed to challenge such assumptions, helped unravel the insidious power of these discourses: "Sarah, why do you think Mike was disciplined for talking, but Sam (his white friend) wasn't?" or "Mike, why do you think your teachers accept a kid as smart as you getting C's? Are they the same way with the white kids? Why?" or "Do you think that Mike is starting to think that he deserves all the trouble he gets into at school, or that doing well in school isn't worth the effort?"

Such questions place personal stories in social context. They generate self-respecting understandings of, and responses to, marginalization. We can open up new considerations by asking how clients' experiences and conflicts might compare if they had a different gender or sexual orientation, more or less money, education, or racial privilege, spoke a different language, or participated in a different spiritual community. Such conversation counters the shame associated with seeing one's struggles solely as reflecting personal failings.

Making Room for Multiple Voices: Toward a Just and Dialogical Clinical Stance

Elise was from a Scottish American working-class family; Olu, from a well-off Yoruba family in Cameroon, had come to the United States for college. They had three children and worked as mid-level professionals. They sought couple therapy for escalating arguments over frequent visits from relatives who would come from Cameroon for school or medical care and stay for months. Elise was outraged that Olu welcomed his relatives without her say, when the house was small and his schedule left her with most of the responsibility for them. She was increasingly overwhelmed and depressed by her in-laws' presence; her friends were urging her to divorce Olu. Many American therapists would have supported Elise's right to a say over the privacy of her nuclear family's home, but Olu's position needed validation as well.

Olu's father, as a well-off Muslim, had two wives who had raised their eight children together, including Olu, the youngest. The Yoruba, like most collectivist societies, do not distinguish between what Americans call nuclear and extended family. Obligation to kin runs deep. After their father's death, Olu's brothers had paid for his professional education. Olu could no more turn away their children and grandchildren than his own young sons. He was mystified by what he saw as Elise's selfish response to her in-laws and embarrassed by their complaints that she was racist as well. Olu and his kin saw the drain on household finances and privacy as minor compared to Olu's collective responsibility to family. They didn't see that, unlike Yoruba wives, Elise did not benefit from mutually helpful relationships with female relatives.

Elise and Olu were both justified in their own respective cultural frameworks, but wrong in each other's. In an old story, a couple asked the rabbi, who served as judge and therapist in the *shtetl* (a walled Jewish ghetto), to resolve a dispute. He listened carefully to the husband's argument, nodded sagely, and intoned, "You are right." The wife protested that he had to hear her side; the rabbi listened to her story and nodded, saying, "You are right." The rabbi's wife strode in from the kitchen (where else?), upbraiding her husband for telling people in total disagreement that they were both right. Ever thoughtful, he heard her out, nodded, and proclaimed, "You are right!" Like the rabbi, I had to understand both Olu's and Elise's perspectives and help each understand and respect the contexts and discourses that guided the other's (and their own) values and perspectives. Neither had seen the other as behaving honorably in a context different from one's own but as willfully flouting presumably shared values.

Healing Relational Wounds of Power and Privilege: Hardy and Laszloffy's Model

The capacity to hurt and be hurt that permeates family and therapeutic relationships is intensified by socially constructed differences among people. Therapists, even when marginalized in some way in the larger world, always have more power than their clients, who come to them in need. Our power to impose meaning is often underestimated and misused. Hardy and Laszloffy (2002) argue that everyone, both privileged and marginalized, is hurt when one group is normalized over others. They propose that we must all take responsibility for healing the relational injuries of power, but the privileged (including therapists and clients) are more responsible for healing *in their domains of greater privilege*. Thus two or more parties may be accountable to each other, but in different domains of privilege.

Hardy and Laszloffy (2002) propose the following steps in healing these relational injuries in the acknowledgment, validation, apology, and forgiveness (AVAF) model. *Acknowledgment* involves accepting that one has committed an injury (regardless of intent) and communicating that awareness to the injured party. *Validation* legitimates the wounded party's feelings about the harm done. *Apology* involves taking responsibility for the harm one has done. *Forgiveness* follows only if the wounded party is ready. If not, whether because of the extent of harm or because the victim perceives the apology as insincere, the offending party must keep validating and accounting for the injury until forgiveness is forthcoming. The AVAF model suggests specific responsibilities of both the privileged and the subjugated in working toward repair and achieving justice in their relationships.

The Tasks of the Privileged in This Model

The tasks of the privileged in the AVAF model include the following:

1. *Resisting the idea that your own suffering is equal to that of the subjugated.* Discourses that equalize all suffering deny power differentials and their ill effects, thereby silencing the subjugated. This task is particularly challenging when people privileged in one domain carry their own pain of marginalization, past or present, in other domains. It is unproductive to fall into a competition over victim status.

2. *Distinguishing between* intent *and* consequences, *because even unintended injuries result in harm.* It is important to acknowledge the suffering you have caused, without asking to be understood and even when feeling misunderstood. Because subjugated people are so often traumatized by both intended and careless "micro-aggressions" (Pierce, 1995) at the hands of the privileged, their pain must be judged more important than the intentions of the privileged.

3. *Resisting the tendency to define or negate the experience of the subjugated.* Two infamous examples of this tendency are the diagnoses of "penis envy," imposed on women yearning to achieve in a man's world, and "drapetomania," a 19th-century race-specific "disorder" that purportedly impelled slaves to keep trying to escape slavery (Tavris, 1989). We laugh (nervously, perhaps) at such diagnoses today, even as, with the best of intentions, *we tell our clients the meaning of their experience.*

4. *Developing the "thick skin" needed to respond compassionately to feedback, even rage, from a subjugated person you have injured.* It is hard (and important) to grow that thick skin if you feel injured in other domains. Painful as it is to live with your own scars of oppression, it is

never productive to ask someone to care about your oppression while you are contributing to theirs.

5. *Allowing feelings of remorse (not paralyzing guilt) to mobilize efforts aimed at establishing justice.* Those pangs are instructive if they help you become accountable to others. The point is not guilty self-flagellation. No one can always resist the discourses or practices of oppression, but remorse can fuel corrective actions.

6. *Staying in the relationship even if you feel that you are not getting the appreciation you deserve for "doing good."* Do it not for the kudos but to heal and strengthen relationships.

The Tasks of the Subjugated or Marginalized in This Model

The tasks of the subjugated or marginalized in the AVAF model include the following:

1. *Resisting narratives of internalized oppression,* including those shaming you and your cultural group; shame precludes critical thinking and action.

2. *Resisting the privileged party's pull to educate them, for their sake,* about your group's experience. (It is important for clients to resist, to avoid being exploited as cultural brokers.)

3. *Resisting "invitations" to take care of, or comfort, the privileged,* for instance, minimizing your discomfort or suffering because of their actions, to protect them. This tendency maps perfectly onto the tendency of the privileged to equalize all suffering. It also relates to the historical strategy of assuaging the discomfort of someone who could easily hurt you with his or her power (as slaves, servants, and women know about masters and some employers and men).

4. *Resisting silencing and learned voicelessness* to be the author of your own story. There is an important difference between educating the privileged for *their* sake and the healing experience of using and hearing your own voice—whether or not you are heard and witnessed.

5. *Channeling rage to make it useful;* when unchanneled, rage is constricting or becomes the stuff of vengeance, which can be as destructive to self as to other—consider the incarceration rates of blacks and Latinos. Channeled rage can give birth to constructive personal and social transformations.

6. If you acquire privilege in one realm (e.g., as a woman of color with class privilege), *do not allow your privilege to turn you away from the struggle against marginalization* for yourself or others, or to say, "I'm too tired to keep fighting for equality" (Hardy & Laszloffy, 2002).

Some Guidelines to Inform a Culturally Respectful Clinical Stance[2]

As healers and witnesses, we confront clients' needs for healing the wounds of oppression, marginalization, and silencing, as well as those of mental illness, trauma, and interpersonal conflict. These wounds, which affect us as the injured, perpetrator, and witness, can last for generations (Weingarten, 2003). Family therapists address the toll of these wounds of oppression on family life by integrating psychological and social healing in therapy. I have developed the following guidelines to inform clinicians striving toward socially just and collaborative healing relationships with family members struggling with injuries of power and subjugation.

1. *Learn about your location in the social matrix.* To understand someone else's social location, you must start by exploring your own (see Vasquez & Magraw, Chapter 3). Understanding the history of our multiple memberships, each of their dominant and marginalized discourses, and their interrelationship helps you understand your relationship to particular theories and clinical approaches, and how you resonate with clients' stories. This is a lifelong process.

2. *Develop sensitivity to clients' experiences of their multiple memberships.* Read, seek consultations, and find pluralistic settings in which to speak openly about divergent experiences, asking respectful questions. Learn from clients, who are the only experts on their own experiences, meanings, and contexts, but avoid exploiting them for their knowledge.

3. *Respond to differences as valuable and necessary learning opportunities, rather than as hierarchies of better and worse or as "us" and "the other."* Llerena-Quinn (2001) suggests that cultural diversity is as important to our survival as is eco-diversity.

4. *Serve as coinvestigator with clients* (Anderson, 1997; White, 1995) concerning different interpretations and meanings for particular behaviors, phrases, and identities, without giving dominant interpretations more weight. This work requires a dual stance of respectful curiosity and "informed not-knowing" (Anderson, 1997; Laird, 1998), in which you cannot know another's experience in advance, but are forthcoming with your own knowledge base. Socially just and clinically astute work requires us to ask our clients and ourselves, "Whose voice is missing in this conversation?" (Llerena-Quinn, 2001) and look for the "not-yet-said" in this conversation (Anderson, 1997).

5. *Pay close attention to details of the language,* the importance of which is recognized by narrative (White, 1995) and collaborative

(Anderson, 1997) therapists. In culturally respectful work this attention is applied to a regular scanning for, and deconstruction of, cross-cultural misunderstandings. When family members (and therapists) participate in different cultural discourses, different interpretations of the same words often reflect important differences not only in value, but also in degree of privilege, as we see with the following family:

> Carlos, a Puerto Rican mechanic, and Yvonne, a French Canadian office manager, consulted me because of bitter conflict over their 16-year-old's behavior. Daniel was leaving home early on Sundays to avoid family dinner at Carlos's parents' house. Carlos was furious at Daniel for disrespecting his relatives, and at Yvonne for condoning his behavior. Mother and son were incredulous that Father thought Daniel, who had an after-school job and basketball practice, should spend every Sunday with relatives. Dan complained that no one else had to see relatives every week. Yvonne was angry that Carlos expected her to support his position. She rebuked Carlos for preferring his parents over Daniel and her, adding that her family was happy with getting together monthly. My speaking Spanish, the father's native tongue, and English, Yvonne and Daniel's only language, helped us out of this tangle. Knowing that the meanings of *respect* and *respeto* are not identical, I asked them to define the term that was getting them into trouble with each other.

> YVONNE: Well, not talking back, doing what you are told, not breaking the rules, you know, just being respectful. And Daniel is a lot better than a lot of his friends at that, so I wish his father would just go easy on him!

> JODIE: Carlos, does Yvonne's description fit what you want from your son?

> CARLOS: Yes, sure, I expect those things, but to me, respect is much bigger than that. If Yvonne and Dan don't show that family is more important than friends or anything, that's a shame, a *verguënza*, to our whole family. If he's too busy to talk to his grandmother or help his little cousin, then he doesn't know what's important and we have failed to teach him devotion and *respeto*. I can't understand why Yvonne and Daniel don't see that hurts us in front of everyone!

> JODIE: Daniel, did what your dad just say surprise you? And what do *you* think respect is?

> DANIEL: Well, yeah. I thought he meant it like Mom does, you know, the *normal* way. I mean, I know he gets mad when I don't go to his parents, but I didn't know it made him feel like such a *loser*. (*turning to his father*) But Dad, you're wrong that I don't

care about the family! I mean, I do what you want, I work hard at school, I don't get in trouble, I do my chores. You expect me to do stuff no one else does and it's embarrassing to always say I have to go to some family thing. (*turning to Jodie*) And then he yells at me when I'm on the phone—that's not respectful to me! I don't want to hurt him, but why should I respect him if he won't respect me?

JODIE: (*after further exploring these different understandings of* respect *and* respeto) So if Father means *respeto* the way *his* family does, and Mother means *respect* the way *her* family does, and Daniel's *respect* combines his mom's and his friends' meanings, it's hard for each of you to get the respect you expect. When important words have different meanings, sometimes the person with the unpopular view doesn't get heard—like a kid's view, a woman's view, or an immigrant's view. How could you all make sure that everyone gets heard and feels respected?

Finding and emphasizing the cultural mistranslation of seemingly similar terms honored the cultural and generational contexts that each person (including grandparents and friends) brought to the conflict. Now we could resist Father's marginalization as a Puerto Rican migrant, Mother's as a wife expected to bow to her husband's wishes, and Son's subordination as a child.

Although it helps to know the culturally contrasting meanings of a word, knowing a family's language and culture is not imperative (and sometimes offers false confidence). What *is* necessary is carefully scanning for cross-cultural misunderstandings. I once offered a family consultation for a family therapy class in Sweden. On hearing that the mother had started staffing a "hot line," I suggested that helping women who, like herself, had been sexually abused might provide her with an avenue of healing. When I noticed my colleague and his class looking first puzzled, then quietly horrified, I invited their unvoiced thoughts—and understood. In Sweden, a "hot line" does not offer succor to the abused, as in the United States, but, rather, telephone sex! Without the group's subtle nonverbal cues and my Swedish colleague's cultural guidance, I could have kept applying a hopelessly inappropriate definition of *hot* to a (very polite) Swedish context, thereby losing both my credibility and utility.

6. *Culturally respectful therapists strive to avoid imposing meanings on clients or allowing clients to impose meaning on them, or on each other.* Therapy can be used to question dominant narratives or to reinforce them. People of color, Jews, refugees and their children, and trauma survivors of all backgrounds can be witnessed respectfully or pathologized and defined as paranoid, always looking for signs of oppression. Therapists routinely

impose goals of individuation and independence on families whose cultural discourses value loyalty and interdependence, criticizing parents for not letting go and young adults for dependence. Teenage girls can be asked if they are interested in anyone special, which opens up the possibility of talking about attraction to girls, or they can be asked if they have a *boyfriend*, which slams shut the door to that discussion. Bacigalupe (1998) describes such imposition as a colonial practice that excludes the voices of the colonized. An Asian American colleague once recounted having met a graduate school requirement by seeing a therapist, a white woman. When my colleague got angry at a racist assumption the therapist had made, the therapist told her she could not be angry because she *knew* that Asian women do not get angry! (Suffice it to say, treatment was *very* brief!) Regularly looking for and questioning one's own assumptions limits the imposition of meaning.

7. *Therapy that involves a culturally respectful stance that makes room for all voices helps move conversations from a monological to dialogical mode* (Kamya & Trimble, 2002). In one form of monologue, one voice and the discourses it reflects prevails over others, which are drowned out (as happened to my Asian American colleague) or silenced. In another form of monologue, conversations become debates ("You're wrong!" "No, you're wrong!"), in which no one hears and considers the other's argument. Dialogical conversation involves a true exchange of ideas and feelings; every voice is heard and considered. It does not require agreement, only careful, respectful listening and response.

8. *Culturally respectful therapists are ready to learn about what they do not know or notice.* Modifying Hardy and Laszloffy's (1995) cultural genogram, I once asked a group of interns to select their two most personally meaningful aspects of cultural identity and present their family histories in a social context. I expected one intern to name her lesbian and Latina identities. In fact, she focused on growing up abroad on naval bases as most salient—a facet of identity I had not considered. I was reminded that to be culturally respectful in relation to multiple discourses, I had to hold my assumptions lightly and be ready to be surprised. Professional class therapists of color are routinely asked to treat racially similar families without regard to other differences. Yet a black woman whose uncle sexually abused her may prefer a female therapist of any race over a black man. A devout Muslim or Orthodox Jewish family in conflict over adolescent sexuality may want a non-Muslim or non-Orthodox therapist for reasons of community privacy, but insist on having a therapist who lovingly observes some religious tradition. A black and Latina lesbian couple may care more about a therapist's commitment to work against internalized homophobia and racism than his or her race, gender, or sexual orientation.

9. *We must be ready to gently raise delicate topics about differences, including in power and privilege, when we join clients in navigating unex-*

plored differences and similarities among themselves, between us and them, and between them and others. When asking about such differences, we should not assume that early reassurances that "differences don't matter" reveal the whole story. When the therapist holds more privilege than one or more of the clients, it is important for the therapist to remember to *earn* trust before assuming that these comforting reassurances reflect clients' actual experience. Trust is gained slowly, by demonstrating cultural respect and continuing to ask about the effects of differences on the therapy. It is not uncommon for clients to say that they were not ready to acknowledge the importance of a particular difference before the therapist "proved" her- or himself trustworthy.

10. *Asking clients questions that place their stories beyond the solely personal and include larger social contexts* adds richness to clinical work. However, when clients offer rehearsed and simple social answers, such as, "That's just what we [or they] are like," pursuing detailed questioning can challenge constricting and stereotyping narratives. A colleague once challenged a Mexican man who justified hitting his wife by saying, "You know, we Latinos all hit our wives when they get out of line." She replied, "Really? That's interesting, because my husband is Latino, and he doesn't hit me!" He asked where they were from and, learning they were Panamanian, countered that all *Mexican* men hit their wives. She replied, "Really? My sister's husband is Mexican, and *he* doesn't hit her either." He responded that maybe it was just men from his province. Ultimately, he acknowledged that maybe the men in *his family* always hit their wives. "Okay, *now* we can get to work!" rejoined my colleague (Y. Flores-Ortiz, personal communication, June, 1995).

11. *Identifying and exploring the multiple and contradictory cultural and class narratives* influencing their (and your) relational experiences, expands the possibilities in therapy. Asking variations on, "How might this situation be different if you/I/she had more/less money, education, racial privilege, were of a different gender or sexual orientation, spoke a different language, belonged to a different faith, were healthy?" can be liberatory:

> Ted, an architect from a working-class family, becomes worried when Dory wants to borrow $8,000 to redecorate their child's room. His anxiety is grounded in memories of his parents skimping on food to pay essential bills. Dory, a business consultant, grew up in economic comfort, but winces to remember her mother "stealing" from her housekeeping allowance to avoid asking Dory's father for clothing money. Dory worries about a man financially controlling her, whereas Ted worries about insupportable debt. Emma, a privileged child, doesn't understand her father's anxiety or her mother's anger at her father. Ted sees Dory's and Emma's class privilege, but not his mother's and mother-in-law's gender-based economic insecurity. Dory doesn't

see how class privilege insinuates itself into her ease with borrowing for luxuries.

12. It helps to *be transparent, acknowledging that both therapists' and clients' ideas are grounded not in "objective truth" but in personal experience* (White, 1995), including experiences of privilege and marginalization. For example, a therapist baffled by her client's anxiety over her daughter's marital problems could wonder aloud if her (the therapist's) response is grounded in life experiences she herself has not had, rather than arguing against her client's anxiety. Such questioning does raise the possibility that clients might ask questions about therapists' lives, which, when answered with care, can help build a shared language and earned trust. This was the case, for instance, when I helped Marla and Jon enter each other's cultural and class-based understandings of disagreement.

13. *Be accountable for any pain or slight you inflict, even if unintentionally, on clients*, particularly when you hold more power in and outside the context of therapy. Create a therapeutic environment in which family members can be accountable to each other (and, as needed, to you as well).

When Denise, a black college student, suddenly stopped coming to sessions after my urging her to get an HIV test to relieve her of her growing fear that she had contracted HIV during a rape years earlier, I realized that I must have pushed too hard. When she didn't respond to phone messages, I wrote to her. I said I must have hurt her, but wasn't sure how, and I wanted to make it right. I invited her to come without charge to tell me how I had hurt her. She came and in this session she reminded me that her black Southern Baptist church elevated Jews as the Chosen People, G-d's most beloved (a painful perception to this Jew, who rejects spiritual inequality). Although she had felt unready for HIV testing, she assumed that I, as "doctor" and Jew, was right. Although I had always considered some non-New Yorkers and non-Jews finding my interpersonal style somewhat pushy to be based on a stereotyped misunderstanding of Jewish-style dialogue (remember Jon and Marla), I had hurt Denise with my approach. She needed, and we engaged in, the AVAF (Hardy & Laszloffy, 2002) process of healing unintentional harm that I had caused Denise. I am glad to say that treatment resumed and benefited from my accountability to her.

Conclusion

The approach offered here helps to heal the harm that complex combinations of power and privilege can inflict on family and therapeutic relationships. Relational healing requires respectful attention to all the layers of difference that shape relationships. People injured by the workings of power and privilege need to experience accountability from those who have hurt them (Hardy & Lazloffy, 2002). When grief and anger are not witnessed and acknowledged (Weingarten, 2003), grieving is cut short and replaced by destructive cycles of retraumatization and vengeance (Kliman & Llerena-Quinn, 2002). Similar approaches apply beyond intimate relationships to local, regional, and global communities injured in large-scale relationships (Botcharova, 2001; Kamya & Trimble, 2002; Kliman & Llerena-Quinn, 2002; Public Conversations Project, 2004; Weingarten, 2003).

Notes

1. Some Jews acknowledge recently acquired white-skin privilege without identifying as white (European American), because European citizenship was long denied to Jews. I identify as white *and* Jewish, because I have white privilege, but connect to my nonwhite Jewish elders and history.

2. I use "culturally respectful," because acquiring "cultural competence" is a lifelong process.

References

Almeida, R.V. (Ed.). (1998). Transformations of gender and race: Family and developmental perspectives [Special issue]. *Journal of Feminist Family Therapy, 10*(1).

Anderson, H. (1997). *Conversation, language, and possibilities: A postmodern approach to therapy.* New York: Basic Books.

Bacigalupe, G. (1998). Cross-cultural systemic training and consultation: A postcolonial view. *Journal of Systemic Therapies, 17,* 31–44.

Botcharova, O. (2001). Implementation of track two diplomacy: Developing a model of forgiveness. In G. Raymond, S. Helmick, & R. Peterson (Eds.), *Forgiveness and reconciliation: Religion, public policy, and conflict transformation* (pp. 279–305). Philadelphia: Templeton Press.

Boyd-Franklin, N. (2003). *Black families in therapy: Understanding the African American experience* (2nd ed.). New York: Guilford Press.

Boyd-Franklin, N., & Franklin, A. J. (2001). *Boys into men: Raising our African American teenage sons.* New York: Plume.

Brodkin, K. (1998). *How Jews became white folks and what that says about race in America.* New Brunswick, NJ: Rutgers University Press.

Comas-Díaz, L., & Greene, B. (Eds.). (1994). *Women of color: Integrating ethnic and gender identities in psychotherapy.* New York: Guilford Press.

Council on Contemporary Families. (2004). Home page. Available at www. contemporaryfamilies. org

Ehrenreich, B. (1989). *Fear of falling: The inner life of the middle class.* New York: HarperCollins.

Falicov, C. (1995). Training to think culturally: A multidimensional comparative framework. *Family Process, 34,* 373–388.

Greene, B. (1994). Lesbian women of color: Triple jeopardy. In L. Comas-Díaz & B. Greene (Eds.), *Women of color: Integrating ethnic and gender identities in psychotherapy* (pp. 389–427). New York: Guilford Press.

Greenspan, M. (1998). "Exceptional" mothering in a "normal" world. In C. G. Coll, J. L. Surrey, & K. Weingarten (Eds.), *Mothering against the odds: Diverse voices of contemporary mothers* (pp. 37–60). New York: Guilford Press.

Hardy, K., & Laszloffy, T. (1995). The cultural genogram: Key to training culturally competent family therapists. *Journal of Marital and Family Therapy, 21,* 227–238.

Hardy, K. V., & Laszloffy, T. A. (2002). Couple therapy using a multicultural perspective. In A. S. Gurman & N. S. Jacobson (Eds.), *Clinical handbook of couple therapy* (3rd ed., pp. 569–593). New York: Guilford Press.

Hare-Mustin, R. T. (1994). Discourses in a mirrored room: A postmodern analysis of therapy. *Family Process, 33,* 19–35.

Hines, P. M., García Preto, N., McGoldrick, M., Almeida, R., & Weltman, S. (1999). Culture and the family life cycle. In B. Carter & M. McGoldrick (Eds.), *The expanded family life cycle: Individual, family, and social perspectives* (pp. 69–87). Boston: Allyn & Bacon.

Kamya, H., & Trimble, D. (2002). Response to injury: Toward ethical construction of the other. *Journal Of Systemic Therapies, 21,* 19–29.

Kliman, J. (1994). The interweaving of gender, class, and race in family therapy. In M. P. Mirkin (Ed.), *Women in context: Toward a feminist reconstruction of psychotherapy* (pp. 25–47). New York: Guilford Press.

Kliman, J. (1998). Social class as a relationship: Implications for family therapy. In M. McGoldrick (Ed.), *Re-visioning family therapy: Race, culture, and gender in clinical practice* (pp. 50–61). New York: Guilford Press.

Kliman, J., & Forsberg, G. (1998). American welfare reform and the Swedish welfare state. *Journal of Feminist Family Therapy, 10,* 47–68.

Kliman, J., & Llerena-Quinn, R. (2002). Dehumanizing and rehumanizing responses to September 11. *Journal of Systemic Therapies, 21,* 8–18.

Kliman, J., & Madsen, W. (1999). Social class and the family life cycle. In B. Carter & M. McGoldrick (Eds.), *The expanded family life cycle: Individual, family, and social perspectives* (pp. 88–105). Boston: Allyn & Bacon.

Kliman, J., & Trimble, D. (1983). Network therapy. In B. Wolman & G. Stricker (Eds.), *Handbook of family and marital therapy* (pp. 277–314). New York: Plenum Press.

Laird, J. (1998). Theorizing culture: Narrative ideas and practice principles. In M. McGoldrick (Ed.), *Re-visioning family therapy: Race, culture, and gender in clinical practice* (pp. 20–36). New York: Guilford Press.

Laird, J., & Green, R. J. (1996). (Eds.). *Lesbians and gays in couples and families: A handbook for therapists.* San Francisco: Jossey-Bass.

Llerena-Quinn, R. (2001). How do assumptions of difference and power affect what and how we teach? *NMTP Notes: Newsletter of the Network for Multicultural Training in Psychology, 5,* 1–2, 4–6. Available at www.nmtp.org

McGoldrick, M. (Ed). (1998). *Re-visioning family therapy: Race, culture, and gender in clinical practice.* New York: Guilford Press.

Pierce, C. (1995). Stress analogs of racism and sexism: Terrorism, torture, and disaster. In C. Willie, P. Reiker, B. Kramer, & P. Brown (Eds.), *Mental health, racism, and sexism* (pp. 277–293). Pittsburgh: University of Pittsburgh Press.

Pinderhughes, E. (2002). African American marriage in the 20th century. *Family Process, 41,* 269–282.

Public Conversations Project. (2004). Home page. Available at www.publicconversations. org

Rosaldo, R. (1989). *Culture and truth: The remaking of social analysis.* Boston: Beacon Press.

Root, M. (Ed.). (1996). *The multiracial experience: Racial borders as the new frontier.* Thousand Oaks, CA: Sage.

Suyemoto, K. L., & Dimas, J. M. (2003). To be included in the multicultural discussion: Check one box only. In J. S. Mio & G. Y. Iwamasa (Eds.), *Culturally diverse mental health: The challenges of research and resistance* (pp. 55–81). New York: Brunner/Routledge.

Tavris, C. (1989). *Anger: The misunderstood emotion.* New York: Touchstone.

U.S. Bureau of the Census. (2000). *Statistical abstracts of the United States.* Washington, DC: U.S. Government Printing Office. Available at www.census.gov/prod/www/statistical-abstract-us.html

Weingarten, K. (1997). *The mother's voice: Strengthening intimacy in families.* New York: Guilford Press.

Weingarten, K. (2003). *Common shock: Witnessing violence every day: How we are harmed, how we can heal.* New York: Dutton.

White, M. (1995). *Re-authoring lives: Interviews and essays.* Vancouver, BC: Dulwich Centre.

CHAPTER 3

Building Relationships across Privilege

BECOMING AN ALLY
IN THE THERAPEUTIC RELATIONSHIP

Hugh Vasquez
Sukie Magraw

Ilana is a 40-year-old African American, blue-collar, lesbian who is depressed, overweight, and has for years engaged in a pattern of self-destruction in regard to her economic and educational situation. She procrastinates on paying bills (even though she has the funds to do so) to the extent that utility services are sometimes threatened or discontinued. She enjoys her work, is satisfied with her career, works hard, but often neglects to collect the money owed to her. Illana is working on a graduate degree in a program that is intellectually fulfilling and stimulating. She is one of the top students in her program, yet she waits until the last minute to work on school assignments and at times accepts an incomplete grade with an "Oh, well, that's just the way it goes" attitude. Ilana is trying to motivate herself to stay on top of things and create success in life, but her actions continue to put her in a bind. She seems to accept the failures as inevitable and copes by not thinking about the past or the future too much. It appears that Ilana has "bought" the larger societal messages that say she is "no good," a "loser," "dumb" and that it is in her nature to be poor. She believes her problems stem from a deep-seated individual deficiency.

Do racism, sexism, heterosexism, and classism have anything to do with Ilana's psychological distress? Are the societal conditions of racism, sexism, and classism at the root of her problems? Is there a link between her difficulties and those of her family members from previous generations? It is our belief that the answer to all of these questions is yes.

This chapter discusses how the therapist can become an ally in the therapeutic relationship to assist the client in healing from the effects of social oppression. As an ally, the therapist designs a treatment plan that moves outside of those aspects of traditional approaches that focus mostly on the individual, or perhaps using a systems approach, still remains individually focused. Moving outside of traditional approaches means the therapist (1)assesses the clients issues through a broader social–psychological lens; (2) sees the manifestation of self-hate as a reaction to the greater social conditions of sexism and racism; (3) understands that self-hate is not intrinsic to the client's personality but an outcome of social oppression; and (4) identifies the existing intergenerational trauma—again recognizing this trauma as social condition rather than as individual pathology.

First we explain why we believe it is important for therapists to identify their own areas of privilege and disadvantage and the psychological effects these have had on their own lives. We, the authors, then locate ourselves, both to serve as examples of how we have thought about this process and to contextualize our positions. Next, we focus on what it means to be an ally to clients. We discuss the effects of internalized oppression, the important role of the therapist as ally in interrupting the oppression, and treatment plans through the lenses of privilege and oppression.

Locating Ourselves on Multiple Dimensions—
from Privilege to Oppression

To be effective therapists, we must have knowledge about, and awareness of, ourselves, including knowledge of our own cultural heritage(s) and its effects on us. Too often, therapists overlook their own culture, especially if they are European American; instead, if they think culture is important at all, they focus on the clients cultural background, especially if the client is an ethnic minority. In order to understand our clients' worldviews, it is essential that we have an intimate and conscious knowledge of our own worldview: that is, our values, biases, priorities, attitudes, and areas of comfort and discomfort. Questions we need to ask ourselves include:

> In what arenas am I privileged and in what arenas am I targeted for oppression?
>
> How is that privilege and/or oppression internalized?

What are the stereotypes about the groups that comprise my cultural heritage and how have those stereotypes affected me?

In addition to reflecting on our cultural heritage, it is also necessary for us to reflect on our specific background and life experiences—some of which are greatly influenced by our cultural heritage—and again, to be cognizant of how these have shaped our values, biases, priorities, and attitudes. These background and life experience factors could include age, sex, socioeconomic status, sexual orientation, religion, physical abilities, degree of family stability, type of childrearing, alcohol and/or drug abuse, mental illness, exposure to violence, education level, and all of those experiences—unique to the individual—that make us who we are.

The Importance of Knowing Oneself

As therapists there are several reasons why it is important for us to know ourselves in these ways. First, the dynamics of oppression can be enacted unconsciously. We can fall back on our stereotypes about our clients; we can be oblivious to the ways our privilege gets used in sessions; we may not give enough credence to internalized oppression—either the client's or our own. The way to be vigilant about these dynamics of oppression is to be able to identify them, and the only way to be able to identify them is to have done work on ourselves in these areas (Pedersen, 2002; Sue & Sue, 1999). Second, we will be asking our clients to look at their lives through the lenses of power, privilege, and oppression. This work can be arduous and scary, but also exhilarating and ultimately liberating. We are in a much better position to help our clients on this journey if it is a journey that we are continually in the process of taking ourselves.

Finally, we must recognize that as therapists we are inherently in a position of power over our clients. There may be other ways in which we are less advantaged than our clients: For example, we may make less money than our client, or we may be female while the client is male. However, in this relationship-defining area—as therapist and client—we always hold the position of power and privilege. We must be constantly aware of the ramifications of that position—that is, of the typical dynamic that gets enacted when two people of unequal power interact. As therapists, our awareness of our power over our clients helps guard against the unwitting abuse of that power (Brown, 1994; Freire, 1970; Miller, 1976).

We use ourselves as examples of how to locate yourself culturally and contextually, and how to think about being advantaged or disadvantaged in several different areas. *Location* means identifying where you reside in this society on a continuum from privilege to oppression in relation to various contextual aspects of the self, such as ethnicity, gender, sexual orientation, religion, and class status.

Our Backgrounds

I (HV) am keenly aware that I am a man, writing this chapter with a woman, for a book that is about a feminist reconstruction of psychotherapy. In all aspects of my life, not only in relation to authoring this chapter, my location in terms of ethnicity, gender, sexual orientation, abilities, and class influences and affects me.

As a male, I walk in a society that awards unearned privileges to men, and I realize that I benefit from these privileges. For example, I know that for the most part, I will be paid $1 when I earn $1, but that women will receive only 76¢ for every dollar earned (U.S. Department of Labor, 2002). In most circumstances, I am not afraid for my physical well-being and I never worry about being sexually assaulted. It is highly unlikely that I will ever be the victim of domestic violence. I believe that I will be taken seriously by an employer and that my leadership skills as a male will be valued. In most corporations, institutions of higher education, and political offices, my gender is highly represented. In a worldwide context, there is no society today where women enjoy the same opportunities as men. A United Nations study reported that of the estimated 1.3 million people living in poverty, more than 70% are female; women work longer hours than men in nearly every country and provide more labor then men, but men receive 74% of the world's income; men dominate the political landscape by occupying 90% of the seats in government; and men receive the greatest share of income and recognition for their economic contributions while most women's work remains underpaid, underrecognized, and undervalued (e.g., since the creation of the Nobel Peace Prize in 1901, only 28 of 634 individual recipients have been women) (United Nations, 1995).

Although unearned privilege came to me as a male, as a Latino from a blue-collar background, I experienced disadvantage on the basis of race and class. This experience affected my health and well-being. In fact, because my experiences of being targeted for racism and classism occurred routinely and pervasively—that is, every day, in every part of my life—I did not always notice areas of privilege. For example, I was afforded male privilege in contexts where the male voice was taken more seriously than the female, but at the same time, my ideas, thoughts, and experiences were devalued as a Latino working-class individual. This devaluing was played out in many college courses and professional meetings where my thoughts and ideas were passed over; when a white person raised the same ideas, however, he or she received praise and affirmation for great thinking. This dynamic caused me to doubt that I truly benefited from male privilege.

Often it seemed to me that race and class disadvantage trumped gender privilege to such a large extent, that I felt I was not the beneficiary of any privilege. I was intimately feeling the effects of racism to such an extent that the privileges I was receiving due to my gender remained invisible to me.

Some of the greatest challenges to considering privilege are the various intersections of cultural and contextual differences. For example, whereas my working-class background produced great internal and external challenges in my life, I recognize that my movement into the middle class places me in a position of privilege over those who are poor. As a heterosexual, I benefit from laws that award me protections that homosexuals do not have. The intersections of these contexts are complex and multiple—that is, none of us is only of one culture. My understanding of the areas in which I have privilege did not come until I was able to understand the impact of oppression—of racism and classism—on my life. As I healed from the effects of racism, my mind and heart opened to listening to, and learning how, women have been devastated by sexism, how the disabled are impacted by ableism, and so on.

I (SM) am keenly aware that I am a white woman. I was and am privileged by being white, in that I know I walk on a playing field that is either level or tilted downhill for me. There are many unearned but assumed entitlements that come my way—for example, that life is basically fair, that if I work hard I will get ahead. And, as a white person, I do not have to constantly wonder if a negative comment, or being overlooked, or overt hostility, is due to my skin color (McIntosh, 1989).

I grew up able-bodied, in an upwardly mobile family, in an upper-middle-class suburb with a good school system that led me to an Ivy League college. I lived in a stable family with no financial concerns, in a community with very little crime—one that was almost entirely white. That, too, was a privilege in that my parents could choose where they wanted to live, and with whom they wanted to associate. My mother was culturally Jewish and my father was Protestant. The children in the family were raised secularly in a largely Jewish community. I grew up knowing I was privileged, knowing I lived in a society that discriminated against some people for the most arbitrary of reasons, and that that was not just. However, my feelings of social injustice, although real, were quite abstract. I, living in my privileged, upper-middle-class white world, did not know many people of color. And when I got older and was with my African American, Native American, or Puerto Rican friends, I did not know how to have discussions about the effects of racism on all of us. It took a long time and a lot of discomfort to get to honest discussions. Listening to others' experiences of racism and then thinking about the effects that racism had on me—ingrained fears, unchecked stereotypes, walls of separation—led me to realize that even though I was privileged, I too was being negatively affected by racism.

I also have attributes that lead me to know what it is like to be a target and to feel oppressed—and these experiences have helped me better understand my role in those areas where I am privileged. I have felt the effects of sexism throughout my life and have been keenly aware of the ways in which I have internalized some of its dictates. I have held jobs in which similarly qualified men have been paid up to three times as much as I. As a lesbian, I have also had to struggle with rampant societal heterosexism and my own internalized homophobia.

Psychologically, it is extremely complicated to be privileged, on the one hand, and to feel oppressed, on the other. Yet that is the situation for all of us. Usually we are much more in touch with our areas of oppression, where we are wounded, and it is harder to be aware of our areas of privilege.

My main reaction to having socioeconomic and racial privilege was guilt. That guilt stifled me. It was not conducive to reaching out to others or to curiosity. There were "right" and "wrong" ways to be with others—especially others of color. It felt safer to stay away than to slip up and be found out as racist. How liberating it was when I understood that I was racist—but so was everyone else! How could we not be, given our intensive social training?

The Journey to Becoming an Ally

Healing leads to recognition of privilege, which in turn opens the door to developing into an ally. Imagine a conversation with a woman in which you ask her questions about her hand. You ask about her hand's experience, how much she likes her hand, a description of her hand, and her feelings about her hand. However, all the while you are asking about her hand, something very heavy is resting on her foot, crushing it a bit and causing a great deal of discomfort and pain. Finally, after enduring many questions from you about her hand, she replies, "I'm having trouble talking to you about my hand because my foot is hurting so much. Will you please help me get this heavy thing off my foot? Then I may be able to talk more coherently about my hand!" Oppression is what is hurting the foot and until the source of that hurt is dealt with and healing occurs, the individual cannot attend to areas of privilege and become an ally. There is a connection, then, between the experiences (1) of being targeted for oppression, (2) healing from the hurts of oppression, (3) recognizing one's privilege, and (4) developing into an ally.

One of my (HV) earliest experiences of learning about the need for healing, recognition of privilege, ally development, and the connections among them came while working with a group on race, gender, religion, and sexual orientation issues. As we were working on racism, I was placed in a small group with two white people with the instructions to talk about how each of us was "hurt" by racism. I was livid and could not fully participate in the discussion, because I did not believe (at that time) that anyone other than a person of color was hurt by racism. Racism targets people of color every day—and being a person of color, I had firsthand experiences of it. How could white people even consider the thought of being hurt by racism? I was not only unable to listen to the other group members, but also unwilling to let them know anything about my experience. After discussing the impact of racism in this manner for a while, the group was then asked to discuss sexism in the same way. Although I did not understand why at the time, I was completely immobilized and unable to participate in the discussions.

What happened in the above situation? First, I had not experienced enough healing on racism to open my mind, eyes, and heart to the possibility that racism hurts white people too, and second, my lack of healing closed my mind to seeing how women were hurt by sexism. I was identifying as a victim of racism and was experiencing it routinely and pervasively—that is, all the time and almost everywhere I walked. The weight of racism was on my foot, and I was unable to listen to or acknowledge another person's experience of racism, or any other "ism," because I had not received the healing I still needed.

As for my (SM) experience, with the advent of the feminist movement, I found a way of understanding my experiences around manifest and internalized sexism, and I felt validated. It was only after that validation and after I had similarly come to terms with being a lesbian that I was truly able to look beyond my own wounding. I became better able to not only acknowledge my many areas of privilege, but to begin to understand the ways those areas affected my relationships with others different from me. It became easier to build bridges across difference: Yes, I hold racist beliefs, and I hold homophobic beliefs. My friends of color do, too. We are united in our desire to eradicate these beliefs and to dismantle the institutions that perpetuate them.

The healing each of us needed, and eventually received, in part came from being listened to and understood by allies. Telling our stories about racism led to healing from the effects of it. As the weight of racism was lifted, we became better able to listen to, and explore the impact of, other oppressions on other people—such as sexism on women, anti-Semitism on Jews, homophobia and heterosexism on lesbian, gay, bisexual, and transgender individuals (LGBTs), ableism on disabled, and so on. In other words, healing from where we were targeted for oppression was a prerequisite for our development as an ally.

It is the ally's role and responsibility to work toward the elimination of oppression, both on individual and institutional levels. Being an ally goes beyond personal awareness and sensitivity; it involves *taking action*. For each of us, we consider the cowriting of this chapter as a form of action.

As allies, we are writing this chapter (1) to take responsibility for raising the consciousness of those who are in a similar place of privilege and to push those with privilege to notice it and use it to work toward dismantling the systems in our society that produce it; (2) because we are committed to action; and (3) because we have to continue working to become an increasingly better ally to women, poor and working-class folks, and others. We are also writing this chapter because each of us has a partner and a daughter who live under sexism and we are continually outraged and saddened by seeing its impact on their lives, such as seeing our daughters suffering from the pressure to be thin, popular, and sexual at a very young age. As a person of color, my (HV) writing comes also from the understanding that if I expect white people to be allies with me against racism, then I must work to be an ally with others in areas where I have privilege. Similarly, as a woman and a lesbian, if I (SM) expect men and heterosexuals to be allies with me against sexism and heterosexism, I must work to be an ally to others in areas where I have privilege. Finally, we are writing this chapter because we know that to be an ally, we have to engage in an ongoing process of developing our skills—one does not become an effective ally by taking one class or training and taking one or two actions. Instead, it is an ongoing process.

Privilege

"Privilege," in this context, refers to the social systems, structures, and societal ways of functioning that are designed to benefit some and not others. Those who belong to the controlling or dominating culture have privileges not accorded to any outside that culture. They do not have to notice how society is set up to benefit them, do not have to earn the benefits awarded to them, and do not have to concern themselves with wondering if their benefits will be taken away. Those with privilege are often unaware of their privilege and simply believe that they worked hard and earned everything they have. To use a sports metaphor, privilege is being born on third base and believing you hit a triple. As the therapist looks at developing an ally relationship with the client, a prerequisite is identifying his or her privilege in society.

Therapists' Privilege

Tony, a psychology student from South America, was training in a clinic in San Francisco that had a large gay clientele. Tony's client, Jorge, was a gay Latino male in his late 60s. Jorge had been diagnosed with alcohol dependence, in remission. He also was depressed about not having a current partner and not having much of a social support group. Tony clearly had the makings of a fine therapist; he was thoughtful and caring about Jorge. He was able to contextualize some of Jorge's feelings about being a Latino man in a society that privileges white men, and he was able to discuss with Jorge what it was like to be gay and Latino. They talked about cultural messages, about Jorge's family's reaction to his being gay, about internalized racism and homophobia. In all these areas, Tony was proving to be a consciously competent therapist. However, as we shall see, one can be competent in some areas and incompetent in others.

Tony had also asked Jorge about his HIV status, which was negative. Given this response, Tony did not pursue this line of questioning any further; he did not ask about the effects of the AIDS epidemic on Jorge's life. As a straight man, Tony had not been confronted with the devastating impact that AIDS has had on men in San Francisco, especially men of Jorge's age. He has a "blind spot" in this area, because he has the privilege of not having to think about this topic. Tony, therefore, missed a significant aspect of Jorge's experience: living through the fear of the "gay cancer" when no one knew what caused AIDS; Jorge's internalized homophobic feelings that perhaps this disease was God's punishment; the effects of having friends who died, many of them early in the epidemic; and the ways these deaths had changed him.

A therapist who is unaware of the forces of privilege will miss dynamics that may very well be a key in a client's healing. Tony's privilege prevented him from implementing interventions that could have significantly helped his client. With supervision, Tony became aware of this blind spot regarding the effects of the AIDS epidemic on Jorge's life and Tony was then able to ask Jorge about it, which opened up rich discussions around Jorge's lack of friends, his survivor guilt, and his internalized homophobia. Through this experience, Tony was reinforced in his belief that supervision can be very useful, and more importantly, he came to the realization that to be a culturally competent therapist, to be an ally to his clients, he needed to be continually aware of his own areas of privilege.

The Therapist as an Ally

Allies continually examine their location in relation to the clients. As Sue (2003) states, "clinicians are not immune from inheriting the biases, stereotypes, and values of the larger society" (p. 5). In developing cultural competency, Sue writes that the therapist must continually build knowledge about racial identity development. Specifically for white therapists, this means knowing about white identity development and white privilege issues. For men, it means knowing about male privilege. For heterosexuals, it means knowing about homophobia and heterosexism, and learning how society continually awards unearned advantage to heterosexuals. For people who are financially well off, it means learning the intricacies of classism, how the class system in our society gives privileges to the owning class.

An ally is someone who gets in the way of oppression. An ally intervenes from a place of privilege to stop mistreatment from occurring. An ally is someone who takes action when witnessing racism, sexism, homophobia, and the like. Kivel (2002), in writing about white allies, states that "being an ally . . . is an on-going strategic process in which we look at our personal and social resources, evaluate the environment we have helped to create, and decide what needs to be done . . . we need to listen carefully to the voices of people of color so that we understand and give credence to their experience" (p. 94).

The therapist puts into practice being an ally in four specific ways: (1) identifying racism, classism, ableism (the privilege of able-bodied), and other "isms" as root causes of mental illness and thinking in terms of social oppression when assessing the client's problems; (2) interrupting internalized oppression; (3) bringing an analysis of institutional oppression, its relevance to the presenting problem, and expanding the treatment plan to include working toward eradicating the social conditions that are at the root of the problem; and (4) acknowledging the effects of intergenerational trauma in the client's functioning.

Understanding Oppression as a Root Cause of Mental Illness

Effects of Social Oppression

The therapist must identify racism, sexism, classism, and other "isms" as root causes of mental illness and must think in terms of social oppression when assessing the client's problems.

> Carrie worked in a child and family community clinic. She was assigned to see a 13-year-old girl, Susan. Susan's parents were in the middle of a divorce. Susan lived mainly with her mother but saw her father on weekends and at other times. Carrie found out that before the breakup, Susan had had a fairly trouble-free life. But since her father had moved out, she was skipping school, her grades had fallen,

and she was behaving in an oppositional manner at home. Carrie's initial hypotheses in formulating this case revolved around Susan's responses to the divorce intersecting with developmental issues—and these were the areas she was exploring with Susan. The therapy was going fairly well, but it really took off when Carrie asked about the effects of having an Iranian father and a European American mother. Carrie had known about Susan's ethnicity from the start, but delving deeper into its ramifications had not been an initial priority. Upon asking, Carrie learned from Susan that her father held some traditional ideas about the role of a woman in the house. He had not wanted Susan's mother to spend much time out of the house. He did not like her socializing or having friends. When her father moved out, her mother felt liberated and was trying to make up for lost time, meeting people, spending time with them, going out a lot. Susan understood her mother's need for more friendships; however, her mother, at this very difficult time, was less available to her than she ever had been.

With this new information, Carrie was able to talk with Susan's mother about balancing her own needs with her daughter's needs. In later conversations with the two of them, they talked more about the ramifications of Susan having an Iranian father and a European American mother. These interventions led to a great reduction in Susan's acting-out behavior, a closer relationship with her mother, and a deeper understanding of her father.

Oppression is a root cause of psychic and emotional trauma and should always be included in a therapist's assessment of a client's problems. Considering social oppression as a root expands diagnosis and treatment plans beyond traditional methods. The client's social, political, and cultural experiences are given primary importance in treatment. Duran and Duran (1995) highlight this point in discussing clinical treatment with Native Americans, stating that "successful clinical interventions are not possible in a Native American setting unless the provider or agency is cognizant of the sociohistorical factors that have had a devastating effect on the Native American family (p. 27)." As the Surgeon General reported at the 2001 American Psychiatric Association conference, there is a strong need to understand both the cultural and sociopolitical factors affecting the life experiences of racial and ethnic minorities (Surgeon General, 2000). When the experiences resulting from a client's gender, socioeconomic class, or sexual orientation are added to racial and ethnic background, a much more complex picture emerges.

The traditional psychotherapy lens through which a client's issues are viewed derives from white, European, monocultural values and belief system. In today's multicultural society, the competent therapist must expand her or his lens to view a client's situation in multiple ways, thereby challenging the assumptions of traditional theories and approaches. Primary filters that the therapist ally uses to grasp fully the life experiences of the client are those of sexism, racism, classism, heterosexism.

If the therapist applies these filters to the presenting problems, what is indicated for treatment? If the social condition of sexism is at the root of a woman's abuse, lack of success, feelings of worthlessness, depression, etc., then what treatment plan would address the root problem? If the therapist combines the experience of being a woman with the experience of being poor, working class, or perhaps even middle class, what treatment plan is indicated when paying attention to gender and socioeconomic conditions? Add yet another filter so that the client is now seen as a woman, poor or working class, and a woman of color, what now are the indicators for a treatment plan, given the life experiences of this client? The therapist as an ally continues to apply various filters of the client's life experiences (e.g., heterosexism, anti-Semitism, ableism) in order to identify the effects of these life experiences on the client.

Interrupting Internalized Oppression

Women, people of color, and poor and working-class clients manifest problems that stem from social conditions rather than from individual deficiency. One of the most devastating effects on the individual level is the internalization of social oppression, that is, internalized racism, sexism, heterosexism, ethnocentrism, and classism. According to Sherover-Marcuse (1988):

> Each group targeted by oppression [women, people of color, poor, etc.] inevitably "internalizes" the mistreatment and the misinformation about itself. The target group thus "mis-believes" about itself the same misinformation that pervades the social system. This "mis-believing" expresses itself in behavior and interactions between individual members of the target group which repeat the content of their oppression. Internalized oppression is always an involuntary reaction to the experience of oppression on the part of the target group. (p. 2)

Myers, Young, and Obasi (2003) focus on the dynamics of internalized oppression, stating that, "anger, rage and sense of inferiority and self loathing turned inward manifest in anti-self and alien self disorders in which one acts in ways detrimental to self and one's group (p. 16)." Internalized oppression not only expresses itself in certain behaviors and interactions between members of the target group, but also within the individual. Self-abuse, eating disorders, depression, unhealthy relationship choices, domestic violence, drug and alcohol abuse, academic failure, gang involvement, hopelessness and despair, and so on, can all be manifestations of the internalization of mistreatment experienced in the larger society. Internalized oppression may, therefore, contribute to clients' beliefs that they are not smart enough, not beautiful enough, not deserving—that they are, in fact, less human than people in the dominant culture.

A therapist can interrupt internalized oppression by bombarding clients with "truths" to counter the lies (also known as misinformation or stereotypes) that pervade their psyches. In treatment, therapists can:

- Teach clients about the origins of their negative beliefs, emphasizing that the origins stem from social forces beyond their control.
- Give examples of positive social contributions from clients' culture(s).
- Help clients see that their behavior, as unhealthy and destructive as it might be, is a resistance strategy to deal with oppression and that their resilience is incredible, given the pervasive, nonstop targeting they receive from the dominant culture.
- Help clients identify how they have tried to resist internalizing racism, sexism, and classism in both adaptive and self-destructive ways.
- Explore with clients how they can replace destructive coping mechanisms with healthy alternatives.
- Give clients positive messages about their true nature.

Institutional Oppression: Expanding the Treatment Plan

Institutions in our social system maintain gender, race, and class advantage for a select few and to the disadvantage of many. Yet a therapist's treatment plan rarely includes consideration of the impact of these institutions on those who occupy the disadvantaged end of the privilege continuum, or interventions to address this root cause of so many problems. What would a treatment plan involve, if it were to include interventions in social institutions?

Focusing on the impact of larger social systems on people of African descent, Myers and colleagues (2003) call for greater understanding among practitioners about how the health of the larger society, its institutions, and the nature of the established social environment affect the functioning of people of African descent. They state that mental illness "represents the disruption of a healthy social context in which institutional structures and other systems of social organization functioned . . . to support individual and collective well-being (p. 13). . . . [The] therapist must take into account the psychological impact of the brutal system of dehumanizing assaults institutionalized to support the exploitative economic agenda of the trans-Atlantic slave trade and maintained today in the global economy" (p. 15).

In other words, even though the slave trade happened many years ago, institutions remain in place that affect the health and well-being of African Americans. Sue states, "Culturally competent therapists must balance their traditional helping roles with understanding and ability to intervene in the larger system" (2003, p. 6).

Extrapolating this analysis to consider the impact of institutional structures and the health of the social context for other people of color, women, and the poor or working class, it is clear that institutional structures do not support well-being for all cultures. Ilana, the 40-year-old African American, blue-collar lesbian introduced earlier, believes that her problems stem from deep-seated personal deficiencies. A traditional therapeutic approach would focus on these personal deficiencies. A culturally competent therapeutic approach would raise questions about the effects of racism, sexism, heterosexism, and classism on her understanding of herself and her actions. It would name the oppression and include teaching Ilana about the effects of oppression on functioning. It would help her view her problems less as a result of personal deficiencies and more as a result of societal deficiencies. From this vantage point, Ilana is in a stronger position to take action on her own behalf.

Expanding the treatment plan involves interventions on institutional issues relevant to the client. A current-day example is the institutionalized "English only" initiatives that are government-endorsed acts of bias that give the message to those whose first language is other than English that their culture and heritage are not valued. At the very least, the therapist teaches clients about institutions and how they contribute to, or may be the root cause of, their problems. As clients understand the impact of social conditions on their well-being, they are able to feel less alone and/or less responsible for their situation. Clients gain understanding that their psychological, social, or emotional dysfunction actually makes sense, given the social conditions. For example, a young woman struggling with eating disorders can learn about the impact of the media on a young girl's body image and understand that her pathology has roots in an unhealthy social construct that promotes unrealistic, unnatural, and unhealthy bodies for women. A Latino/a, Native American, Cambodian American, or African American clients who are failing in school and perhaps becoming involved in destructive behaviors can see that the educational system's low expectations for students of color and its European monocultural focus foster feelings of worthlessness and low intelligence, which lead ultimately to dropping out of school. Teaching clients about oppressive social conditions and their relevance to their situations does not constitute an abregation of individual response or responsibility for getting well. Although clients did not produce the social conditions, they are charged with taking individual actions to cope with the consequences of those conditions. However, being taught the root causes of their problems releases the client from believing that they are the sole cause of their predicament.

A deeper level of therapeutic intervention involves encouraging clients to become advocates and activists in "taking on" the institutions in question. The therapist ally assists clients in strategizing about how to intervene in the system and to build the skills and confidence to do so. Education may involve helping clients organize others to join with them in the intervention so that they are not doing it alone. An even more involved therapist may become an advocate and intervene with an institution (e.g., social services, school officials, law enforcement, employers) on clients' behalf. In this case, as Barcus (2003) states, "the role of a mental health worker is more broadly defined . . . and may include being an advocate, serving as a consultant, and providing psycho-education to clients, agencies, and the community (p. 25)."

Effects of Intergenerational Trauma

It is our assertion that an aspect of privilege within the profession of psychology is the power and practice of divorcing a client's psychological problems from the trauma experienced by past generations. Privilege allows the profession to define at what point an individual's functioning is related to his or her past, which means dictating the onset of a particular dysfunction as well as the relevancy or irrelevancy of the client's cultural history and experience. Privilege allows the profession to ignore trauma that occurred before the client was born and, therefore, ignore the impact of that prebirth trauma. Privilege focuses the attention on the individual and his or her current life conditions without connecting his or her current state of affairs with past generational traumas. If the therapist is to become an effective ally to the client, he or she will need to recognize the intergenerational trauma of the past as it continues its harmful impact in the present.

Various researchers have documented the effects of intergenerational trauma. Iwamasa (2003) describes this phenomena as "transgenerational psychological trauma" when looking at the Japanese Americans interned during World War II and Asians who have come to the United States from war and economic upheaval in their home countries. She states, "Although their progeny may not have personally been tortured, raped, or beaten, their parents who did experience those atrocities may pass down the psychological trauma to them" (p. 10). Duran and Duran (1995) write that Native Americans experience intergenerational posttraumatic stress and exhibit similar dynamics to the Jewish experience with the Holocaust. Genocide and ethnocide were perpetrated on Native Americans; however, unlike the Jewish Holocaust in Europe, "the world has not acknowledged the Holocaust of native people in this hemisphere. This lack of acknowledgement remains one of the stumbling blocks to the healing process of Native American people" (p. 30). Again, it is privilege within the profession of psychology that allows for past trauma to be dismissed as irrelevant to current problems. Myers and colleagues (2003), working with clients of African descent, say that "the group is unique by virtue of the nature, quality, and degree of socially sanctioned violence, hostility, and aggression practiced by the dominant culture towards them generation after generation" (p. 17). Calling the phenomena multigenerational trauma, they state that the "long history of socially sanctioned abuse has not been dealt with" (p. 15).

Thus we believe that historical contexts are just as important to consider as contemporary sociocultural contexts in order to assess and intervene effectively.

Assessment: Using a Cultural Genogram

Although there are many activities, techniques, and tools to help a therapist locate his- or herself in relation to various cultural issues and understand the impact of oppression on clients, a particularly useful one is the cultural genogram (Hardy & Laszloffy, 1995). This technique helps people learn how cultural treatment and mistreatment have affected them. In the genogram, people answer questions such as the following:

What have your group's experiences been with oppression?
What significance does race, gender, etc., have in your experience?
Have you experienced sexism and racism, and what was your response to it?

This tool can be adapted for clients and therapists alike to use as they identify their location on various issues. In addition to answering the above questions, the therapist can answer the following:

Which groups in our society have unearned privilege and which ones suffer from unearned disadvantage?
Where are you (the therapist) located in relation to these groups?
What is your understanding of the existence of a system that awards privilege to some and disadvantage to others?
What role do you play in these systems?

Four Processes of Development as an Ally

Becoming an ally demands intention, consciousness, and action. We suggest a four-process model by which a therapist can develop into a therapeutic ally. These processes are not linear; that is, a therapist does not complete process one, then advance to process two, then to process three, and so on. Instead, the processes form more of a spiral. As the therapist moves from unconsciousness to consciousness, he or she develops new awareness, skills, and insights in that particular area, but must then start over in another area and move through the processes again. These processes are as follows:

Process 1: Unconscious Incompetence (UI)

This process is characterized by a state of "I don't know that I don't know." The therapist is not aware of the existence or relevance of privilege, oppression, or its impact on clients. Therapists in this process are not only oblivious to their privilege, they do not know that they are oblivious to it. Hence they are not aware that they have a particular deficiency in this area. If this deficiency is pointed out, therapists might deny the relevance or usefulness of becoming multiculturally competent and forming an ally relationship with the client. Until their consciousness about their incompetence is raised, UI therapists will be ineffective in forming meaningful and deep therapeutic relationships with clients whose difficulties or life experiences are strongly affected by oppression.

Process 2: Conscious Incompetence (CI) as an Ally in Therapy

This process is characterized by an attitude of "Now I know that I don't know very much, and I know I need to learn." The therapist is now aware of the existence and relevance of multicultural competence and of the importance of developing an ally relationship, although he or she is not sure how to do it. CI therapists become aware of their deficiencies in looking at the therapeutic relationship through the lenses of oppression and privilege, and they realize that by increasing their knowledge and improving their skills in thinking contextually, their effectiveness will improve. These therapists make a commitment to learn and practice new ways of thinking, and to move into the "conscious competence" process.

Process 3: Conscious Competence (CC) as an Ally in Therapy

In this process therapists bring their knowledge of privilege and oppression into their practice. Clients' problems are assessed through a variety of cultural lenses and treatment plans include addressing issues of privilege and oppression in clients' situations. However, this ability is not automatically a part of the therapeutic repertoire; therapists need to remind themselves to bring this way of thinking into the room with the client. Ongoing practice of doing so is the single most effective way to move from process 3 to 4, that is, from conscious competence to unconscious competence.

Process 4: Unconscious Competence (UC) as an Ally in Therapy

In this process working contextually becomes so practiced that it is now part of the way in which therapists see the world; it would be impossible not to think contextually, not to see through a multicultural lens, not to act as an ally in therapy. Being UC does not mean that learning and further development are over; rather, therapists continue to grow by pursuing an ongoing study of cultures, holding study sessions with colleagues in which analysis and insights about client situations can occur, and conducting rigorous self-evaluation of their actual practice of multicultural skills.

Conclusion

In conclusion, there are several ways in which therapists can work as allies across privilege with clients. However, for many therapists, discovering ways to raise these issues in therapy is moving into largely uncharted therapeutic terrain. Our advice: Give yourself permission to delve into these new arenas. Experiment with different ways of exploring issues of class, gender, and related areas within yourself and with clients. Speak openly with colleagues about your self-reflections and interventions, asking them to think multiculturally with you and critique cases with this filter in place.

Therapists must be knowledgeable about their own cultural heritage and their own areas of privilege and oppression. Use supervision time or discussions with other therapists to talk about your cultural backgrounds. Therapists must be able to intervene with clients on multiple levels. For example, addressing issues of heterosexism with a lesbian is not enough— although it might be a good beginning. Individuals are complex entities with many areas of oppressions and privilege that therapists can identify for their clients. Therefore, in addition to addressing heterosexism issues with the lesbian client, issues of class, age, abilities, and ethnicity are identified and explored as well. When working multiculturally, the therapist has the opportunity to educate clients about the effects of oppression, including the effects of internalized oppression and how it results from overt and covert oppression. Clients can be helped to distinguish internalized oppression from the institutional or systematic effects of oppression and see connections between these to the legacy of oppression and how intergenerational oppression operates in their life. Finally, in becoming allies, therapists need to find ways of becoming activists—fighting oppression—both with their clients and in the wider world.

References

Barcus, C. (2003). Recommendations for the treatment of American Indian populations. In *Psychological treatment of ethnic minority populations* (pp. 24–28). Washington, DC: Association of Black Psychologists.

Brown, L. (1994). *Subversive dialogues: Theory in feminist therapy.* New York: Basic Books.

Duran, E., & Duran, B. (1995). *Native American postcolonial psychology.* Albany: State University of New York Press.

Freire, P. (1970). *Pedagogy of the oppressed.* New York: Continuum.

Hardy, K., & Laszloffy, T. (1995). The cultural genogram: Key to training culturally competent family therapists. *Journal of Marital and Family Therapy, 21,* 227–237.

Iwamasa, G. Y. (2003). Recommendations for the treatment of Asian American/Pacific Islander populations. In *Psychological treatment of ethnic minority populations* (pp. 8–12). Washington, DC: Association of Black Psychologists.

Kivel, P. (2002). *Uprooting racism.* Gabriola Island, BC, Canada: New Society.

McIntosh, P. (1989, July/August). White privilege: Unpacking the invisible knapsack. *Peace and Freedom,* pp. 8–10.

Miller, J. B. (1976). *Toward a new psychology of women.* Boston: Beacon Press.

Myers, L. J., Young, A., & Obasi, E. (2003). Recommendations for the treatment of African descent populations. In *Psychological treatment of ethnic minority populations* (pp. 1318). Washington, DC: Association of Black Psychologists.

Pedersen, P. (2002). Ethics, competence and other professional issues. In P. Pedersen, J. Draguns, W. Lonner, & J. Trimble (Eds.), *Counseling across cultures* (5th ed., pp. 3–28). Thousand Oaks, CA: Sage.

Sherover-Marcuse, R. (1988). Liberation theory: A working framework. In H. Vasquez & I. Femi (Eds.), *No boundaries: A manual for unlearning oppression and building multicultural alliances.* Oakland, CA: Todos Institute.

Sue, D. W. (2003). Cultural competence in the treatment of ethnic minority populations. In *Psychological treatment of ethnic minority populations* (pp. 4–7). Washington, DC: Association of Black Psychologists.

Sue, D. W., & Sue, D. (1999). *Counseling the culturally different: Theory and practice* (3rd ed.). New York: Wiley.

Surgeon General of the United States. (2000). *Mental health: A report of the Sur-*

geon General: Disparities in mental health care for racial and ethnic minorities*. Washington, DC: U.S. Public Health Service.

United Nations. (1995). *Human Development Report, 1995*. New York: United Nations Development Programme.

U.S. Department of Labor. (2002, May). *Highlights of women's earnings in 2001*. Washington, DC: Bureau of Labor Statistics.

PART II

Women in Interpersonal Relationships

CHAPTER 4

Immigrant Mothers

MOTHERING IN THE BORDERLANDS

Roxana Llerena-Quinn
Marsha Pravder Mirkin

I (RLQ) am sitting in my office, trying to integrate so much information about mothering across cultures. I am trying to hear the concerns of the mothers whose voices are marginalized in their adopted country as I listen to the all-too-familiar argument between Josefa and her daughter.

JOSEFA: You won't believe what Priscilla has been telling me. She says that when she is 18 she will go!

PRISCILLA: Yes, when I am 18; I can do whatever I want. It is the law!

JOSEFA: See what she is saying! For us, they [our children] are always our babies, even if they have a white beard. We don't throw them out when they are 18 or have a job. (*turning to her daughter*) You do what you want. What do you want?

PRISCILLA: I want to go out and chill.

JOSEFA: What is *chill*?

PRISCILLA: Going out with my friends.

JOSEFA: Well, it is 3:00 P.M., be back by 6:00 P.M. Where is out?

PRISCILLA: Boston. And 3 hours is not enough time. It is crazy, she is crazy.

JOSEFA: Boston!! And for so many hours!

PRISCILLA: Mother! What are you afraid of?? I am a mature kid. My friends are good kids—you know them.

JOSEFA: Yes, I am afraid. I trust you, but the devil plays dirty tricks. They [friends] can change.

JOSEFA: (*addressing me*) After she goes out mad at me, I question myself. I wonder if I am being a good mother. I try. I am so much more flexible than my parents were with me.

What happens to a mother's voice and her best intentions when delivered in a foreign land and in a borrowed language? How do we make meaning of the differences that emerge in the privacy of the home or in the public places? What contexts do we need to explore, to notice, to hear the true meaning of her most deeply felt intentions and how they are received?

Looking like a "good mother" may be easier when the mother's ideals, needs, and preferences match the dominant culture or she has sufficient privilege to fulfill or challenge the role. For others, the choice is more limited. Immigrant mothers raise their children from the cultural borderlands—the place where different cultural worlds meet to delineate their similarities and differences (Anzaldúa, 1987)—knowing well that differences are seldom neutral. From the borderland space, mothers need to protect, guide, and launch their children into a world they, the mothers, may not fully understand, be a part of, or even allowed to enter.

Although this chapter cannot cover the experience of all immigrant mothers, we do explore the experiences and meanings of women who are faced with the task of mothering children in a land different from the one in which they were born; in a place where their individual and collective histories, and other important aspects of their identity, are largely unknown; and in an adopted country whose dominant culture marginalizes their race or ethnicity. Focusing on the postmigration experience and its impact on mothers and mothering, our goals are to provide clinicians with (1) an understanding of the impact of culture on mothers and mothering, (2) a respect for the multiple contexts that affect mothering, and (3) specific skills for working with women who are mothering across culture.

Situating Ourselves

Roxana's Story

I was born at home, in a seaside village in Peru, with the help of a midwife. Marujita was introduced to me as the woman who helped my mother bring me into this world. Although I was connected to her by the circumstances of my birth, this smiling woman seemed more connected to my mother than me. A large circle of women surrounded my mother, including grand-mothers, aunts, cousins, *madrinas*,[1] *comadres*,[2] neighbors, friends, and the ever-present *trabajadoras domesticas*.[3] I understand now how our well-being was closely dependent on that circle of women. Subtly and not so subtly, I was being taught how to be a woman, about the power of collective processes and the dangers associated with its loss. Indirectly, I was also learning about mothering, mothers, and their power in the home. These women showed how they understood this power, the proper ways to express it, disguise it, or share it.

Women were not the only ones shaping the meanings I learned about gender and gender roles. Men, fathers, and grandfathers reduced or expanded these meanings through their way of validating the role. Messages were delivered in different languages: Spanish, Italian, and the Quechua symbols of the inhabitants of my world. Embedded in these languages were other complex messages. How does a *mestiza*[4] child understand why the indigenous language is not as valued as the European language(s) and the costs imposed on women and mothers because of these differences? Later, in the United States, I would ask the same question about other languages: English and Spanish. Like others in the circle of women, I was not an equal participant until I was older and slowly allowed to participate more intimately. It was as if throughout my whole life I had been preparing to benefit from their collective wisdom. And then everything changed. . . .

I was to spend my senior year studying in Boston. Leaving was harder than I had anticipated. I remember my mother holding me reassuringly tight after I had said good-bye to the large group of family and friends who came to the airport. "Before you realize it," she said, "we'll be here again to greet you." I did not know then that this would be the last time I would see her.

After 35 years, images of my departure are still clear in my mind, for they marked the turning point that divided my life into the *before* and *after*. The home I had hoped to return to in a year abruptly disappeared while I was on my first venture away from that home. Five months after my departure, a car accident killed my mother, stepfather, and baby brother. At 17, I became acutely aware that life can change suddenly and unexpectedly, linking forever my trip to the United States to these events, and vice versa. Both introduced discontinuity, outsider experiences, and the challenge to re-create a coherent sense of self and belonging amid the change. A military coup brought further social changes that transformed the country I had left, so that truly *returning* home was possible only in my mind. (Llerena-Quinn, 2004).

I share with many immigrant mothers a legacy of losses, but for many there are other stresses from which I am protected. Resources available to me before and after immigration, due to my social class, age of migration, educational level, skin color, and language skills, served as protectors relative to other Latinas with less privilege, but not compared to the dominant population. Like all women who become mothers, I have had to adjust my identity to include the role of mother, waging a battle between what has been handed down to me by my mother, society's projections about this role, and my needs and preferences. My dilemmas, though, always play themselves out in two distinct cultural contexts, the *old* and the *new*. For I always see the *new world* through the eyes of old memories and the *old world* with "American" eyes. I struggle to balance a desire for intimacy and connection to the group, the family, and the extended family with the values of autonomy, self-determination, and privacy demanded by the context in which my 17- and 20-year-old children are growing up. I must launch my children to adulthood on paths I have never walked before, without the support of the old circle of women, while trying to protect them from the shadow cast by the circumstances in which I left home.

Marsha's Story

My grandmother Sadie, a Polish Jew from Lodz, arrived at her tenement on the Lower East Side of New York already traumatized by the spring of 1921. I imagine that she prayed a silent prayer of gratitude when she, her husband, her baby son, and my 7-year-old mother-to-be reached shore. After all, they had escaped the pogroms that had claimed the lives and threatened the safety of so many of her friends, neighbors, and family. Yet, at the same time, she was drowning in a grief from which she would never completely emerge. The Polish government required that she leave her teenage son in Poland until he had completed serving in the army—and she never saw him again. He remained in Poland, and he, his wife, and his children, along with most of Sadie's brothers, were killed in the Holocaust.

Unlike many other Polish Jewish immigrants, including my paternal grandparents, whose poverty in the *shtetls* was unbearable, Sadie moved from a life of middle-class comfort in Poland to the poverty of the tenements. Although she had assumed anti-Semitism would be left in Poland, she entered a country where anti-Semitism remained a powerful force through the 1940s. Furthermore, although my mother picked up English easily, and quickly learned the subtleties of the new culture, Sadie's primary language remained Yiddish. She grew to depend on her daughter to navigate this new world, especially when her husband's job took him away for several months at a time. This dependency contributed to a loss of parental authority within her household that added to her confusion and hopelessness. How could she mother in a land where she did not understand the language, customs, regulations, unspoken assumptions? At the same time,

Sadie had settled in a Jewish area where her belief in her religion and the associated traditions and rituals remained strong. In addition, Sadie was not culturally constrained by some of the assumptions entrapping many U.S.-born women at the time. Both in the *shtetl* and in her middle-class environment, Polish Jewish women often worked, and earning a living and utilizing her skills in math were part of Sadie's history. Eventually she and her husband opened a small store and offered a model of a proud working woman that her daughter would later emulate.

My grandmother's losses carried over to my own mother, leaving her feeling both depressed and responsible, waiting always for the "other shoe to fall." Her witnessing of her mother's loss of authority made her claim unyielding and total household authority. Although she was a brilliant community activist, she never overcame an intergenerationally transmitted fear of loss, an issue with which I too would have to grapple. As her daughter I was both the recipient of the sacrifices they had made that allowed me the privilege I have, and the witness of the depression, anger, and fear that my mother carried as part of her Jewish immigrant experience—an experience I would have to understand and resonate with in order to carry the pride and hope without taking on the depressive, angry, scared parts of the legacy.

Multiple Contexts That Impact Immigrants' Mothering in the Adopted Land

Latina immigrant mothers whom I (RLQ) have met formally through my practice or informally through friends, have shared with me what they found helpful in raising their children in the United States. They seemed to agree that they must be ready to fight for their children and believe in them even when others do not. They encouraged the children—and themselves— to learn English well, but not to lose the language of origin, because it is a connection to their roots and the extended family. They were clear that children need love, discipline, and investment in their education. They believe that mothers should encourage pride in their ethnic identity and awareness of the environmental forces that influence their experiences. Community activism and joining forces with others like themselves diminished the isolation and promoted hope. When everything else failed, they reported finding strength in their spiritual beliefs and religion.

The voices of these mothers can help guide clinicians. Immigrant mothers experience unique challenges and dilemmas borne out of their cultural displacement. Their sense of empowerment in the new world can influence how their children perceive them and how they (the mothers) negotiate the dilemmas of the home or the outside world on behalf of their children. Immigrant mothers must overcome a number of cultural, linguistic, economic, and institutional barriers that are invisible to those who have citizenship or class privilege. To notice, we must listen as they speak to us about the impact of immigration on family support systems, the environmental forces that often place in conflict the collectivist culture of origin and the dominant individualistic culture of the United States, struggles in larger systems, class, acculturation, language differences, and the experience of racism.

The Family Context: Support Systems and Worldviews

Questions for clinicians to consider when meeting with immigrant mothers include the following: Who is this mother? In what kind of family did she grow up? What was she taught about being a *good* mother? How is "family" conceived in her culture of origin? Is the family here? Are *all* family members here? Are there taboos or sanctions associated with membership in a family form that is different from those of the country of origin? Or from the new country? It is also important for clinicians to note any relevant family events or stressors, such as death, loss, separations, chronic illness, and so on, that may have taken place before, during, or after migration and that impact the well-being of the mother and the family. For example, many immigrant mothers come from families that were part of large extended family networks. These networks provide a means of support and nurturance for their children's children (Flores, 2000). The extended family works for the young and for the mothers because it includes a variety of adults who can help with mothering and child care activities. Studies have shown that a greater number of healthy social connections is a key element in resistance to disease, healing, and a long life (Ornish, 1998). An immigrant member of a group of depressed Latina mothers that I (RLQ) co-lead contrasted her experiences in the two contexts:

> "*Here* you are alone, isolated inside your apartment walls . . . you are sad and no one notices. *There*, everything is open with people around to talk to you, distract you, give you *animo* [encouragement]. If you don't come out one day, they go knocking at your door. *Busybodies*, my kids would say . . . but I felt cared for."

Losing this support system can have a significant impact that may not be fully appreciated by clinicians raised primarily in nuclear families. In addition, clinicians trained in the medical model may focus primarily on the experience of the *illness*, whereas the mothers want to focus on the losses and life stressors. We have learned from many immigrant Latina mothers who are depressed that they seldom label their experience as *depression*, although they meet diagnostic criteria. For example, a Dominican mother in the same group stated:

> "The doctor says I am depressed and I say '*Lo que yo tengo una pena profunda* [what I have is a profound sadness].' I miss my family! But they don't understand that, they change the subject as if I am talking about the wrong thing, feeling the wrong things."

Using the mother's language for meaning making can help clinicians understand the woman's experience and join with her in constructing hope.

Healthy individuals can be raised in all kinds of family forms (Carter & McGoldrick, 1999). Depending on one's culture, privacy may be sacrificed in exchange for the mutual support of the extended family, or support may be sacrificed for privacy in the nuclear family. Both forms can become dysfunctional in their extremes. However, labeling the differences as dysfunctional because they do not match the clinician's family preference or that of the dominant culture can be problematic to all involved.

Many immigrant families carry a collectivist orientation that is misunderstood at times. A common misunderstanding is to confuse mutuality with parentification in families who strongly prioritize responsibility to family. The responsibility of the individual is to contribute to the group, and it is seen as ungrateful and sinful not to do so (Shorris, 1992). We have seen countless families who seek help because a child "won't help around the house." These mothers are further upset that clinicians born in the United States often respond to the parental request that the children pick up their rooms by saying "just shut the door." These clinicians completely miss the point, which is responsibility to the larger group and the family. This response also fails to address the underlying fear that the mother is raising selfish children.

Another common misunderstanding occurs in adolescence. Some immigrant mothers may view adolescence as a process of "joining" the adult world; as an apprenticeship period for assuming increased responsibilities for self and others, rather than as one of separation or detachment. Clinicians sometimes confound *differentiation* with *distance*, and *cohesiveness* with *enmeshment*. This conflation can lead to a view of closeness, cooperation, and caregiving in relationships that identifies these attributes as a negative form of enmeshment, thereby pathologizing what are actually competence-enhancing processes (Green & Werner, 1996). Customs of ethnic minority families and women's relational styles may be particularly vulnerable to such mislabeling (McGoldrick, Anderson, & Walsh, 1989; Weingarten, 1991). If the adolescent pursues a more "American" course, mother and child can become entrenched in conflict that arises from different worldviews and that will need to be negotiated by the therapist, emphasizing the positive elements of both experiences and focusing on common goals.

Experiences with Larger Systems

Many of the functions fulfilled by the kin system in the countries of origin are replaced in the United States by distant, impersonal, governmental institutions. Although social supports are needed, immigrant mothers report a sense of fear, confusion, and disempowerment when their values clash with the agencies that are meant to help them. The most common misunderstanding between professionals and immigrant mothers occurs in the area of discipline and child abuse. Although there is no uniform discipline pattern that can be attributed to all immigrant mothers, there are differences in discipline practices between immigrant families and the dominant American culture that can be misconstrued as abuse. Of course, immigrant children deserve the same protection from harsh physical punishment as all other children. However, national research studies repeatedly have found that children from poor and minority families are more likely to be labeled "abused" than children with comparable injuries from more affluent and majority homes (Hampton, Gelles, & Harrop, 1989), and more likely to be removed from their homes, as compared to white children (Child Welfare Watch, 1998). A study by the U.S. Department of Health and Human Services in 2003 demonstrated a lack of racial, cultural, and class awareness on the part of child welfare workers. For example, respondents suggested that a white or middle-class worker might not be aware of the cultural foundations of some modes of corporal punishment. Poor and minority parents are more likely to use control-oriented forms of discipline than are middle-class and white parents (Steinberg, Dornbusch, & Brown, 1992). Some longitudinal research has suggested that this type of parenting style may result in more favorable outcomes for poor and minority children (Deater-Deckard & Dodge, 1997; Steinberg et al., 1992). Aronson Fontes (2002) noted that loving and devoted parents who practice traditional forms of childrearing may include an authoritarian style and corporal punishment side by side with high levels of intimacy and support. As in all families, stress and isolation can increase the risk for maltreatment among immigrant families. Poverty, fear of deportation, isolation stemming from cultural and language differences, and loss of family networks are among many social stressors experienced by immigrant families. Helping mothers reduce stress and isolation is an important step to prevent child maltreatment. Counselors can help mothers expand their discipline repertoires through systemic interventions that provide validation and support to the mothers. Investing time in understanding each mother's situation, her hopes and concerns, can help her take the lead on this issue.

Migration and Social Class Context

Suarez-Orozco (1998) hypothesizes that the impact of immigration is moderated by social class. In general, upper-middle-class women sustain the fewest losses because they are able to retain their status and prestige and are able to travel back and forth to maintain their valued relationships. Middle-class women may suffer a downward trend in jobs and are often cut off from loved ones, with infrequent opportunities to visit. In addition, their quality of life may suffer, as they may no longer be able to afford the domestic help to which they were accustomed. They may also experience, for the first time, the pain of discrimination in the new country. The poorest immigrants, who are largely members of the lower classes in their country of origin, suffer a great deal of adversity, including racism, xenophobia, and competition for lowest paid jobs; however, at the same time, they may also experience an improvement in their economic situation. The social disparagement they may experience here may not necessarily be a new experience to them. Among them, mothers who are undocumented are the most disempowered, most vulnerable to all kinds of abuses, and most unlikely to have access to, or be willing to seek, services. Undocumented immigrants often take lower-paying jobs, work longer hours, and are not entitled to any of the benefits and rights of their documented counterparts. Fear of deportation silences them and increases their vulnerability and that of their families.

Although many families come to the United States in the hope of escaping severe poverty, others find that their economic circumstances deteriorate when they arrive here, after changes in their governments made life unsafe in the country of origin.

> One mother, who had a medical degree in her country of origin, had to, by U.S. law, train again in the United States. Unable to do that and raise her children, she took a more menial position. Her teenage daughter blamed her for taking her away from friends and from their comfortable home, infuriating the mother who knew that her daughter's opportunities would be more limited and her safety compromised if they had stayed in their country of origin.

Therapists can help bridge such a gap by opening space for the mother's and daughter's wishes to be voiced: They both wished that they could have lived safely and with opportunity in their country of birth. They both missed the material comforts that had been available. They both missed their friends, language, familiar foods, scents—all that is familiar and holds meaning. What they need to mourn is a loss that has impacted both of them.

Acculturation Differences in Context

"Acculturation" refers to the changes that groups and individuals undergo when they come into contact with another culture (Berry & Kim, 1998; Williams & Berry, 1991). Studies reveal that first-generation immigrants experience greater acculturative stress than later-generation individuals, with each succeeding generation experiencing lesser stress, and first-genera-tion individuals who move before the age of 12 experience less accultur-ative stress than individuals who move after the age of 12 (Mena, Padilla, & Maldonado, 1987; Padilla, Alvarez, & Lindholm, 1986; Padilla, Wagatsuma, & Lindholm, 1985).

One of the most common concerns that contributes to the intergenera-tional conflict of immigrant mothers is the difference in pace and degree of acculturation between mothers and their children (Mirkin, 1998; Szapocznik, Rio, Perez, & Kurtines, 1986). There are many determinants of acculturation differences. Generally, the children are in school and have opportunities to gain familiarity with the dominant U.S. culture and with the English language. Conversely, many low-income immigrant mothers work in situations that do not support contact with non-immigrant popula-tions, so it is difficult for them to learn the dominant language (English) and customs (European American Christian customs, values, and tradi-tions). In other families, women find jobs and have more access to the adopted culture, whereas the men have the greater difficulty in obtaining work or are in job situations that provide no access to English. Many immi-grant parents, therefore, not only learn English more slowly than their chil-dren, but also are less familiar with the customs of their new country. Eng-lish classes are limited and are often given during times when the parent is working or cannot attend because of lack of access to child care.

Further, many immigrant parents who value their culture of origin find the acculturation issues disturbing: They migrated because of political threat or economic poverty, not because they were unhappy with the cus-toms, traditions, and people in their country of origin. Most of our immi-grant friends and clients call their country of origin "my country," and do so with pride. They do not come to the United States to give up what they value from their country of origin, but rather to provide greater safety and security for their families. They maintain and value many of the rituals and ways of life from their home country. So, when their teenagers want to wear the style of clothing popular among U.S. teenagers, or go to parties, or argue with them, many mothers are appalled by what they see as the poor moral values of this new home. In response, some mothers pull the reins tighter in an attempt to protect their children from what they see as negative influences. As a result, the children, often longing to fit in with their peers, may feel more estranged and embattled.

Although working-class immigrant mothers often work long hours in poor conditions to help provide for the family, what the children may see is a woman who looks, speaks, dresses, and acts differently from the mothers of their American-born peers. Some children feel embarrassed by the difference between their mothers and the mothers of their peers. This awareness of their children's humiliation, which is often unspoken, can be very painful to the mothers. Therapists can help mothers who personalize their children's shame understand that the children's attitudes come from the pull of a new culture and the children's attempts to make this new place their home, rather than their failings as mothers. In general, families that are able to maintain their language of origin and ties to the home culture, while acquiring elements of the new language and culture, seem to have the best outcome (Falicov, 1998).

An argument exploded when Julia, a 15-year-old immigrant from Colombia, insisted on going to the school end-of-year dance with a European American boy in her ninth-grade class. When her parents refused to let her go, citing the lack of chaperones and their distrust of American values, Julia came up with an elaborate ruse to get to the dance. Her parents, suspicious that her peers had distorted her values, caught her, further cementing their belief that Julia is being corrupted by U.S. culture. When I (MPM) consulted about this case, we discussed the need to reframe the argument from one between parents and children to one of cultural emphasis. Julia and her parents agreed that they wanted Julia to adjust to her new country while maintaining what they valued about Colombia. The discussion then became how the family could achieve that goal, given some of the cultural conflicts.

The flip side of the coin was a consultation concerning 15-year-old Manuel, whose anger about leaving Chile to come to the United States fueled his refusal to participate in any social activity—much to the concern of his mother, who saw the move as one that enabled their son to have greater opportunities. She also reported enjoying a relative degree of freedom that she had not had as a woman in her country of origin. Allowing space for both parents and children to mourn the losses they experienced through the migration process can repair the connections that may have been damaged due to family members' different responses to the move.

Language Differences in Context

An immigrant mother's ability to speak the new language largely impacts the degree to which she will be able to negotiate the outside world. Latino families living in primarily Latino communities or barrios usually do well until they venture outside that circle. Immigrants tend to live in segregated communities with others who speak the same language. They may work in similar settings where the new language is not needed, and their shift times may reduce the opportunities for attending ESL classes. A promising alternative is the provision of ESL classes in the workplace, as some institutions have initiated (Wilson, 2003).

A common problem for immigrant families is that parents often rely on their children to interpret for them, creating family role reversals that can impact parenting and unbalance the power dynamics of the family system. Therapists can encourage mothers to develop a network of trusted adults to interpret for them, rather than relying on their children, who have different generational perspectives. Providers, too, need to be sensitive to this issue and avoid relying on the children for translation. Many factors influence language acquisition in the new country: the mother's level of literacy prior to migration, her age at migration, and opportunities available to learn the new language. In general, research studies do not support the claim that immigrants resist learning English (Suarez-Orozco & Suarez-Orozco, 1995). Portes and Rumbault (1996) found that the majority of children of immigrants knew English and that the children who maintained both languages had higher self-esteem, higher educational aspirations, and higher test scores in both English and math in junior high school. English-only policies at schools further impede mother's and children's access to each other's world. A mother's limited language skills results in many misunderstandings in the family, restricted access to her children's world and schooling, and diminished capacity to get to know the world her children now occupy.

The loss of language is closely associated with the immigrant's loss of voice within families, communities, and the larger social context. To overcome this tradition of silence, mothers must reclaim their voices.

> Carmen is a widowed Costa Rican woman who has been in this country for 7 years. She lives with her 13-year-old daughter, Lucia, and her 8-year-old son, Samuel. Lucia takes care of Samuel after school while their mother works in a nearby factory. Carmen has not been able to learn English because of her work hours and her need to take care of her family after work. She understands a little but avoids speaking her broken English because "people make fun

of" her. Lucia is fully bilingual but prefers to speak in English. Samuel, who started school after the English immersion law was passed, speaks only English. Samuel and Lucia communicate with each other in English, but Samuel and his mother cannot communicate with each other without Lucia's help. Lucia hates to translate for them, but most of all, she hates the resulting family dynamics. After discussing as a family how the situation was affecting their relationships, all agreed to work on reclaiming their voices—their links to each other—even if the message is to be delivered in an imperfect, accented, broken language. A plan was made for Carmen to learn English and for Samuel to learn Spanish, working around institutional barriers and limited financial resources to do so.[5]

Unsafe Contexts: Internalized and Institutional Racism

Racism—which is a combination of prejudice and power—is connected to loss of voice and limited access to resources. Along with ethnocentrism and anti-immigrant bias, racism hurts a mother's identity and mental health and interferes with her capacity to advocate for her children.

Aylin came to Boston from El Salvador as a young child. She never graduated from high school because she fell in love and became pregnant before finishing her last year of school. At the time, she also wanted to get away from her traditional immigrant parents who did not understand her needs. Her parents have not forgiven her for not taking advantage of the opportunities that they had never experienced, for betraying their Latino values, and for becoming another "statistic." Aylin has promised herself to have a better relationship with her daughter, Andrea, and to avoid the cultural conflicts she had with her immigrant parents. She works in a beauty salon. Andrea participates in a desegregation busing program and is bused from her urban home neighborhood to a suburban school system; Aylin wants her daughter to have a better education and safer environment than the one in which she grew up. Aylin's salary supports the family and allows her to pay for Andrea's music lessons in the suburban community. When a classmate from the affluent community played a prank on the music teacher and hid the teacher's music book, Andrea was suspected and questioned. Although she knew who was responsible for the prank, Andrea would not tell anyone except her mother. She was hoping her classmate would tell the truth. When this did not happen, Aylin was called into the school, and she became intensely distraught about the experience:

"I get along with my daughter," Aylin told me. "I talk to her, I am honest with her, I tell her about my life so it will be different for her— but I have trouble in the 'outside,' I can't always defend her when she is unjustly blamed because out there, my voice doesn't count. Out there, I am no one, I am a nobody. (*with tears*) If I had money or more education, I would be somebody and they would listen. I feel ashamed that I can't protect her. *Yo no soy nadie* [I am a nobody]."

In this situation, the therapist's facilitation of a conversation between key school personnel and the family helped resolve the problem and enlisted the support of sympathetic personnel at the school to be available to Aylin and Andrea, as needed. The women in the group that I (RLQ) facilitate challenged Aylin's construction of self as a "nobody" and helped her connect with her strengths in carrying out her best intentions for her daughter in the context of unaffirming environments. She is learning how to pass this sense of empowerment on to her daughter.

Unsafe communities are one of many consequences of poverty and racism. For many, the danger that they tried to escape in the country of origin follows them here. When violence occurs, mothers feel trapped in communities they cannot escape because of the unspoken and prevailing racism that exists in the housing market today (Walsh, 2002).[6] Renting an apartment is a not easy for families who do not look like the dominant majority or do not project the right stereotype.

Yolanda's son, for example, was threatened by a gang. Fearful for the safety of her only child, she decided to move: "I want to move out of here, but it is so hard to find an apartment. No one wants to rent to us, and I don't want to go where I am not wanted. It is not my credit, it is perfect. Then why do they refuse?" Yet, even those who succeed in getting their children away from unsafe environments, as in Aylin's case, discover that *other* environments are not so safe either because of the stereotypes we hold about each other.

Immigrant mothers see education as a means to guide their children away from danger and toward a better future. Sometimes this education can also bring a sense of estrangement as the children become separated from their mothers by a *privileged distance*. The language to close the gap between these social worlds often falls short.

Some immigrant children are terrified of leaving home for college because to them it risks a permanent disconnection from their families. Sandra Cisneros finds a more compelling solution: "You live *there*?" the outsider comments about Esperanza's home in *The House on Mango Street* (Cisneros, 1984), and for the first time she realizes that *home* is a place from which she has to get away. But she leaves home only to come back to it empowered—to come back for the ones who cannot get out.

The Invisible Mothers: Transnational Mothering

> Contemporary transnational motherhood continues a long histori-
> cal legacy of people of color being incorporated into the United
> States through coercive systems of labor that do not recognize
> family rights.
>
> —HONDAGNEU-SOTELO and AVILA (1997, p. 568)

No chapter on immigrant mothers could be complete without a discussion of transnational mothering (Hondagneu-Sotelo & Avila, 1997). This
term was developed to describe a trend in migration in which mothers leave
their countries of origin to come to the United States in an effort to support
their families back home. Although statistics are unavailable, many transnational mothers are *domesticas* from Latin America and Mexico.
Ironically, in order to support their children, they must leave their children
to take care of someone else's children and house.

Demeaning, arbitrary, and exploitative behavior toward *domesticas* is
common: They are often paid below minimum wage, required to work long
hours, and given no benefits. Hondagneu-Soelo and Avila (1997) describe
three levels of *domestica* work, each progressively more difficult and
exploitative for the worker. The most lucrative, although still oppressive, is
working as a housekeeper for a number of families. Next are the live-out
nannies and caretakers, and finally the live-in *domesticas*. Many Latina
families assume that the mother will come to the United States for a short
time and then return home, but the stays become protracted because of the
low wages. Both immigration rules and job requirements make it almost
impossible for a mother to bring children to the United States while she is
working at a live-in job. Further, many mothers feel that they want to protect their own children from the daily microaggressions of racism,
ethnocentrism, and other structural oppressions that they suffer; therefore,
they do not try to bring them to the United States. The intersection of race,
class, and immigrant status leaves them marginalized within the homes of
primarily wealthy, white, English-speaking employers. Instead of bringing
their children to the States, many transnational mothers work to acquire
the financial security to educate their children in their home countries so
that if the children ever come to the Unites States, it would be for higher
education and not for a low-paying, demeaning job.

Whereas families often migrate for political reasons, transnational mothers typically migrate alone, leaving their families behind for financial reasons:

> I (MPM) met Claire, a black Caribbean[7] woman, when she was taking
> care of an ill, elderly woman whom I knew. A hard worker with a very
> upbeat attitude, Claire spent long hours lovingly attending to her

infirm employer. With deep pain and strong resolve, Claire told me about her two children who stayed in her country of origin when she came here. She hadn't seen the children in a year and longed to visit them. Claire was adamant that she wanted to work as many days as possible with few days off, so that she could earn money to help her children live a different life from the one she had experienced so far. Claire reported that in her country, and many others throughout Latin America and the Caribbean, high school education is not free. In her case, it cost far more than her family could afford. She knew that her children needed to have both high school and college educations in order to have opportunities for better lives. So she was here, and they were home, living with their father. Claire worried much of the time because her mother and sisters lived in different parts of the United States and Canada, also doing domestic work, so there were no close relatives, other than her husband, to look after her children. Several months after I met Claire, she was finally able to return home for a visit, a rare and much longed-for event. She encountered a crisis at home and needed to make alternative plans for her children before she returned to the United States. In the interim, she lost her job to another woman with a similar story—who, when and if she ever returned to visit her small children, might also lose her job to yet another woman with yet another similar story.

Claire and other mothers like her have had to find a way to mother from a distance, not knowing when they will see their children again and yet remaining emotionally close to, and financially responsible for, them. To accomplish this challenging task, these mothers have developed a whole new idea about mothering. Both the dominant U.S. culture and Latina culture view mothers as the ones responsible for taking care of their children. As Hondagneu-Sotelo and Avilla (1997) note, the Virgin Madonna figure and the Virgen de Guadalupe support this prescribed mothering role. Yet circumstances have always made it impossible for women in financial need to stay home in spite of cultural mandates. So low-income Latina women have historically developed networks of child care. These include *comadres*, *madrinas*, grandmothers, and especially the mother's mother (Hondagneu-Sotelo & Avila, 1997); mothers' sisters and other kin as well as fathers and oldest children are also involved. The hope is often to make sure that someone in the kinship network has primary responsibility for the children when the mother cannot, and the belief is that family will take better care of the child than a stranger.

Whereas on one hand, the dominant Latina culture sees a good mother as one who takes care of her own children, the experience of women through the years of childrearing is that kin take on a major role in mothering. These values have supported transnational mothers, but at a cost, because it is often guilt provoking to behave in a way that counters the socially ingrained ideals of a good mother. In addition, given economic circumstances, many transnational mothers such as Claire are daughters and sisters of other transnational mothers, and therefore the kinship network itself is sometimes uprooted, making alternative childrearing networks more difficult to put in place.

Although there is a strong support system for alternative mothering, this does not diminish the pain the mothers feel when they are physically separated from their children. Mothers often try to bridge the gap through phone calls, letters, and continued advice-giving and financial support. They do not abdicate their maternal responsibility because they move to another country, but the physical absence is felt by both children and parents.

While dealing with the pain and the logistics of mothering across borders, transnational mothers might also be dealing with aging parents. In many cultures, it is customary for aging parents to live with extended families. However, this way of life is being disrupted by the migration experience; one study shows a two-fold increase in numbers of elderly living alone in 52 Mexican villages (Kanaiaupuni, 2000). While many U.S.-born women with class privilege are experiencing the stress of the "sandwich generation," immigrant mothers are dealing with these emotional pulls with a cultural value that elderly parents should live with family but without either the financial or the geographical opportunity to provide that care. Therapists need to bear witness to the pain and guilt induced by this situation and help the mother identify the multiple and conflicting cultural expectations. It can be helpful to connect the individual to others from her adoptive country and/or church group to see how they are handling the situation, receive new information that might be helpful, and experience some support as she is dealing with the situation.

It is unlikely that therapists will encounter transnational mothers while they are separated from their children, because therapy is expensive, time consuming, and often culturally dystonic; many of these mothers are undocumented, do not have insurance, and/or the time to leave work. However, it is more likely that families reunited in the United States will be seen if the child is having trouble with the transition.

In a longitudinal study of 385 youths who immigrated to San Francisco and Boston from Central America, China, the Dominican Republic, Haiti, and Mexico, Suarez-Orozco, Todorova, and Louie (2002) reported that 85% of their sample were separated from one or both parents during migration, with a much higher percentage of separation in Haitian and Central American groups. Children separated from their parents during migration were more likely than those who were not separated to report depressive symptoms. However, there were no other differences on any other psychological symptom scales. Suarez-Orozco and colleagues interviewed parents and children, who movingly reported the difficulties of the separation. Parents were able to acknowledge the difficulties that their children encountered when separated from other relatives in the country of origin, as well as the difficulties in their family relationships after reunification.

Even when children are able to join their mothers in this country, the transition may be difficult. On the one hand, reunion is positive. On the other hand, the child may be uprooted from other loving family members as well as from friends, neighborhoods, and a familiar culture, which leads to a sense of loss (Sciarra, 1999) and often to conflict with the mother. Some mothers reported having difficulty asserting authority with a teenager after years of separation; others felt that the closeness they remembered was not there, and a cutting distance aggravates the already painful wound of having left the child. Mothers and children often felt like strangers upon reunion (Forman, 1993). Other mothers reported that their children acculturated quickly, and they feared that the children would lose the important traditional values of their country of origin (Mirkin, 1998). In other cases, because mothers have been in the country longer, they have acculturated and the children feel less integrated into the new culture (Sciarra, 1999).

Clinical Implications

Immigrant mothers who seek consultation are often treated by providers from a different ethnic background than their own. Clinicians see the world through their own cultural lenses and through the lenses of the mental health culture, which is often monocultural and lacks context (Hardy, 1989). Therefore, many of the cultural imperatives impacting mothering may be invisible to us. It is a challenge to us as therapists as well as to our clients to recognize and name these cultural imperatives, especially as they clash with the values and belief systems of the immigrant families.

To a large extent, the cultural fit between the mother, the family, and clinician will depend on the level of acculturation of the mother, the clinician's attitude toward and familiarity with the mother's culture, the mother's preferences, the mother's past experiences with the mental health system, and the history of the relationships between the clinician's and the mother's cultural groups (Cultural Consultation Service, 2004). As clinicians, we need to help these mothers and children contextualize their problems. The issue is not intrapersonal or even interpersonal between mother and child. Instead, we need to externalize the problem and explore differences in rates of acculturation; ease of new language acquisition; differences in beliefs about the necessity of the separation; and social, political, and economic contexts that led to the separation. We need to pull strength from the currently painful situation and help them co-create a bicultural experience that includes sources of strengths from both the culture of origin and U.S. culture.

The therapeutic relationship can be further impacted by language differences. The use of interpreters is preferable to using children, but we must be aware that some of what the mother says is lost in translation, and that can take a toll on the therapeutic relationship.

It is important to be able to see immigrant mothers as they see themselves if we are to help them expand their narratives to include their power. We need to give back the *good mother* to their children so that they can be *filled* rather than *depleted* by the differences. As therapists, we can help transform the legacies of loss and trauma to legacies of hope and resilience. Therapists working with transnational mothers must challenge their own cultural understanding of what it means to be a mother so that they can include the form of transnational mothering. Examining their own classism may help in this context. For example, many wealthy white women employ live-in nannies who raise their children. Blaming transnational mothers for leaving their children, while not challenging the lifestyle of the wealthy women who employ them, bears reflection.

Reunification between mother and child will often be smoother if the child lived with family that was supportive of the transnational parent (Suarez-Orozco et al., 2002). It is critical to find out about the relationship between the caretakers at home and the mother. The therapist needs to normalize the awkwardness between mother and child, as well as some of the stage-appropriate behaviors.

> I (MPM) was called in to consult with a Mexican immigrant, Yolanda, and her daughter, Elena. When Yolanda was finally able to bring Elena to the United States, Elena was 14, and Yolanda had not lived with her for 6 years. She expected to pick up where they had left off; she expected Elena to be the loving, cuddly, wanting-to-be-with-mom 8-year-old for whom she had waited all these years. Elena, however, was eager to be accepted by her new American friends and had no desire to be cuddly or to stay home. Yolanda was heartbroken, and Elena felt that she was living with some Old World autocrat.

We need to bear witness to the sadness of separation while still holding the psychological strengths that many of these children and mothers possess. Sadness is a normal response to these difficult situations, and bearing witness to the stories and normalizing the responses can be useful to some families. Sometimes rituals that involve reviewing and saying goodbye to old stages and moving into a new stage can be helpful. One ritual is for the child to bring, or for the mother and child to create, an object that represents each year they have been apart. These objects may include dolls, toy trucks, report cards, old clothing, and so on. Starting with the first year of separation and going until the present, mother and child bring out the object, share stories, hopes, regrets, joys, and longings about the item, and then place each item into a memory box, to be taken out whenever needed.

Domesticas tend to be very isolated because their jobs often require them to live with a family, and they do not have time for friends. Once their children come over and they are often no longer in live-in jobs, it is helpful to assist them in developing a support system. Against the odds, some *domesticas* already have such a system. Claire told me (MPM) about using her brief break during the day to sit outdoors with other caretakers. She moved in with other immigrants when she left her job, and later had newer immigrants move in with her. Not every *domestica* is that fortunate; many leave their jobs in order to live with their newly migrated children and have nobody to turn to for support.

To work successfully with immigrant and transnational mothers, we as therapists must be able to bear witness and convey the message that we can tolerate hearing their stories. We need to be humble; we cannot possibly know as much about clients' cultures of origin as they do, but we also must take the responsibility of educating ourselves in a basic way, rather than expecting our clients to wholly educate us. We need to listen carefully to each mother's story and to learn as much as we can about her migration history: loss, trauma, and "culture shock" as well as strength and resilience. We need a working knowledge of the current sociopolitical, sociocultural context in which immigrant mothers parent their children. We need to challenge ourselves constantly to see and hear the larger context—that is, the contexts of race, gender, class, and religion/spirituality, to name a few—as we listen to the mother describe her mothering experience (Mirkin, 1998). Thus a parent's decision not to send her child to a potentially beneficial summer program offered at a local community center may not necessarily reflect a "cultural belief" of the family but a structural, financial issue. Low-income working families may not qualify for subsidies, be able to afford day care, or may need to send money home to the extended family. Identifying these issues and situating them in the proper context is an important first step in avoiding inappropriate labeling. Helping mothers identify and advocate for resources are important next steps. Therapists can also tap into the strength that many mothers derive from their faith by inquiring about religious beliefs and how those beliefs can help them through the hard times.

Conclusion

We end with excerpts from a poem by Grace Lopez, MD, a 2004 graduate of Harvard Medical School:

You brought us to this country;
a country of hope, prosperity, new beginnings and new struggles
You worked endless hours;
sweating, struggling, fighting to subsist . . . dodging not bullets but the
pain and price of ignorance—for how could an elementary school
education protect you and us?

You gave up your lives for ours to prosper;
. . . to escape the shackles of poverty that the U.S. greeted us with . . .

My key to liberation was education
I soared to new heights that you were never able to reach. . . .

Yet,
I've paid a price
A privileged distance now separates us
. . . for how can you comprehend how far I am?
. . . do you comprehend me?
. . . my struggles are not comparable to yours. . . .

. . . for where do I begin to tell you of all the complex theories I've
learned and how I view the world and my surroundings
. . . you never have time
. . . you're too tired
. . . my Spanish is too colloquial or my thoughts too complicated
I am torn between two separate worlds without knowing where the
bridge is to close the gap
The distance may be too great . . .

Yet . . .
I thank you for your sacrifices
I thank you for loosening the cultural reins that bind Latinas
I thank you for letting me go
. . . for letting me fly
¡*Gracias a ustedes estoy aquí*!

Notes

1. *Madrina*: godmother
2. *Comadre*: relationship between mother and godmother. It can also be used informally, without being godmother to a child, to indicate the same close bond between two women.
3. *Trabajadoras domesticas*: domestic workers
4. *Mestiza*: mixed race resulting from a blending of Spanish and indigenous races
5. This case example, as well as all others mentioned in this chapter (unless otherwise specified), represents a composite of many individuals and families.
6. On June 22, 2002, the *Boston Herald* published a study that showed that Latino renters in the Greater Boston area were more likely than whites to find doors closed when they tried to rent an apartment. Out of 100 phone calls, 50 from Latinos and 50 from whites responding to housing ads, more than 40% of Latinos were not given a chance to see an apartment, whereas those in the white sample were shown it. In some instances, Latinos were quoted a higher price than whites for the same unit.
7. We are not identifying the specific country not only because this is a composite story based on several transnational mothers, but also because this story is similar across a number of countries.

References

Anzaldúa, G. (1987). *Borderlands la frontera: The new mestiza*. San Francisco: Aunt Lute Books.

Berry, J. W., & Kim, U. (1988). Acculturation and mental health. In P. Dasen, J. W. Berry, & N. Sartorius (Eds.), *Health and cross-cultural psychology: Towards application* (pp.207–236). London: Sage.

Carter, B., & McGoldrick, M. (1999). Overview: The expanded family life cycle. In B. Carter & M. McGoldrick (Eds.), *The expanded family life cycle: Individual, family and social perspectives* (3rd ed.). Boston: Allyn & Bacon.

Child Welfare Watch. (1998, June). *The race factor in child welfare*. New York: Center for an Urban Future. Available at http://www.nycfuture.org/content/reports/report_view.cfm?repkey=9

Cisneros, S. (1984). *The house on Mango Street*. New York: Random House.

Cultural Consultation Service, Department of Psychiatry, McGill University. Available at www.mcgill.ca/ccs/handbook/assessment/

Deater-Deckerd, K., & Dodge, K. A. (1997). Externalizing behavior problems and discipline revisited: Nonlinear effects and variation by culture, context, and gender. *Psychological Inquiry, 8*, 161–175.

Falicov, C. J. (1998). *Latino families in therapy: A guide to multicultural practice*. New York: Guilford Press.

Flores, M. T. (2000). La familia latina. In M. T. Flores & G. Carey (Eds.), *Family therapy with Hispanics: Toward appreciating diversity* (pp. 3–28). Boston: Allyn & Bacon.

Fontes, L. A. (2002). Child discipline and physical abuse in immigrant Latino families: Reducing violence and misunderstandings. *Journal of Counseling and Development, 80,* 31–40.

Forman, G. (1993). Women without their children: Immigrant women in the United States. *Development, 4,* 51–55.

Greene, R.-J., & Werner, P. D. (1996). Intrusiveness and closeness-caregiving: Rethinking the concept of family "enmeshment." *Family Process, 35*(2), 115–136.

Hampton, R. L., Gelles, R. J., & Harrop, J. W. (1989, November). Is violence in black families increasing? A comparison of 1975 and 1985 national survey rates. *Journal of Marriage and the Family, 51*(4), 969–980.

Hardy, K. (1989). The theoretical myth of sameness: A critical issue in family therapy training and treatment. In G. W. Saba, B. M. Karrer, & K. Hardy (Eds.), *Minorities and family therapy* (pp. 17–33). New York: Haworth Press.

Hondagneu-Sotelo, P., & Avila, E. (1997). "I'm here but I'm there": The meanings of Latina transnational motherhood. *Gender and Society, 11*(5), 548–571.

Kanaiaupuni, S. M. (2000). *Leaving parents behind: Migration and elderly living arrangements in Mexico.* Madison: University of Wisconsin–Madison, Center for Demography and Ecology.

Llerena-Quinn, R. (2004). Naming the tears: The multiple contexts of loss. In M. McGoldrick & F. Walsh (Eds.), *Living beyond loss: Death in the family* (2nd ed.). New York: Norton.

McGoldrick, M., Anderson, C. M., & Walsh, F. (Eds.). (1989). *Women in families: A framework for family therapy.* New York: Norton.

Mena, F. J., Padilla, A. M., & Maldonado, M. (1987). Acculturative stress and specific coping strategies among immigrant and later generation college students. *Hispanic Journal of Behavioral Science, 9,* 207–225.

Mirkin, M. P. (1998). The impact of multiple contexts on recent immigrant families. In M. McGoldrick (Ed.), *Re-visioning family therapy: Race, culture, and gender in clinical practice* (pp. 370–384). New York: Guilford Press.

Padilla, A. M., Alvarez, M., & Lindholm, K. J. (1986). Generational status and personality factors as predictors of stress in students. *Hispanic Journal of Behavioral Sciences, 8,* 275–288.

Padilla, A. M., Wagatsuma, Y., & Lindholm, K. (1985). Acculturation and personality as predictors of stress in Japanese and Japanese Americans. *Journal of Social Psychology, 125,* 295–305.

Portes, A., & Rumbault, R. (1996). *Immigrant America: A portrait* (2nd ed.). Berkeley: University of California Press.

Ornish, D. (1998). *Love and survival: The scientific basis for healing power and intimacy.* New York: HarperCollins.

Sciarra, D. (1999). Intrafamilial separations in the immigrant family: Implications for cross-cultural counseling. *Journal of Multicultural Counseling and Development, 27*(1), 31–41.

Shorris, E. (1992). *Latinos: A biography of the people.* New York: Norton.

Steinberg, L., Dornbusch, S. M., & Brown, B. B. (1992). Ethnic differences in adolescent achievement: An ecological perspective. *American Psychologist, 47*(6), 723–729.

Suarez-Orozco, C. (1998, Winter). The transitions of immigration: How are they different for women and men? *DRCLAS News.*

Suarez-Orozco, C., & Suarez-Orozco, M. (1995). *Transformations: Migration, family life, and achievement motivation among Latino and white adolescents.* Stanford, CA: Stanford University Press.

Suarez-Orozco, C., Todorova, I. L. G., & Louie, J. (2002). Making up for lost time: The experience of separation and reunification among immigrant families. *Family Process, 41*(4), 625–641.

Szapocznik, J., Rio, A., Perez, Z. A., & Kurtines, W. (1986). Bicultural effectiveness training: An experimental test of an intervention modality for families experiencing intergenerational–intercultural conflict. *Hispanic Journal of Behavioral Sciences, 8*(4), 303–330.

U.S. Department of Health and Human Services, Children's Bureau Administration for Children and Families. (2003). *Children of color in the child welfare system: Perspectives from the child welfare community.* Washington, DC: Author.

Walsh, T. (2002, June 22). Study: Latino renters often find doors closed. *Boston Herald*, pp. 1, 16.

Weingarten, K. (1991). The discourses of intimacy: Adding a social constructionist and feminist view. *Family Process, 30,* 285–305.

Williams, C. L., & Berry, J. W. (1991). Primary prevention of acculturative stress among refugees: Application of psychological theory and practice. *American Psychologist, 46,* 632–641.

Wilson, R. (2003, Spring). *Massachusetts extended care career ladders initiative.* Gaston Institute Report, University of Massachusetts–Boston. Available at www.pbs.org/kcet/publicschool/roots_in_history/bilingual. html

Race, Gender, Class, and Culture through the Looking Glass of Interracial and Intercultural Intimate Relationships

Maria P. P. Root
Karen L. Suyemoto

Robert and Sarah had been married for 2 years when they came to therapy to discuss their relationship. Robert came from an upper-middle-class African American family; he had graduated, like his parents before him, from an Ivy League college and currently worked in business. Sarah was a second-generation (first U.S. born) Vietnamese American woman from a poor refugee background. She was the first in her family to obtain a college degree. Robert and Sarah had met at Sarah's state university, when Robert was taking summer classes. They dated for a year and then married. Neither Robert nor Sarah's families were pleased with the marriage. Sarah's family had strongly encouraged her to marry a Vietnamese man and initially threatened to disown her when she made it clear she intended to marry Robert. They were, however, pleased with Robert's job in business and his plans to get an MBA. When Sarah recently told them that she was pregnant, they were pleased and excited, but Sarah noticed that they never invited Robert's family members to any events. Robert's family made it clear that they would have preferred an African American daughter-in-law. They continued to invite Robert and Sarah to all family holiday events, but Sarah frequently felt out of place, because she did not always understand the language used, the shared references, or the relational undercurrents within the family.

Initially, Robert and Sarah felt united in their relationship, and both felt that the problems were with their families (who would eventually "come around"). Over the 2 years of their marriage, however, issues began to emerge between them. Sarah wanted to spend many weekends with her parents and siblings, in spite of the fact that they didn't fully accept Robert because he was black. Robert highly valued his own immediate and extended family connections, but felt that seeing them on holidays and special occasions was enough. Robert was angry at Sarah for encroaching on their time together and passively accepting her family's "racist" rejection. Robert also felt that Sarah downplayed the effects of racism on both of their lives, whereas Sarah felt that if Robert would be a little more tolerant and less suspicious, then life would be much easier for both of them. Both Robert and Sarah wanted Robert to enroll in an MBA program, but they had been fighting about how to pay for such a program. Sarah wanted Robert to take a loan from his family (which, she argued, they could pay back over time because they had the money to do so) or from hers (although she acknowledged it would be difficult for them to come up with the money, she knew that her parents and siblings would find a way if necessary). She also wanted them to move in with her family, who would support them and provide child care once the baby was born. Robert wanted to take out student loans, attend school part time, and take advantage of the day care offered at his company.

Personal and social constructions of race, culture, sex, gender, sexual orientation, and class are frequently made clearer and more salient through the experience of loving someone who is different from oneself. Sarah's cultural experiences of interdependence with her family (socially and financially); her class and cultural experiences that contributed to avoiding bank and government loans; and the intersection of class, culture, and racial understandings that contributed to her desire to acculturate and accommodate rather than challenge racism and ethnocentrism are all highlighted by Robert's very different experiences of greater individualism from his culture, greater self-reliance and willingness to accept temporary debt, and greater awareness of the existence and impact of racism, both from the dominant white society and from Sarah's Asian family. This chapter examines the connections, disconnections, and intersections of race, culture, sex, gender, and class within heterosexual and lesbian relationships that are interracial, intercultural, and interclass. We also offer suggestions for helping clients identify and bridge these differences.

As multiracial Asian American women, we have experienced love across differences from our families of origin to our current relationships. I (MPPR) was born in the Philippines to a Filipina mother from an educated middle-class family. My parents met when my white American father was stationed in the Philippines during the Korean War. Given that they were not married at the time of my birth, our subsequent immigration required some of the common subterfuge when the immigration quotas were so small. My mother and I crossed the ocean to British Honduras, then traveled to Guatemala, where we stayed until the necessary papers were arranged and my mother and father were married. My first language was a mixture of Spanish and Tagalog. Eventually, my languages were Spanish and English and then English only, though the mixture prevailed around me at family gatherings. My father came from a working-class family, the most recent origins of which were Oklahoma. No relative had completed high school before him. His father, divorced from his mother, attempted to dissuade my father from marrying my mother by posing him a very difficult choice: His father would pay either for my mother's and my passage by boat, or he would pay for his son's college. The choice to send for us resulted in a classic family estrangement. Growing up, class differences emerged, in addition to the clear cultural differences, whether it came to gift giving, rules and interpretation of gender and age-appropriate behavior, childrearing practices, to whether or not college would be financed by my parents. Every week seemed to produce some source of values- or world-view-related tension. I was raised Catholic, the predominant religion of the Philippines, and attended Catholic school for several years; my father was an atheist. My views of religion were influenced by Philippine Catholicism and by the U.S. Catholic Church, which excommunicated my mother because she had not married in the church. Attributions of divine interventions, guardian angels, and reincarnation were not a subject of discussion with my parents, but not uncommon in the larger family gatherings that were composed of relatives on my mother's side. Because of the presence of several maternal relatives living lives now identified as bisexual or homosexual, the discussions of difference and the lived experience of overwhelming similarity and mutual love have also influenced my experience and view of sexual orientation and identity. As I grew older, I came to see that at the root of the differences between my parents that caused and still cause pain are aspects of personality style, some of which are clearly rooted in responses to familial and war trauma. This understanding has helped me in my work with cross-cultural and interracial couples.

I (KLS) come from a family rich with different experiences: My father is a Nisei (a second-generation Japanese American) who experienced the Japanese American concentration camps of World War II and rose from poverty to an upper-middle-class social standing; my mother was a devout Baptist from a poor rural Southern background; my stepmother is from a Russian Jewish background. When my mother died 4 years ago I found a letter in her papers from her mother (my grandmother), stating that my grandmother had consulted her minister about whether it was okay for my mother to love a Japanese American man. The minister (who was clearly ahead of his time, as this was in the mid-1950s when anti-miscegenation laws were still common), said that it was all right to marry across racial lines *as long as the person was Christian.* My father wasn't, but that wasn't as obvious. When my father and my stepmother married in the 1970s, religion was again the stated issue: My father was not (and is not) Jewish. Whereas my stepgrandparents eventually reconciled with and actively embraced my family, it took time for acceptance and understanding to grow.

Within my own relationship, our differences have created challenges and contributed to a richer experience. For example, my partner identifies as heterosexual but I identify as bisexual; the meaning of my identity claim and whether I should or should not "come out" in social conversations became part of our relationship conversations several years ago, as I challenged him to see how not doing so would not only negate my own identity, but also maintain heterosexist oppression. Within our relationship, my race has been an issue with particular members of my partner's white family, our class differences and values became part of our discussions over time as we merged our financial and career realities and aspirations, and the values and interaction styles rooted in our differential experiences with privilege related to the intersections of gender, race, and culture have had to be named and negotiated within our relationship. Over time, and with much effort, we have bridged our differences in ways that contribute to and sustain our partnership.

Romance and falling in love are almost universal parts of life's journey, perhaps because love promises happiness and wholeness. Love serves as the imagined compass keeping people on a constructive and transformative path. Couples believe that they—and the world around them—will be better with them together rather than apart. But it is not always the case that families, communities, and societies agree with couples' conclusions about their united destiny. Root (2001, p. 1) observes, "Families support this ideology of love so long as their children uphold two conventions in their choice of partners. *Marry within your own race. Marry someone of the opposite sex.*" Until recently, adult children who were seen as violating these conventions were commonly disowned or rejected due to taboos about with whom one could partner appropriately. Although many families and communities have become more tolerant, in some cultures or families, adult children may still be disowned for loving someone of a different race or culture or class, or someone from the same gender. The recent passage of laws prohibiting gay marriages (or even civil unions) in 11 states during the 2004 elections makes it clear that as a society, we have a long way to go before we achieve acceptance of different forms of love and partnerships.

The taboo against loving someone of a different race is as old as the idea of race itself. Root (2001, p. 72) summarizes Gordon's (1997) analysis of structural power based on the linkage between race and gender:

> Gordon points out that from a White point of view, the assumed race of the human race is White. To be non-White is to be racialized in an anti-Black world. To be raceless is to be "pushed up" towards Whiteness. Gordon also notes that for centuries the Western tradition has configured the gender of the human race as male. So although power may be defined as genderless and raceless, the default values for power are male and White.

Those in power (white men) have historically and currently used that power to maintain the social boundaries of race and gender that support the hierarchy and limit the associated privileges to the few, rather than the many. Restricting "acceptable" relationships by race, gender (which, relationally, intersects with sexual orientation), and class is a powerful way to maintain these boundaries. The myth of disturbed, alienated, confused, and/or "defective" children reflected in the question "What about the children?" has been used effectively throughout centuries to maintain race boundaries in relationships. Although there is a recent burgeoning literature about the children themselves, clearly locating difficulties they may encounter in the discrimination they experience from outside their families, rather than in the families themselves (see, e.g., Clunis & Green, 1988; Root, 1992; Root & Kelley, 2003; Tasker & Golombok, 1997; Wehrly, 1996; Zack, 1995), the myth and taboos continue.

The taboo against interclass relationships can be just as strong as the taboo against interracial relationships, but goes more frequently unspoken. Whereas we think of race and gender as permanent statuses (despite their socially constructed nature), we seldom think of the signature or imprint that class origins have on individuals' worldviews. Differences in class origins, particularly when they are disguised by current social achievements or economic standing, may be minimized. Sarah and Robert are both college-educated professionals at this time. They may not recognize that their different attitudes toward money, achievement, and careers are rooted in class values and experiences, in addition to those of culture.

The intersection of class and gender illuminates (1) double standards predicated upon the gender roles and values in a patriarchal society, (2) the value of gendered social capital, and (3) the premise that a woman's social status is dependent not upon her own achievements but upon the status ascribed to her by her relational connection with a man. European-based fairy tales, for example, suggest rescue from cruel working-class families, such as in *Cinderella*, or an uplifting of class ranking through (heterosexual) relationships such as in the movies *Pretty Woman, My Fair Lady*

(Pygmalion), and *Sabrina*. Because in a patriarchal society such as ours, wealth has been typically inherited through the male side of the family, heterosexual marriage patterns are predicated on the normality of male partners having their choice of female partners. The class standing of the woman is not as important in a patriarchal society because the woman usually assumes much of the material standing of her husband. Families therefore become particularly interested in preserving their capital of property, money, and social connections by making sure that their daughters marry someone of equal or greater rank.

What happens when we examine class in same-sex pairings? Do we have the same gender-socialized expectations? Perhaps not in relation to the interaction of gender, social status, and class. That is, the expectation that the male will be wealthier or of a higher class rank than the female does not translate well to relationships between two men or two women. But this does not mean that class differences do not have significant impact on same-sex couples:

> Francis came from a fifth generation of college-educated African American women. Having attended privileged schools, she was used to certain entitlements. She grew up with private tennis lessons and skiing in resorts amid wealthy people. Her partner, Nancy, a multiracial Filipina American woman, grew up middle class with two parents who worked hard to provide their children a comfortable, though not luxurious, existence. One week of summer camp by junior high was a sign that the family had achieved some economic stability. Nancy and Francis met at a professional conference and started their relationship. Living together for less than a year, the once "perfect" relationship developed tensions. Francis noted that she did not understand why Nancy picked on her for being wasteful of household supplies, such as paper towels. It bothered Nancy that Francis bought clothes that then hung in the closet for months and were never worn.

These nitpicking complaints are ensconced in class differences and the deeply internalized and frequently unspoken values attached to them. Therapy can help decode the source of conflicts and explore whether there might be structural, experiential differences resting underneath or alongside the concrete issues. In therapy, Francis pointed out that they could afford not to watch every cent, because they had more than enough money, and both women were good money managers—so money itself could not be the issue. However, the therapist pointed out that the treatment of money as limited or infinite may be a symbolic marker of their class values and hence, of their class differences. And indeed, Nancy disclosed that she had refused to join the upscale athletic club that Francis enjoyed not because of the money, per se, but because she perceived the people (perhaps stereotypically) as snobby and acting as though she was not good enough for them. The therapist helped them recognize that their conflicts were not just small complaints that had emotionally escalated, but were instead rooted in value systems and well-established patterns related to their class backgrounds. This understanding increased the empathy each partner could offer to the other: Francis could now understand that wasted paper towels felt like a lack of care and prioritization of what was important, and Nancy could see that Francis's actions stemmed from an assumption of having more than enough, rather than a feeling of not caring for Nancy's needs. Labeling the class conflicts and recognizing the social system of class also helped Francis and Nancy externalize their difficulties, so that they could ally with each other to overcome them.

Race, class, and gender clearly interact. In a society where individuals may be able to change their class standing economically, race may serve as a caste status that imposes a glass ceiling in terms of social acceptance, credibility, or status (Coe, 1993; Essed, 1990). Robert Merton's (1941) classic sociological studies of black–white intermarriage predicted most common to least common pairings based on exchange theory and the understanding that women should marry "up" in terms of their future partner's occupation or the social status of his family, and that women's choices are therefore more limited. However, Merton's (1941) predictions were largely incorrect because he had not considered that race has a master status that acts in many ways as a caste status (Root, 2001). Despite the class standing of the African American man, racism does not allow him equal status with white men. The frequency of pairings between white women and black men and between black women and white men suggests that black men occupy a standing more similar to white women than white men. However, in a patriarchal society, male gender is still privileged, and thus, within the African American community we see much higher proportions of black men pairing up with women who are not African American. In contemporary times, some of this pairing is due to unequal sex ratios, which allow the members of the sex in smaller proportion (black men) to go outside their cultural community or even resist marrying. However, other communities with unequal sex ratios but different cultural imperatives and meanings, such as the Vietnamese community with its shorter supply of women, underscore the cultural gender difference in cross-racial pairings. Although black men and Vietnamese women are both in shorter supply within their respective communities, Vietnamese women do not have the freedom to marry outside their race or resist marrying that black men have: As women, they are watched carefully and socially pressured to prevent their marriage to outsiders. Thus different variables influence the values and norms that govern intermarriage for men and women within specific races and cultures.

Families and communities have demanded that couples conform to particular social norms not only in relation to race and class but also in relation to the gender of who may be coupled. Heterosexual couples are socially as well as legally sanctioned, whereas lesbian couples are clearly ostracized legally and, in many cases, familially and socially as well. Again, the cry of "what about the children?" is frequently used to maintain the taboo against lesbian relationships, in spite of research that repeatedly shows that it is not the sexual orientations of the partners raising children but the environment parents provide that is correlated with the well-being of the children (Clunis & Green, 1988; Root, 1998). However, even for a lesbian couple who is not yet (or never) considering having children, the legitimacy of their relationship is often legally, socially, and familially challenged, leading to differences in the impacts of racial, cultural, and class differences within lesbian relationships.

By examining the experiences of courtship and commitment within interracial, intercultural, and interclass heterosexual and lesbian relationships, we have the opportunity to explore the lived intersections of what research finds to be a tangled web. Exploring notions of romance and courtship and definitions of healthy relating and "family" in relationships across differences offers moments of awakening and insight into meanings of race, culture, class, and gender.

Meeting and Courtship

Brown has noted that we are a homosocial society, even though the expectation is that we will engage in heterosexual romantic alliances (L. S. Brown, personal communication, 1988). People tend to meet and partner with other people similar to themselves in education, class, and religion. Although schooling, technology and the women's movement have played a significant part in increasing the diversity of the "eligible dating pool" (except in most religious settings, which tend to be one of the most segregated sectors of our society), intimate relationships that cross differences in race, culture, or class are still the exception rather than the rule. Those who are attracted to potential partners across differences may have very different reasons for their unconventional response, ranging from curiosity, defiance of stereotypes, practical convenience, or attraction to what is seen as complementary or similar experiences of difference.

Curiosity is a normal part of initial sexual and interpersonal attraction in any relationship. In interracial and intercultural relationships, it may be an even greater part of the initial attraction, as individuals are invited to explore and experience new values, foods, languages, experiences, etc. Curiosity and attraction to difference may interact with fantasy and practical constraints or challenges to bring couples together across differences. Hopeful fantasy in romance is not only the purview of men. All romantic relationships involve some projections based upon the needs of an individual. However, when the relationship is based more on projections about differences than on the actual lived experiences and meanings of these differences, it is likely to lead to considerable misunderstanding and distress as the couple moves past the courtship stage.

When curiosity, fantasy, and projection are rooted in cultural or racial stereotypes, a courtship is embedded in discrimination and ultimately will become problematic, if not destructive, to the participants. Asian or multiracial women may be sought out as "exotic," Latina women may be perceived as "passionate," African American women may be seen as particularly nurturing, and Native American women as particularly spiritual. African American men may be sought out for sexual prowess, and white men or women may be sought out to provide access to white privilege. Racism becomes apparent in multiple ways both within and across racial groups: when a woman is deemed beautiful because she is light skinned, or desirable because he is an object through which to rebel against parents, or sought after because the person's race or culture provides social capital with a desired group or individual. Although these stereotypes may also affect lesbian relationships, they operate quite differently because the race–culture–gender power dynamic is not present. However, race stereotypes may intersect with stereotypes of lesbians, affecting courtship choice and expectations, as when an Asian American lesbian is expected to behave passively rather than "butch" (Lee, 1996). Relationships based on stereotypes are unlikely to last long beyond courtship (if the couple members have choices and are not constrained by challenges such as finances, immigration status, family expectations or pressures, etc.), because real people are inevitably more complicated than stereotypes. However, these relationships may damage the individuals within them, particularly those who have less power and privilege. Furthermore, relational stereotypes and their associated damage fuel community suspicions of relationships across difference, making the social climate even more difficult for couples who are courting or building relationships in more positive ways.

Fantasy and projections may interact with practical needs and necessities to create relationships across differences that are not based on racial discrimination, but actively reflect stereotyping of other sorts, such as gender stereotyping or nationalism. For example, many projections are involved in the correspondence marriages between Filipinas seeking to leave an economically devastated country and (primarily) white men from the United States, Australia, and Germany. The men's hopeful fantasy is that the women they "rescue" will uphold many of the traditional or conservative roles and conventions of womanhood; they will not challenge the man's role and privileges, even if he is not a socially skilled or economically successful man by, say, American standards. The women's hopeful fantasy is one of a better life with more money and social standing, and perhaps a more equitable "American" relationship. Thai (2002) describes an example of an arranged marriage between an older, well-educated Vietnamese woman lawyer and a poorly educated Vietnamese American assistant cook. Thanh was "unmarriageable" in Vietnam due to her age and high education; her hope was that her U.S. husband would have an egalitarian approach to marriage that respected her education and career. Minh had been in the United States for 16 years and considered many Vietnamese women in the United States to be disrespectful; he was seeking a wife who did not want to be equal, but would be supportive of her husband, as occurs in a traditional Vietnamese relationship. Although Thanh and Minh are both from Vietnamese backgrounds, their relationship crossed cultural and class differences, creating similar issues related to discrepant expectations as those in interracial overseas relationships. Many overseas brides are disappointed once they find out that their "prince" is not considered much of a prize in this country. Many of the men are disappointed when the women find their footing and begin to assert rights and voice new expectations of their husbands.

Projections and idealization are a normal part of courtship, including those that are unrelated to stereotyping or systemic differences such as race, culture, or class. Although projection and idealization are normative beginning processes, through courtship couple members gradually come to adjust their views of each other in relation to more realistic understandings of each others' backgrounds and current experiences. However, in courtships occurring across difference, this process can be more difficult or lengthier because of a lack of understanding of the lived context and experience of someone different from oneself. Therapists are more likely to see couples who have encountered difficulty with this process of moving away from projection and idealization toward a shared and realistic understanding of each other and the relationship.

> Pat, a European American woman, met Aki, a Japanese man, when she spent a year abroad teaching. Pat was not a conventionally physically attractive woman by American standards; she had dated infrequently and was in her mid-30s when she met Aki, who was 7 years younger than she and the older of two sons. Aki was an engineer. He courted Pat by suggesting ideas for dates, giving her gifts, and sharing his country and culture with her. He literally swept her off her feet with his devoted attention to her. He told her that she was beautiful, so fair skinned and smart. Aki also saw Pat as relatively dependent and deferential to him, as a man. In fact, as an American, Pat was aware of her

cultural inexpertise in Japan and regularly deferred to Aki because he was her liaison to a culture with which she was unfamiliar. As was congruent with his culture and developmental process (cultural prescriptions encouraged him to woo a woman and get married), Aki placed their courtship as a priority in his life. Those same cultural prescriptions decreed that once married, Aki's priority should become work, to be a good provider and a loyal company employee.

Pat was unaware of these cultural mandates. She thought Aki was the perfect man: educated, affectionate, and doting. She expected his attention to diminish only minimally after they had married. Within the year they married and moved to the United States, and Pat and Aki found themselves in very different circumstances. Although Aki spoke English, he had a second-class status in this country and found that the prescribed gender roles that worked in his country did not apply in his current situation. Aki was dependent upon Pat to be the culture broker, and she was now in charge of much of their personal and social life. He was uncomfortable being dependent upon Pat and resented her for no longer deferring to him. Simultaneously, because Pat had misunderstood Aki's courtship behavior, she now felt put aside by the time and energy he spent on work. Pat wondered if Aki had married her just for a green card. Aki stated that he was very hurt by her doubt of his love for her.

Pat and Aki met in Aki's native culture that was foreign to Pat and moved to Pat's native culture that was foreign to Aki. This shift in circumstances made their projections and disconnections clearer.

Couples may also meet in special environments, such as school or in a country foreign to both of them, that creates a "third culture" that may minimize their cultural differences and provide a particular (and usually temporary) context for equality and sharing. The expectations for teamwork may temporarily override conventional gender norms. Furthermore, the excitement or loneliness of a new environment may bring people together and fuel romance.

Mohamed, a Somali immigrant, met Kytrina, an African American woman, in business school. Both of them were from professional families. Though they were both well liked by their peers, they felt isolated for different reasons. Kytrina felt conscious of being one of only two black students in their cohort. The other students, primarily white, made many false assumptions about her, so she adopted a watchful demeanor. Mohamed felt homesick and was the only foreigner in his class. He and Kytrina ended up working on a group project together and enjoyed each other, which led to a relationship. Kytrina found Mohamed's cultural differences interesting. With her mother's side of the family from Jamaica, she had always felt a little different from many African American students she met. She felt some kinship with Mohamed as an immigrant and a black person who was not African American in the usual U.S. meaning (i.e., descended from slaves). As the end of school approached, Mohamed and Kytrina both received job offers but in different cities. After 2 years of dating during business school, the relationship was at a crossroads: In one direction was termination, and in the other, making a further commitment toward permanency. Although in their romantic bid to connect, they had minimized their differences in values, such as the immediacy of starting a family, religion, and where they would live if they stayed together, these issues now became hard to ignore, and the couple entered counseling. As they explored areas previously avoided, Kytrina was shocked that Mohamed, who had always treated her as an equal in school, was espousing values that asserted his right to expect her to stay home to raise their children, as his mother had done. Mohamed was stunned that Kytrina, who had always been curious about his religion, would not convert.

For Mohamed and Kytrina, school had created a context in which they could experience an idyllic interlude of romance and courtship. Both had been able to suspend the reality of their nonnegotiable differences. But as they contemplated moving into a different context, with very different demands, they were confronted with the depth of their differences. Therapy helped them express these differences to each other, consider which were deeply rooted in their cultural and family value systems, and evaluate the possibility of compromise.

Same-sex relationships may allow for quicker clarity on cultural differences, due to the lack of gender differential. However, as with different-sex couples, lacking familiarity with the cultural context of a partner, it is difficult to understand which behaviors that are part of courtship are likely to last. Without a good insider understanding of the culture, an individual may not know whether or not some of the behaviors or personality traits are problematic in the individual's culture. One may not know whether certain behaviors convey serious intent or transitory/passing attraction. Thus there is much room for misinterpretation of the other.

Making a Commitment

At some point, relationships move from courtship and romance to commitment. As couples move toward commitment, they are often explicitly confronted with the knowledge of their disconnections and miscommunications related to projections and idealizations across differences. Making a commitment means considering more than the romance and the immediate good time; it means considering and experiencing the daily interactions that make hidden differences visible. And it means integrating long-term goals and visions in ways that make previously inconsequential differences suddenly relevant and important. Making a commitment is frequently accompanied by a change in circumstances: a move, a job/career change, or a change in living circumstances (e.g., living apart vs. living together). These circumstantial changes may emphasize relational dynamics that were less obvious in the more distant or less dependent circumstances of courtship. For example, Pat and Aki's relationship illustrates the difficulties of out-of-context interpretations of the cross-cultural "other." In his home country, Aki was very much in charge, but in the host culture he was dependent—not a quality that most women are socialized to view as attractive in men. In contrast, Pat, an otherwise very independent woman, was dependent on Aki when she was in his country. Mohamed and Kytrina's job offers in different cities forced them to actively consider how they would integrate their lives, making salient their values and views of family and career, gender and religion. Nancy and Francis began having greater difficulty with their class differences when they began living together, sharing space and resources, as a result of their decision to make a commitment to each other.

McGoldrick (1982) noted a dynamic that plays into cross-cultural relationships and the decision to make a commitment in heterosexual relationships:

> Couples who choose to marry are usually seeking a rebalance of the characteristics of their own ethnic background. They are moving away from some values as well as towards others. As with all systems, the positive feelings can, under stress, become negative. The extended families may stereotype the new spouse negatively—often a self-protective maneuver—reassuring themselves of their superiority, when they feel under threat. During courtship, a person may be attracted precisely to the fiancé's difference, but when entrenched in a marital relationship the same qualities often become the rub. (p. 21)

McGoldrick (1982) notes that people are frequently attracted to others who seem to offer something they lack or something they want. For example, the attraction to a partner from a different race or culture may reflect an attraction to their partner's valuation of family intimacy and connection. The family model of their own family of origin may not accommodate their partner (as in the corporation model) or the connections are not as deep, extensive, or unconditional—sort of a distant franchise. A white woman, Kylie, reported that she and her other two siblings had all partnered with people racially and culturally different from themselves: Kylie married an Alaska Native man, her older brother partnered with a Vietnamese woman who had emigrated at a young age, and her younger brother married an African American man. When asked to offer some ideas for this consistency in her family, she suggested that she and her siblings were neither very close nor attached to each other or to other family members, but that all of them wanted this intimacy. They found it with people who came from cultures that were more collective, family oriented, and intimate. Their partners' families "took them in" and provided the family intimacy and cultural connections that they craved.

Although the desired characteristic may be clearly seen, what is frequently not clearly visible are the numerous other characteristics, values, and experiences associated with that desired characteristic. Difficulties may arise not only because these associated characteristics may not be similarly desired, but also because they are simply not recognized or anticipated; they do not meet expectations. Sometimes these expectations have to do with what people do in exchange for someone who loves them. Often the actions and words that convey love are not understood in intercultural relationships. Aki's focus on work and achievement felt to Pat like a rejection, but to Aki it is a culturally and gender congruent way of expressing his love and care. In these cases, therapists can create "cultural translations" that help the partners express their intentions and identify disconnections between intentions and interpretation.

Class differences, which interact both between and within cultures, also create conflicts due to different expectations. They can be correlated with whether or not, as well as when, a person operates from an individualistic versus a collectivistic worldview (Singelis, 1994). Thus, although women in this (U.S.) culture may be thought to operate more collectively than men, the reality of that assumption depends on class origins and current status. Relative to other cultural groups, women from European backgrounds are thought to be more individualistic than women from other cultural groups. However, that assumption may prove incorrect in individual cases. Marian, for example, originally from Canada, and Jasmine, originally from Afghanistan by way of England and now living in the United States, found that some of the tensions in their relationship came from Jasmine's "selfishness" (i.e., individualism):

> Jasmine came from a professional family, had obtained a professional degree in the United States, and made more money than Marian. Although Jasmine would buy Marian luxury gifts on occasion, she insisted that they keep their money separate. Marian came from a working-class family in which multiple generations lived within the same household and pooled resources to benefit the well-being of all. Together for 5 years, Jasmine and Marian have talked of buying a house together. Jasmine felt that they should contribute equally to the

significant down payment needed, in spite of their different resources and incomes. Marian questioned whether or not this was reasonable and felt that if Jasmine really loved her, she would not insist on the 50/50 share of financial responsibility.

Although Jasmine, from Afghani culture, may be assumed to be more collectively oriented, and Marian, from Canada, to be more individualistically inclined, their cultural worldviews were turned around by their class experiences and backgrounds. Marian and Jasmine had to sort out their expectations, cultural stereotypes, internalized beliefs about gender socialization, and class differences to determine if their relationship would last and how they should move forward with the dilemma of how to buy a suitable house. Both Jasmine and Marian needed to become aware that their expectations about how money and resources were shared were not "normal" or universal but were, instead, connected to their particular backgrounds and circumstances. Their therapist helped Jasmine and Marian recognize that Jasmine's socialization in her family of origin had contributed to an expectation that her partner would take care of her emotionally and financially. This expectation contributed to Jasmine's feeling that Marian needed to contribute 50% so that she would feel cared for. But Jasmine had not explored how this formula was evolved for a patriarchal society in which men had more income-earning power and a big part of their role was one of provider. Marian was emotionally attentive and showed her care for Jasmine in multiple ways, but it would take her a long time to be able to save her 50% of the down payment for the type of house Jasmine would be comfortable and proud to own.

Family Matters

Making a commitment to a long-term relationship is not a decision done in a vacuum, affecting only the two people in the couple. Particularly in couples connecting across differences and for lesbian couples, families' values and their acceptance or rejection are particularly relevant. Definitions of family are culturally based. Culture affects who is considered family, how resources are shared, what obligations take priority based upon relationships, and what sacrifices are made. Same-sex couples and interracial, intercultural couples face additional challenges when they are required to begin their own families without the support of their families of origin.

Root (2001) outlines how families define and operate in a manner that is similar to business models as a result of culture and class origins. Some families operate as clans. When two people make a commitment to each other, the clans merge and resources are merged, to some degree, if someone is in need. These families usually come from recent tribal or clan-based communities. A second type of family operates as a franchise. These families usually have more of a European base, and if not, are a bit more detached from their culture-of-origin values and definitions of family. The franchise families keep some connection with their sons and daughters, but see them as a related but separate enterprise. The last type of family is one that recognizes only the partner of their son or daughter. The family life of the couple must garner the approval of the persons running this corporation. Thus, when the new partner is acquired, little is known about his or her family members other than if they have the right pedigree or if they would be a hindrance to the reputation of this family "corporation." The new partner must switch allegiance from his or her family of origin to the family of his or her partner.

The implications of Root's (2001) theory for intercultural and interracial relationships, whether involving same- or different-sex partnerships, are tremendous. If heterosexuality or sameness of culture, race, or class is required, partnerships that do not meet this requirement will not be recognized to varying degrees. The clan/merger family will recognize the couple but regard their son or daughter as the "black sheep" of the flock as justification for distancing them. Sarah's family operates as a clan: They expected to merge resources with Sarah and Robert, such as loaning money for his MBA or providing housing or child care; however, they resisted socially "merging" with Robert's family because of his race. The franchise family requires the couple to start a separate enterprise of a very different nature, which should not reflect on the family of origin: The couple may or may not be recognized, although frequently the inclusion of children (through birth or adoption) brings franchise recognition. Robert's family may be a franchise family, or alternatively a clan family, whose distance was also related to Sarah's race and class. The corporation family will not recognize the couple and may disown their son or daughter because the partner does not have the appropriate pedigree:

> Raj, a South Asian American man, and his white American girlfriend, Kim, had been in a relationship for 5 years. Although Raj was a professional, he lived at home, which Kim understood was not odd from his culture's perspective. What had become a point of contention as Kim's safe childbearing years were coming to an end was that Raj could not or would not make a further commitment to her because his mother did not want him to marry her. Kim was willing to learn to cook Indian food and had made enthusiastic attempts to learn about his culture. What she found difficult to understand was Raj's mother's shift in treatment from friendliness to rudeness. Originally, Kim was Raj's sister's friend and was well liked by the family; Raj's mother started treating her rudely only when her son started dating Kim. For

example, whereas she used to speak directly to Kim, now she only speaks to her through a third party, even in her presence.

The therapist's work was to help this couple define their limits and priorities in light of the cultural differences, Raj's closeness to his family, and Raj's inability to defy his mother's wishes, despite professing that he wanted to be married to Kim. The therapist encouraged them to explore ways he could address his mother's rudeness with her differently, and if he could not address it and her behavior continued as it had for years, what Kim wished to do. In therapy, Raj expressed his mother's fears that the children would not be "Indian enough" and that Kim was "beneath the family" in terms of education, job, and class origins. Raj also expressed his inability to go against his mother, given these fears, and his hope that she would eventually come around to accept Kim. Kim came to understand that Raj would not marry her against his mother's wishes; she then had to determine how long she could and would wait. Kim decided to end the relationship with Raj.

Culture is often highlighted with some interface with class in compromises about commitment and intimacy that couples make in response to families of origin's expectations and cultural definitions of family. These compromises may be related to sharing resources, giving up certain goals, and/or suppressing individualistic needs for the good of the collective:

> Linda, a Filipina now residing in the United States, taught at a private school. Her partner, Glynis, was a white woman from a middle-class family who worked as a contractor. Together for 7 years, Glynis still did not understand why Linda would sacrifice buying things she wanted or needed for herself to send money home to her sister and parents, who lived together in one of the provinces outlying Manila. Although she did not understand, Glynis had mostly resigned herself to the fact that Linda sent all her spare money to her relatives. However, at points in time, Linda's choice bothered Glynis, who paid for much of their recreational endeavors. Occasionally Glynis complained. Linda would respond that Glynis need not spend her money, because they could find things to do that did not cost anything. Recently, Glynis had started to insist that Linda needed to let her family fend for itself. Linda tried to explain that "out of sight was not out of mind" and that she must continue to help them to be a good daughter and be true to herself.

The attractive quality of caring, integrity, and dedication that Glynis loved in Linda was now part of the difficulty in their relationship because of their different cultural understandings of the meaning of family. Although Glynis felt that Linda had a choice about where to spend her money, Linda did not experience a choice, because spending her money on herself or on Glynis, rather than on her family-of-origin, would change her basic self-understanding and cost her, her own self-respect.

Although this chapter focuses primarily on courtship and the decision to commit, interracial, intercultural, and interclass couples continue to face challenges related to their differences throughout the development of their relationship. As couples make longer-term commitments to each other, they also need to negotiate the different meanings of different types of rites of passage and family transitions. Cultural differences may arise particularly around major family transitions, such as births, marriages, and death. Having children frequently creates major changes (beyond those common to all new parents) in meanings and negotiations of racial, cultural, and class differences, particularly as the partners consider what cultural legacies they would like to pass on to their children and how to prepare their children for potential discrimination. The attitudes of parents and other family members may also change with the birth of children. Cultural differences affect other life transitions as well. For example, culture guides the behaviors around death and grieving, including ways to cope with loss, appropriate length of grieving, and the roles that different people should play. Religion and religious culture may also play a significant part in these rituals:

> Esmerelda, a Catholic Latina, had always assumed that she would be cremated, as her mother and father had been. Now in her 60s, she and her Jewish American partner of 20 years, Phyllis, were making their wills. Phyllis said that she could honor just about anything Esmerelda wanted, but she did not think she could cremate her. She told her that cremation made her think of relatives burning in the concentration camps, and that this association is part of why Jews do not like to be cremated. Throughout their relationship, Esmerelda and Phyllis have honored each other's religious traditions, though neither of them would say they are very religious. But at this point in time, talking about death, they found it hard to separate culture and religion.

Legal, social, and institutional meanings of commitment and family are also particularly relevant to interracial, intercultural, and lesbian relationships. Interracial and intercultural couples still need to deal with stares, comments, and other social stigma, although there are no longer legal restrictions on their ability to marry and to therefore access the legal privileges and benefits of that institution. There are, however, legal restrictions on the relational commitments of lesbian couples. Esmerelda and Phyllis will have to be careful about creating explicit legal documents to ensure that they will each have a say in what actually does happen upon their deaths (unless they live in Massachusetts and have chosen to marry). And, given the recent (2004) bills passed in some states, even the creation of such legal documents and contracts between them may be challengeable by members of their biological families. Therapy with interracial, intercultural, and lesbian couples must address not only the internal meanings within the couple and their families, but also the social and legal discriminations that affect their relationships.

Helping Couples Reflect:
Recommendations for Therapists

As illustrated above, many different types of cultural differences can be sources of tension. The successful negotiation of these differences requires good communication. But communication itself may be one of the major cultural differences. For example, one partner may feel that hinting is the appropriate way to intimate a preference for something, whereas the other partner may experience hinting as very indirect and frustrating—especially when conflicts arise because he or she did not hear the hints as forms of request or information about needs. In some cultures (particularly more collective cultures), people are expected to carefully observe and perceive others' needs without request. This form of "high-context communication" requires sensitivity to the implicit rules of a relationship, the implications within a particular situation, and a large amount of knowledge about the people and the interaction. In contrast, "low-context communication" requires a direct and explicit message (see review in Sue & Sue, 2002). A person used to low-context communication interacting with a partner used to high-context communication may feel frustrated at the apparent expectation that he or she should be able to "mind read" what the partner wants, given the implicit information. At the same time, the partner that is used to high-context communication may feel that his or her partner is not attending to his or her needs, is insensitive, or is uncaring about what he or she is "saying." The therapist can help make explicit the implicit messages within high-context communication as well as also help the couple see the different cultural backgrounds and communication styles that are contributing to the difficulty in even talking about their differences (Root, in press).

Another cultural disconnection related to the ability to communicate about differences is the use of go-betweens. In many minority cultures it is normative to have close and frequent contact with parents and extended family members, to consult with and defer to parents and elders, even as adults, and to use mediators or go-betweens to discuss difficult topics and maintain harmonious relationships. Often the person chosen to be the mediator has certain skills or status that allow him or her to wield personal power in the role as go-between (Root, in press). However, if one person in the couple is accustomed to using a mediator and the other is not, this too can contribute to increasing difficulties in bridging differences. These dynamics can be further exacerbated by situational acculturation, wherein one person in the partnership operates from one cultural stance in some situations and from another in others. For example, Raj could see how Kim would be frustrated by his mother's rudeness, and he agreed with Kim that it was wrong. The therapist helped him talk about how he had asked his sister to discuss with his mother how hurtful it was to him and to Kim that she treated Kim this way and thus was not supporting Raj. Kim could not understand why, if Raj could see that it was wrong and ask his sister to intervene, he could not confront his mother himself. This type of acculturative code switching (applying one understanding or behavioral rule in one situation or with one person and another understanding or behavioral rule in a different situation or with a different person) can confuse a partner. It is the therapist's job to be able to point out, and at times decode, this code switching (Root, in press). However, in family therapy, therapists themselves frequently misinterpret normative cultural practices of family closeness and informal mediation as enmeshment and triangulation. The therapist must have insider knowledge of the cultures in order to avoid pathologizing normative relationships in context (Falicov & Brudner-White, 1983). Knowing what forms culturally functional "triangles" helps the therapist in this role.

Interracial and intercultural couples may also have difficulty in coming to therapy, recognizing when therapy maybe helpful, or agreeing about what is helpful in therapy. The ways in which people ask for and give help may have significant cultural and gender differences based upon socialization. One person's form of help may seem intrusive and too effusive. Another person may give help by doing rather than talking. Therapists working with interracial and intercultural couples need to be aware that the differences that brought the partners to therapy will also affect how they view the therapy itself.

When things go awry in an intercultural, interracial, or interclass relationship, it is often for the same reasons that they go awry in other couples' relationships. Sternberg (1998) discusses how seemingly different people *can* make a relationship last forever, whereas others who seem so well matched will dissolve it after many years and to many people's dismay. He suggests that one of the explanations for such dissolution is that the story that brought the two people together ultimately changes for one or both partners, whereupon they begin to forge different journeys rather than traveling together. Couples having difficulty and contemplating separation may find it helpful to identify the story that bonded them and the changes in their lives that have shifted the story. The particular challenge with interracial, intercultural, or interclass couples is to figure out the compounding tensions that occur at the intersections of gender, race, class, culture, and sexual orientation. Although it is complex, it is real life.

Usually, a couple's contemporary story is different from the original story, and that difference helps identify the sources of tension arising from disappointments and hurts. Disappointments may arise from the decay of exoticness or other stereotype-based projections, non-negotiable value differences, misinterpretations of love and commitment, or differences in how to negotiate new challenges related to family and individual developmental transitions. Clarifying these issues requires patience and understanding of why people came together and if they are still on the same journey. If not, can they negotiate a new journey? Sometimes, as was the case with Mohamed and Kytrina and Raj and Kim, this is not possible, because it becomes clear relatively quickly that the initial story was vastly incomplete or that the future story of each partner cannot be integrated with that of the other. In some cases, it is a longer process to explore the current story, locate where it diverged from the original story, and evaluate whether a new story can be created. Therapy can be helpful here, because the differences in the beginning story versus the current story may be much more obvious from the outside, as in the example of Pat and Aki. Therapy helped Pat and Aki identify these differences and then attempt to weave together their current stories so that they became collaborative authors again. Pat and Aki worked steadily over a year to identify their expectations of each other. The therapist helped them sort out which issues were related to culture, class, or gender as well as their various intersections; this clarification enabled them to consider what they would want to, or were able to, change in the ways in which their backgrounds affected their current thoughts, feelings, and behaviors toward each other. Pat and Aki each had rigidities in their relationship interactions that resulted in the partner feeling harshly judged. They each also had a self-centeredness that was difficult to transcend. Interestingly, the self-centeredness in Pat's case originated clearly in white privilege, language privilege, and an oppressive attitude of American superiority over her husband. In contrast, Aki's self-centeredness seemed to stem from the interaction of his culture-of-origin and gender, whereby he was privileged as the oldest male with the expectation that he would ultimately have the authority in the relationship. From their new understandings of each other, Pat and Aki each made significant attempts to alter behavior. However, this was difficult work, and their rigid judgments combined with their self-centeredness to make it difficult to empathize and stop criticizing each other. The criticism eventually eroded their openness to each other, which subsequently eroded their intimacy with one another, and they separated.

Some partners may find that they *can* create a contemporary collaborative story. In these cases, partners frequently find that seeing how perceived "individual" differences are actually related to racial, cultural, and class backgrounds helps them understand how their stories began to disconnect, as well as the rich opportunities offered by developing a collaborative story that integrates these differences. Robert and Sarah had an initial story that located the problematic aspects of their differences within their families. Creating a new story was a long process that included recognizing how these differences were also within them; exploring the racial, cultural, and class experiences that were the contexts for developing these differences; and actively working to understand how these different experiences had led to different meanings and interpretations of small, everyday occurrences that, in turn, built into big emotional conflicts. To help Robert and Sarah, the therapist had to understand both African American and Vietnamese American cultures and families; how race was experienced and framed differently by educated African Americans and by refugee Vietnamese within the racialized Asian American group; and how class (not just economic resources and education) had shaped Robert's and Sarah's social experiences. The therapist also had to understand the dynamics between African Americans and Asian/Vietnamese Americans, and the historical contexts that had led to the current dynamics. With this help, Robert and Sarah were able to explore the social influences on their worldviews, better see how each partner's view was developed, and ultimately focus on how their different perspectives could be used to bring different skills that would contribute to meeting their shared goals (raising a child, supporting Robert's career goals, developing closeness with their extended families).

In this chapter we have provided a beginning glimpse of the juxtapositions of differences in class, race, culture, and religion as they affect intimate relationships, both heterosexual and lesbian. In order to effectively understand interracial, intercultural, or interclass couples, the very real complex social contexts of race, culture, and class must be understood, in and of themselves, and in relation to each other and to gender and sexual orientation, as well as other variables. To add to this grounded complexity, we attempted to provide glimpses of how values, worldviews, and coping styles of individuals within couples are the daily real-life dimensions that fuel relational differences; social contexts are not abstractions within people, but are lived through these seemingly small differences in thinking, feeling, and relationship styles. With flexibility in coping and communication style, a grounded sense of the reality of possible tensions that cultural, class, gender, and religious values introduce, and a firm sense of commitment, people can transcend these formidable differences. This transcension may mean that people learn to cope with ongoing tensions in a way that provides an opportunity for mutual personal growth. Love can be transformative.

References

Clunis, M., & Green, D. (1988). *Lesbian couples.* Seattle, WA: Seal Press.

Cose, E. (1993). *Rage of the privileged class.* New York: HarperPerennial.

Essed, P. (1990). *Everyday racism: Reports from women of two cultures.* Claremont, CA: Hunter House.

Falicov, C. J., & Brudner-White, L. (1983). The shifting family triangle: The issue of cultural and contextual relativity. In J. C. Hanse & C. J. Falicov (Eds.), *Cultural perspectives in family therapy* (pp. 51–67). Rockville, MD: Aspen.

Gordon, L. R. (1997). Race, sex, and matrices of desire in an antiblack world: An essay in phenomenology and social role. In N. Zack (Ed.), *Race/sex: Their sameness, difference, and interplay* (pp. 119–132). New York: Routledge.

Lee, J. (1996). Why Suzie Wong is not a lesbian: Asian and Asian American lesbian and bisexual women and femme/butch/gender identities. In B. Beemyn & M. Eliason (Eds.), *Queer studies: A lesbian, gay, bisexual, and transgender anthology* (pp. 115–131). New York: New York University Press.

McGoldrick, M. (1982). Ethnicity and family therapy: An overview. In M. McGoldrick, J. K. Pearce, & J. Giordano (Eds.), *Ethnicity and family therapy* (pp. 3–30). New York: Guilford Press.

Merton, R. (1941). Intermarriage and the social structure: Fact and theory. *Psychiatry, 4,* 361–374.

Root, M. P. P. (Ed.). (1992). *Racially mixed people in America.* Newbury Park, CA: Sage.

Root, M. P. P. (1998). Experiences and processes affecting racial identity development: Preliminary results from the biracial sibling project. *Cultural Diversity and Mental Health, 4,* 237–247.

Root, M. P. P. (2001). *Love's revolution: Interracial marriage.* Philadelphia: Temple University Press.

Root, M. P. P. (2005). Filipino families. In M. McGoldrick, J. Giordano, & N. Garcia-Preto (Eds.), *Ethnicity and family therapy* (3rd ed., pp. 319–331). New York: Guilford Press.

Root, M. P. P., & Kelley, M. (Eds.). (2003). *Multiracial child resource book: Living complex identities.* Seattle, WA: Mavin Foundation.

Singelis, T. M. (1994). The Measurement of independent and interdependent self-construals. *Personality and Social Psychology Bulletin, 20*(5), 580–591.

Sternberg, R. J. (1998). *Love is a story: A new theory of relationships.* New York: Oxford University Press.

Sue, D. W., & Sue, D. (2002). *Counseling the culturally diverse: Theory and practice* (4th ed.). New York: Wiley.

Tasker, F. L., & Golombok, S. (1997). *Growing up in a lesbian family: Effects on child development.* New York: Guilford Press.

Thai, H. C. (2002). Clashing dreams: Highly educated overseas brides and low-wage U.S. husbands. In B. Ehrenreich & A. R. Hochschild (Eds.), *Global women: Nannies, maids, and sexworkers in the new economy* (pp. 230–253). New York: Metropolitan Books.

Wehrly, B. (1996). *Counseling interracial individuals and families.* Alexandria, VA: American Counseling Association.

Zack, N. (Ed.). (1995). *American mixed race.* Lanham, MD: Rowman & Littlefield.

CHAPTER 6

Love in (at Least) Two Cultures
DILEMMAS OF INTIMACY, GENDER, AND GENERATION IN PRACTICE WITH IMMIGRANT FAMILIES

Ester R. Shapiro
Eileen Santa

Transplanting the Territory of Love: A Clinical Example

Gregorio and Carolina Vargas[1] came to their community health center because their 10-year-old son, Francisco (Frankie), was having difficulty concentrating in school, and his teacher insisted that he be evaluated. Carolina came in with Frankie and his baby sister, Sylvia, for the first session; Gregorio worked long hours as a janitor and feared that if he asked for a change in schedule, he might lose his job. Carolina and Frankie agreed that he had experienced long-standing difficulties in school, which had been evident to Carolina since he started preschool, but had intensified after their recent immigration to the United States from Colombia. Frankie presented as a sensitive, affectionate boy who felt deeply connected to his mother's loneliness and worry, longed for time and attention with his distant, preoccupied father, and missed the warmth of his grandparents and extended family. When Gregorio attended a family session, it was clear that he and Carolina were completely at odds in their understanding of Frankie's problems. Gregorio believed that his son was spoiled by his mother and simply did not work hard enough at his schooling or in his responsibilities at home. In a brief intervention oriented toward cultural and developmental systems, Carolina and Frankie were seen in 12 individual and family sessions designed to help them voice their shared immigrant experience of loss, while also redirecting their relationship from mutual sensitivity to loss toward a reconstruction of culturally meaningful, practical resources and shared understandings supporting their transplanted development. Frankie used the therapist's support of his mother, as well as his own opportunity to share worries about his mother and his thwarted needs for his father's affection, to turn his attention toward schooling and his peers. His therapist connected Frankie with a Latino community mentor who encouraged his efforts in school while engaging father and son together in community athletics, thereby enlarging their opportunities for intimacy. Sessions with Carolina explored her struggle with depression, triggered by their economic difficulties, family isolation, and marital problems, as well as by her fears that Frankie's school difficulties might prevent him from achieving academic success in this country. Although she shared Frankie's dream of returning home, she knew that Colombia's economic instability and chronic violence made this impossible, and shorter visits were unaffordable. Carolina had always found Gregorio to be an impatient, authoritarian father and a distant husband, but her close relationships to her parents and rich extended family network had offered ample satisfaction of her intimacy needs. She loved her children but feared she would be unable to guide them competently through the hazards of schooling and growing up in a foreign society. The therapy helped Carolina articulate her goals as a wife and mother in her new U.S. context, identify useful community resources, and advocate for herself and her child with her husband and with Frankie's teacher. Carolina joined a community center's support group for recent Latina immigrants. At the end of this brief therapy, both mother and son experienced decreased depression, increased coping competence, and a redefinition of their mother–son intimacy that preserved their closeness while enhancing the ways in which their relationship supported individual and family development in the context of their new cultural circumstances.

Immigration and Developmental Transitions: Cultural and Ecological Resources That Promote Resilience for Immigrant Women

The Vargas family's brief therapy illustrates how we work with immigrant women and their families using a culturally based, resilience-building ecological model to support them in achieving their own goals for personal and family development. The cultural and developmental systems approach we present in this chapter highlights the ways in which intergenerational family life cycle transitions offer opportunities to support immigrant women. We draw on ecological and multisystemic approaches to assessment and intervention developed by women of color to help evaluate intersections of structural social and cultural characteristics as they impact life experience and dilemmas of intimate life (Boyd-Franklin, 2003; Comas-Díaz & Greene, 1994; Espin, 1997, 1999; Falicov, 1997; Wyche, 2001).

Immigrant women in the United States arrive from all over the world and for a variety of reasons.[2] Some come to attend graduate school, whereas others come to save their family from starvation. Some come under circumstances of choice, some are coerced, some come with partners, others are alone; some are seeking economic opportunity, whereas others are fleeing violent conflict; some are accompanied by their children, whereas others leave their children in the care of others (usually family members). These immigrant women often experience extraordinary new freedom from the burden of poverty or gender oppression, while simultaneously experiencing overwhelming longings for their lost worlds of intimately rooted cultural connections. The conditions of immigration include the presence or absence of material resources; educational opportunities; kinship networks and close-knit ethnic enclaves. The polarization of race that characterizes U.S. society offers both stressors *and* resources to immigrant women. These stressors and resources will be interpreted uniquely by each woman, in light of her subjective experience of these intersecting forces. These intersecting forces include her movements through different settings of home, work, school, and neighborhood; her dealings with diverse groups within the United States; and her freedom of movement across settings and borderlands—those contexts within which she engages, responds to, and transforms her sense of self within worlds.

Work with the Vargas family began with a respectful family-based inquiry exploring each member's culturally based understanding of how gender and generation positioned their mutual obligations in giving and receiving love. Therapists working within U.S.-based assumptions about family relationships might have focused on Gregorio and Carolina's conflicts over Frankie's learning difficulties, Gregorio's authoritarian distance within both his marital and paternal relationships, and/or Frankie's subsequent burden of responsibility for his mother's emotional well-being. Demonstrating a lack of cultural awareness by insisting that Gregorio Vargas attend family therapy sessions might have resulted in his temporarily yielding greater authority to his wife and/or softening his harsh expectations of his son. We believe that therapy emphasizing values contradicting his paternal authority would have run a significant risk of losing the family while intensifying Gregorio's isolation, vulnerability, and need to coercively control his family. This need to control his family most likely counters other areas involving lost affirmation and control. We understood the Vargas family as confronting dilemmas of poverty, language learning, social isolation, and cultural dislocation. These dilemmas are shared with many immigrant families. As therapists, we appreciated the Vargas family's struggle to meet the challenges of family development under new social rules regarding gender and generation. Working within the family's own account of their presenting problems and practical goals, therapy leveraged the close, loving relationship between mother and son as a generative resource that could help both expand their circle of love within broader ecologies of family, school, and community. Although many Latinas and other immigrant women reject a U.S. feminist emphasis on women's individual rights, they become more motivated to take care of themselves once they can see how doing so will help them better care for others (Shapiro, 2000).

This chapter focuses on how the discontinuities in family life cycles that may be created by immigration can disrupt intimacies and connections, yet can also open new opportunities for growth and connection. A cultural and developmental systems approach can help immigrant women to maximize these new opportunities. This integrative ecological approach views gendered development as emerging from negotiated, interdependent adaptations to individual, intergenerational, organizational, and cultural stressors and resources as families face and solve problems of everyday life (*lo cotidiano*) in their particular cultural locations. The intervention style as well as its content must respect individual and family differences, the realistic circumstances, and the uniqueness of each immigration journey. Without a respectful, culturally based approach that nurtures family strengths and helps members articulate and meet their own goals for interdependent development, immigration dilemmas of love and loss, such as those experienced by the Vargas family, might be intensified, rather than alleviated, by therapy.

The Impact of Our Own Migration Experiences on Our Practice Models

We write this chapter in cultural and intergenerational harmony and counterpoint, as teacher and student, colleagues and friends, as Latinas sharing cultural and ecological developmental frameworks for clinical practice with immigrant women, yet in very different places in our journeys of growth within families and nations of origin. I (Ester Shapiro) learned from personal dilemmas of love across cultures in my own Cuban Eastern-European Jewish family. Forty-four years of immigrant life and thirty years in practice has helped me transform my clinical practice by using resilience-building health-promotion models that mobilize immigrant women's considerable strengths as foundations for family and community transformation. I

(Eileen Santa), offer insights and questions from my cultural crossings as a Puerto Rican clinical psychologist in training who has lived on both the island and the mainland, experiencing different definitions of relationships across ethnicity, language, race, and nation and in their expressions within worlds of professional practice. We both share a commitment to understanding immigrant women in family and sociocultural contexts through a stance of appreciative inquiry that helps us listen for the cultural creativity and unique burdens immigrant women bring to the challenging work of transplanting intergenerational relationships across cultures.

To understand how immigrant women negotiate love, intimacy, and generativity within and across cultures, we must come prepared to carefully interrogate our own culturally based assumptions. The process of self-questioning requires an ecological and relational definition of culture that recognizes the importance of our disciplinary training, our practice contexts, and our culturally based, gendered life experiences. Later in this chapter, readers will meet Nancy Haddad, whom I (Shapiro) first saw in a family bereavement consultation as a guilt-stricken college student whose younger brother was killed by a hit-and-run driver while she was babysitting. Five years later, Nancy sought individual therapy to help her make a decision about marriage; her Armenian family's culturally based obligations to live with her mother had intensified with her brother's death, and she was facing a crossroad. As a therapist trained in "individuation," a feminist encouraged to assert my individual rights, and an immigrant daughter who had struggled to establish my rights to independence, I indignantly responded that Nancy was entitled to move forward into her own married life. Nancy respectfully insisted that her obligations to her mother remained a priority in her own decisions, reminding me of the need to more carefully monitor my culturally based clinical assumptions and their roots within my life experience. Person-centered, collaborative approaches to therapy as mutual dialogue help us honor the profoundly transformative experience of learning from difference, even when our patients challenge cherished personal or professional assumptions (Shapiro, in press).

As part of our family-based inquiry, we ask immigrant women and their families to tell us what they desire in their loving relationships, how they view their own needs for sexuality, intimacy, and affection, how they hope to replenish their nurturance and generosity, and how they cope with their frustrations, losses, and thwarted hopes. As we listen and learn, we carefully monitor our own personal, professional, and political history, subjectivity, and potential biases emerging from professional training or U.S.-based feminist beliefs that emphasize individualism and celebrate independence. Our conversations concerning love across cultures are also framed by the culture of the U.S. health and mental health systems, which emphasizes the pathologies of love for which we offer our costly cures. The

case examples offered in this chapter highlight brief therapies and emphasize the clinical relationship as a multisystemic ecological consultation,
designed to make family life cycle transitions across cultures into opportunities for growth and change.

Love, Loss, and Growth in Translation: Overview of a Cultural and Developmental Systems Approach to Integrative Practice

Whereas our ability to form loving relationships is fundamental to our
humanness, our relatedness emerges within a very particular cultural chore-
ography of gendered caretaking as we solve fundamental problems of
growth and change, surviving and thriving, in everyday life. When we
speak of love, we do so within the assumptions of our culture, community,
current relationships, and lived experience. In most cultures, gender is a
powerful factor that organizes roles, relationships, and resources. Regardless of a society's location in individualistic or collectivistic orientations,
women bear a greater responsibility for the care of those who have fewer
resources throughout the life cycle. What happens to love for immigrant
women when economic hardships, educational opportunities, or violent
conflicts alter the words, relationships, meanings, and settings for giving
and receiving love? The integrative framework for assessment of, and intervention with, immigrant women offered by a cultural and developmental
systems approach leverages strengths and resources to help immigrant
women identify their dilemmas of attachment and identity between cultures, and to meet their own goals for both cultural continuity and innovation. We focus on how immigrant women solve problems of everyday life
through culturally meaningful explorations of change and continuity in self
within relationships.

We use integrative concepts to argue for a goal-oriented reflective
practice with immigrant women that emphasizes the creative processes and
potential burdens of carrying primary responsibility for making loved ones
feel "at home" in unfamiliar spaces. This approach appreciates the complexity, specificity, and creativity of life journeys across diverse cultures,
contextualizing a previous generation of clinical literature on immigration
that overemphasizes separation, loss, and grief (Perez-Foster, 2001). This
approach helps us explore how new forms of loving emerge through conflicts, contradictions, and creative confrontations encountered by immigrant women as they strive to reconcile the U.S. emphasis on individualism
and agency with their own ethnic cultural backgrounds, which emphasize
harmonious interdependence.

Construction of a collaborative therapeutic relationship that is responsive to immigrant women's culturally based understanding of suffering, thriving, and healing, and that is accountable to their own goals for treatments, is foundational to promoting resilience in clinical practice. Therapy is designed as a developmental consultation about resources and barriers in multiple systems that promote or impede immigrant women's attempts at caring for their loved ones and themselves. This consultation unfolds through dialogue that explores culturally based assumptions and goals for interdependent development (Boyd-Franklin, 2003; Falicov, 1998). Our approach draws broadly from (1) relevant research literatures studying the role of cultural complexity and "selective biculturalism" in fostering positive coping with the stresses of acculturation and racism (Leadbetter & Way, 1996; Phinney, Horenczyk, Liebkind, & Vedder, 2001); (2) research on developmental pathways that result in positive or symptomatic adaptive outcomes throughout the lifespan, and research that emphasizes resilience in coping with adversities such as death, divorce, poverty, exposure to racism, or community violence (Luthar, 2003; Masten, 2001; Sandler, 2001); and (3) clinical intervention that approaches that emphasize positive psychology and health promotion using ecological, person-centered approaches (Bohart & Tallman, 1999; Brown & Ballou, 2002; Hubble, Duncan, & Miller, 1999). Lastly, our approach recognizes the scientifically demonstrated power of the sacred healing arts (Koenig, McCullough, & Larson, 2001) and includes a cultural and spiritual inquiry as part of a basic assessment.

Speaking of Love in Translation: Learning to Listen against the Grain of Cultural Assumptions

Our customary tools for theory and practice strive for scientific objectivity and speak an individualistic, medical language of personal diagnosis and private experience of distress. Yet the sciences of health promotion and resilience in response to adversity teach us that love given and received within culturally based, spiritually informed frameworks for understanding life's value and meaning offers our most powerful protection, promoting health and well-being throughout our lives. An ecological, multisystemic approach to therapy with immigrant women requires a practical poetics of listening (Katz & Shotter, 2004), in which women's everyday lives, with their often mundane tasks of daily survival, challenge us to perceive the embodiments of lived experience in novel, unexpected ways. Therapists can be most helpful by working within clients' cultural frameworks and traditions for changing gender roles in multiple spheres, rather than imposing U.S. cultural expectations.

Misrek was a 28-year-old Ethiopian Orthodox immigrant who worked as a secretary in a family-owned business. She was referred by her internist for a behavioral medicine consultation because she suffered from frequent headaches that did not respond to medication. These headaches were making it increasingly difficult for her to work or leave the house. Misrek had immigrated at age 16 with her parents and her married older brother, fleeing the war with Eritrea and the subsequent economic and political instability. Misrek graduated from a local high school and completed an associate's degree under the watchful eye of her parents and brother's family, who discouraged her from social contacts with anyone outside their small, close-knit Ethiopian Orthodox community. The family had been especially concerned when Misrek had developed a friendship with an African American neighbor who attended their church, because they feared this relationship would open the door toward her assimilation into a U.S. black community. Misrek's therapist, a white male who was sensitive to her cultural expectations of modesty in relationships between men and women, conducted a brief therapy focusing on Misrek's understanding of her headaches as they emerged within her resentment of her family's control and mandated isolation. Misrek acknowledged that the headaches prevented her from confronting her parents about her desire for experiencing a wider world. She added that she felt trapped in the growing certainty that she would never marry and have a family of her own. Working within the referring context of brief behavioral medicine, her therapist helped Misrek learn to identify signs of an incipient headache and use self-hypnosis and relaxation techniques, likening them to meditation and prayer. At the same time, he helped her identify culturally sanctioned allies who could assist her in negotiating an expansion of her social world with her parents. Misrek decided to consult their priest, who supported her participation in church activities. Misrek also decided to return to school, because furthering her education was a goal her parents endorsed that would also expand her social life, excuse her from babysitting duties, and open a pathway toward greater employability outside the family business.

As Misrek traced the story of her headaches with her therapist, she discovered how her embodied pain resulted from family conflicts she dared not confront. Yet Misrek could not have been helped by a therapy that took a U.S.-based position concerning her right to live her own life without the constraints of her family obligations.

When we speak of love's dilemmas with women from diverse national, cultural, religious, and racial backgrounds, we use a multidimensional assessment of gender, politics, and culture while keeping our inquiry anchored to clients' representations of their lived experiences and problems in everyday life. We are forced to respectfully recognize the limitations of our academic education and the need for a framework that places us in the position of world travelers and lifelong learners. Prepared to listen deeply with a curious mind and a compassionate heart, we open up new channels for learning from others, in which points of difference and of connection harmonize, educate, and heal us. The Gurung communities of the Himalayas use the word *sae* to describe the territory of the heart/mind, which expands with love, peace, joy, belonging, and honor and contracts or shrivels with worry, grief, rejection, and shame (McHugh, 2001). In this space of shared learning, we expand our understanding of love and intimacy to connect the acts of everyday life survival, the passage of time with its cycle of seasons, and the passage of intergenerational time connecting our ancestral past and our generative future.

The Challenge of Family Life Cycle Transitions for Immigrant Women: Love as a Cultural and Spiritual Resource for Shared Development

The collisions of politics and history with women's lives leave their marks within the family life cycle. Some of these marks include the time of immigration (childhood, adolescence, or adulthood), the leaving behind of children or elders, and the experience of adolescence across cultures. Clinicians can help these women organize their experiences of immigration while weaving losses and discoveries, grief and innovation into the fabric of their family's future. Clinical accounts of immigration have focused on yearning for the lost community and unacknowledged grief (Perez-Foster, 2001). Yet immigration can also feel like a great adventure and an opening of doorways to freedom, as it did for my (Shapiro) two Polish Jewish grandmothers, who discovered in Cuba's rural communities an accepting curiosity about newcomers and were welcomed into a racially tolerant society. Successful immigrants adapt through the arduous work of making the strange familiar. It helps to have an optimistic attitude, an ability to channel loss into positive pathways of aspiration and purpose for one's sacrifices and strivings. It also helps to have obedient children whose future represents both family continuity and family achievement. In some families, negotiation of love and loyalty resonates to past traumatic losses and places a greater burden on intergenerational relationships. For example, my paternal grandmother, Basia (renamed Bertha when she immigrated to Cuba), was 10 years old when her father and brother died in a flood, leaving her the oldest daughter in a family of women with limited means of support at the start of World War I. She grew up to be a revered matriarch who brilliantly outsmarted Cossacks, Nazis, and Communists across languages and continents, yet whose grief enduringly shaped responses to the family's multiple uprootings. Basia had three children and named them variations on her father's name, Nachemie ("consolation" in Hebrew), favoring her youngest while coolly rejecting her oldest daughter, Consuelo ("consolation" in Spanish), whose rebellious adolescence coincided with the family's precarious passage from Poland to rural Cuba one step ahead of the Holocaust (Shapiro, 1999). Nearly a century after her father's death, and a decade after Bertha's, I attended Consuelo's 80th birthday party, where, surrounded by her doting daughter, grandchildren, and great-grandchildren, she spoke of her thwarted longings for her mother's love and her closeness to her own daughter, even as her 56-year-old son lamented how his mother's stressful life resulted in her failure to love him. The intertwining of love and loss across gender and generations strengthened Consuelo's resolve to achieve closeness with her own daughter while creating the context for the distance and loss experienced by her son.

Therapy creates what anthropologists call a space of "liminality" or ritual transformation and transition, in which the rules and constraints of everyday life are suspended and a goal of creating a new, more favorable developmental adaptation takes center stage. A supportive therapeutic relationship can help clients create a new "ecological niche" by exploring new and existing symbolic and material resources for continuity and stability. Within a cultural and developmental systems model of health-promotion practice, interventions using positive material involving relational and meaning-making resources are designed to build resilience. Resilience researchers emphasize the "ordinary magic" (Masten, 2001) of positive processes, such as caretaking stability or loving parents who balance authority with structured expectations, to protect development under circumstances of adversity. In supporting the resilience of immigrant women and families, we must translate the developmental systems identified through research with U.S. families and carefully evaluate the "practical magic" of culturally based protective factors conjured every day by women who strive to solve realistic problems of daily survival while making the strange and unstable feel safe and familiar. For example, immigrant families in clinical settings are often viewed as exercising overly harsh and restrictive parenting or physical punishment. Yet immigrant families' strictness can be better understood as protecting development within cultural definitions of loving parenting that remain adaptive, given new ecological realities of sexual risk and community violence within poor immigrant-receiving communities (Luthar, 2003). An emphasis on "practical magic" (Sandler, 2001; Shapiro, in press) views adaptation to adversity as emerging from the realistic problem solving required for everyday survival within optimal, ordinary, and traumatically stressful environments. This perspective means mobilizing creative, culturally complex coping resources to counter the specific stressors presented by distinctive ecologies of adversity while protecting family continuity, stability, and flexibility.

A supportive therapeutic dialogue helps immigrant women reflect on immigration and its impact on their close relationships and interdependence. Interventions that respect cultural differences and are responsive to age and stage of the family life cycle are designed to promote the capacity for strategic reflection on values and goals. This reflection contributes to the immigrant's ability to rebuild the life routines, meanings, and intimacies that have been disrupted by the timing and circumstances of the relocation. Therapists join immigrant women to help them identify and mobilize the many protective factors in individual experience, family relationships, and social ecologies that can generate "upward spirals" of self-reinforcing nurturing images and positive emotions and competencies, instead of "downward spirals" that amplify violent images, distressing emotions, or destructive coping. This model can help both clinicians and immigrant women make the best possible use of available and new resources to meet the many challenges of love and loss that are inherent in the circumstances and consequences of immigration experiences.

> Clara was referred for evaluation at her elite college's counseling center during her freshman year because her roommate and her faculty advisor were quite concerned about her deep depression and difficulty concentrating on her studies. Clara had emigrated from El Salvador as a 9-year-old to a mixed-race immigrant community outside of Boston, rejoining her parents and two younger siblings (who were born in the United States). Her parents had been forced to flee their rural village because their work as community organizers in land reform had made them the target of death threats. Clara had lived from age 6 with her maternal grandmother, who did not approve of her parents' political activity and never spoke of their lives before their immigration. Grateful for the opportunity to join her parents in the United States, Clara had excelled in school and chose to attend a local university so that she could still return home on weekends.
>
> In the first session, Clara could not bring herself to admit how depressed she felt but talked instead about her homesickness and concern about her family, which made it difficult for her to concentrate on her schoolwork. Her home and family were just a short bus ride away from her college, and the lives of her mostly privileged peers seemed worlds apart. Clara found herself thinking a lot about her mother, who alongside her father worked two cleaning jobs, and she worried that her younger, more rebellious, sister was giving the family more trouble than ever, now that Clara was away at school and unable to help keep an eye on her sister and mediate between her and their anxious parents. Clara understood that her parents were old-fashioned in their expectations for their daughters as compared to their only son, but

Clara's sister deeply resented their brother's freedom to walk around town unsupervised.

The college counseling center's brief therapy model discouraged direct family interventions. Clara's Latina therapist used a multisystemic, ecological, and developmental framework to address Clara's dilemmas of love and family loyalty through both brief individual therapy and family coaching. She helped Clara create a culturally meaningful way of expressing her family loyalty that recognized her relationally based understanding of her own interdependence and helped her expand the space for concentrating on her transition into college while remaining a participant in her immigrant family's development. Her therapist began by expressing appreciation of Clara's deep sense of loyalty, rather than emphasizing her right to independence or "individuation" as a task for her age group. The therapist understood that for many immigrant college students, family loyalty is a prime motivation for excelling in school, even in the face of considerable barriers and, in some communities, disapproval from peers. The therapist respected Clara's self-defined role within the family as the good, responsible daughter, while seeking to expand her space for learning within the new college environment and in relation to her evolving family role. She asked Clara to describe her realistic worries about the family's developmental dilemmas and to explore possible resources that could help support her mother and family during this transition, so that Clara could feel freer to concentrate on her schoolwork and live up to her family's dreams for her success. During a weekend family visit, Clara invited her mother and sister to join her at an event at the adolescent resources center where Clara had worked as a peer counselor during high school. She encouraged her rebellious sister to join the center by showing her that most of the participants shared her love of hip-hop culture and used the center to escape the family's watchful eye and gain some freedom of movement with peers. At the same time, she reminded her mother that the center had helped her prepare her college applications and receive her scholarship. Clara also encouraged her mother to join a mother's group, in which other women from the community shared strategies for communication with their hard-to-reach teenage daughters. On the college campus, the therapist encouraged Clara to join the multicultural student center where she would find other young women from immigrant families who shared her search for culturally based family and community connections in their elite white university environment.

During this brief therapy, Clara shared her concern that her mother carried burdens not only of fatigue and family worry but also of some unspoken secrets concerning their political activities and experiences prior to leaving El Salvador—something she was learning about in school but was never discussed in her family. She was beginning to suspect that some violent experience beyond the hardships of immigration and separation had transformed the young, lively, affectionate mother she remembered from early childhood into the withdrawn, worried woman who did not want her daughters to leave her sight. The therapist encouraged Clara to begin a conversation with her mother and sister about their positive shared memories of childhood and home and about her parents' political values and participation during their own college years, before they had to leave the country. Recognizing the possibility that her parents had experienced violent trauma, Clara's therapist also suggested they consider a family-based evaluation within their local health center, so that her parents could receive support as they decided which experiences they wanted to share with their children and which best belonged in the sphere of their relationship.

Immigrant college students often experience intense conflicts at the crossroads of family expectations and acculturation into U.S. society. For many immigrant families, their children's academic success represents the future on behalf of which all their many sacrifices have been made. However, as the young adults leave home and enter college, they may encounter contradictory expectations between their academic environments and their enduring family obligations. As we could see in Clara's case example, the college counseling center mandated a brief therapy model within which family contacts were administratively outside their scope and viewed as undermining age-appropriate separation–individuation processes. Yet the Latina therapist found ways to work within the constraints of the college counseling setting and within Clara's own definition of her difficulties as emerging from a shared family life cycle transition. The therapist had considerable knowledge of Latina culture and was able to appreciate Clara's deep sense of family loyalty as a positive personal and family resource. Their clinical work used the therapeutic relationship as a supportive partnership and new resource within which Clara could reflect on her dilemmas of love and growth between cultures, to identify existing and new resources in the family and community that could affirm their familial relationships and support their individual growth. Planning for and introducing new realistic resources in both home and college communities made it possible for Clara to continue her studies while using school as a space for exploring her own cultural complexity with like-minded others. The therapy helped Clara (and, through Clara, her family) to utilize the familial, cultural, and practical resources that contributed to the "upward spirals," and it interrupted the possible "downward spirals" that would focus on loss, depression, and trauma.

Although Clara was the "identified patient" and clinical point of entry for this example, we could just as easily have seen Clara's mother, who might have been referred by her internist for her experience of fatigue.

Often, immigrant women who have endured traumatic migration histories or traumatic current experiences (e.g., poverty, racism, community violence, family separations) convey their psychological distress through the culturally sanctioned vehicle of somatic distress in the form of fatigue, headaches, or more culturally specific seizure-like syndromes such as *ataques de nervios* (nervous attacks). In families where harmonious relationships are valued and women's anger is viewed as unacceptable, the seizure-like syndromes offer an outlet for self-expression that draws from the cultural cosmology or explanatory system. For example, *hwa-byung*, listed in DSM-IV-TR (American Psychiatric Association, 2000) under culture-bound syndromes and translated from the Korean as "fire disease," draws from traditional oriental medicine in which fire is understood as one of five elements with which we must remain in harmony to sustain health. In working with women who are expressing culturally embodied idioms of distress, we can best support an expansion of possibilities within their changing gender roles by respecting their cultural framings of experiences (Torres & Cernada, 2003).

Even within a family, immigrant adolescent siblings differ by age, developmental status, temperament, and family role in their tolerance of their parents' demands, which invariably seem excessive to them when compared to the greater freedom of their North American peers. Clara's rebellious younger sister is an example of this phenomenon. Although immigrant families worry about the possibility that their sons might be pulled into the street and the school violence that plagues so many communities, their sons enjoy far greater freedom of movement than their daughters, who may deeply resent the control or be embarrassed by their family's differences. In working systemically with immigrant families struggling with a rebellious adolescent, it is useful to introduce new narratives that recognize the struggle to adjust under arduous new circumstances, and to help parents save face while expanding the world within which they and their children establish sources of safety and continuity to balance overwhelming processes of change.

During periods of change most of us cling to continuity and familiarity. When external resources fail us, psychological and relational sacrifices offer resources of last resort. The Vargas family intensified their familiar reliance on culturally based gendered definitions of Gregorio's paternal authority, Carolina's maternal tenderness, and Frankie's responsibilities as an older son. These gendered roles and meanings were mobilized as coping resources and then systemically amplified as last-resort attempts at maintaining continuity and stability in a time when they had lost many cultural and community connections and were experiencing economic and social stressors because of immigration. Clinical interventions with immigrant women such as Carolina need to reflect a careful consideration of the generative and abusive dimensions of gendered power relationships within families, while working within culturally congruent definitions of generosity and generativity to expand family complexity, creativity, and accountability. Carolina Vargas was helped to rebuild her extended network of community relationships and to use therapy as a way of receiving the emotional backing (*respaldo*) she needed to permit her to care for herself, stand up for herself, and relieve her son of the burden of worry, instead helping him to turn toward replanting his own uprooted relationships in new soil. This health-promotion model of clinical practice highlights culturally based strengths that build resilience while clearly articulating the burdens to health and mental health imposed on immigrant women, who, like women all over the world, carry greater responsibilities for the care of others with less power and fewer resources.

Our work with immigrant women and their families requires assessment of family life cycle transitions as markers of gendered development that place unique burdens on women. Immigration itself is a major transition. Carolina Vargas, mother of a toddler as well as a 10-year-old son, experienced a depression linked to the absence of her extended family and community networks for childrearing. Life cycle transitions may include children's movement toward creating extrafamilial relationships, as illustrated by Misrek's efforts to cultivate a friendship with a person from outside of her family's cultural enclave, and her parents' restricting response; or children's movement away from home, as illustrated by Clara and her family. Absorbing the blow of a loved one's death is yet another family life cycle transition that presents significant challenges for immigrant women, whose struggle with grief requires a redefinition of self within relationships and cultural understandings of the death and its meaning.

> Arlene Haddad, an Armenian immigrant who had come to the United States as a teenager and had married within an immigrant Armenian enclave, came for a family consultation initiated by her husband Mark, the son of Armenian immigrants, 3 years after their youngest son was killed by a hit-and-run driver. Her husband was concerned that her deep depression had completely immobilized her and kept the entire family immobilized within their great loss. Arlene kept an altar in Danny's memory in her and Mark's bedroom, which only intensified her emotional unavailability to other family members. Arlene, Mark, and their three surviving children participated in this brief three-session family therapy, in which all spoke of the overwhelming tragedy of Danny's death and the ways in which it had shattered their family. Danny had been the most affectionate member of the family, always smiling and sociable, and without him each member of the family had descended into a deep isolation. First, Arlene listened as her two college-age daughters and her younger son Greg, a junior in high school

and now the youngest family member, talked about their suffering at the tragic loss of Danny's loving presence, their family's heart and soul. Her older daughter Nancy, who had been in charge of her younger brothers that day, shared how deeply responsible she felt that she had not been able to stop Danny as he ran out the door with friends. Greg spoke wistfully of how much he missed coming home from school to the activity of their home before Danny's death, to the kitchen smells and lively sounds of jokes and arguments.

Arlene, startled from her deep communion with Danny's spirit back into the world of her living, surviving children, disclosed that every day when she visited the cemetery she thought of driving her car into an embankment and ending her own life. Yet as she listened to the love in her children's stories of grief and loss, and heard the ways they needed her, their mutual love offered a lifeline connecting her to the love that was still abundant in their everyday world. As her children shared with Arlene how much their loss of Danny had been compounded by her descent into her private grief, Arlene decided to move her altar to Danny's memory from her bedroom into the living room, creating a family space where all could share Danny's enduring spiritual presence and affirm their loving connections beyond death. This act signaled Arlene's return from the world of the dead to the world of her living family. After this brief family intervention, Arlene and Mark were referred for couple therapy in their community, to work more intensively on marital conflicts that were intensified by Danny's death.

Five years later, Arlene's daughter Nancy sought therapy to explore her reluctance to marry her fiancé. In the intervening 5 years, after an unsuccessful marital therapy, her parents had decided to divorce, and her father had moved in with his mother while Nancy remained with Arlene. Nancy felt deeply distressed about leaving her mother alone, now that the other children had left. Nancy's brief therapy revisited and recontextualized her self-blame for Danny's death through openhearted remembering, in which Nancy lovingly recalled how Danny's irrepressible energies usually sent him sailing out the door in spite of her attempts to hold him back. Nancy decided to marry her fiancé, and her father helped them find a house within the same neighborhood, close to both parents and extended family.

Danny's death delivered a shattering blow to the Haddad family, whose life course was redirected in ways that corresponded to their culturally based assumptions about the enduring spiritual presence of the deceased. Although Danny's death intensified preexisting marital problems, the Haddads remained strongly committed to their collaboration as parents within their extended family and community. Helping Arlene connect to the suffering of her surviving children offered a culturally congruent bridge between her spiritual bond to Danny and her concern for her surviving children, which she expressed by moving her altar to a public space in the household, where all could openly share their loving memories. For both Nancy and her parents, marital intimacy was negotiated within a set of expectations to maintain strong extended family kinship ties rather than the privacy of romantic love. The ability of this bereaved immigrant family to restore their loving connections did not necessarily conform to our clinical expectations regarding resolution of grief. Clinical models of bereavement combine biomedical assumptions of psychopathology, illness, and cure with a secular, individualistic approach that misdefines psychological, time-limited, private experiences as "normal" grief (Shapiro, in press). The Haddad family's therapy built on their culturally meaningful intergenerational ties and spiritual understandings of enduring bonds to restore their shared capacity to give and receive love, freeing this family to go on with life in the presence of grief.

Review of Intervention Principles

Each of the clinical examples in this chapter used a cultural and developmental systems framework that views developmental challenges not just as private passages but as interdependent, intergenerational transitions in the shared family life of immigrants. The ways in which families experience these transitions are inevitably shaped by their specific cultural backgrounds and immigration experiences. The clinical examples presented here illustrate the following principles of therapy with immigrant women:

1. *Therapy with immigrant women offers a developmental opportunity for facilitating positive adaptive processes of cultural complexity and creativity within an interdependent passage or transition in the family life cycle.* With all the immigrant women and families described in this chapter, culturally responsive therapy focused on solutions to dilemmas of love and translation that helped honor intergenerational obligations while creating new spaces for mutuality and interdependence in response to new cultural circumstances. Misrek, an Ethiopian immigrant whose headaches "voiced" fears that her family's restrictions would prevent her from finding a life partner, sought support from her church and used education as an accepted vehicle for expanding her personal strivings and relationships outside their community enclave in culturally acceptable ways. Clara, a Latina immigrant entering an elite college environment, experienced significant tension between demands for independence and her own understanding of family obligations and needs. The shadow of her own and her family's migration experiences intensified Clara's dilemmas of love and loyalty, and the therapy focused on supporting her developmental transition into college while seeking new resources that would support her family in her absence.

2. *The goals of therapy are constructed in the context of a collaborative relationship and a strengths-based appreciative inquiry into the immigrant woman's understanding of her life passage, desired goals, and dilemmas as she experiences the crossroads of relationships and culture.* Therapy considers the perspective of both the individual and the family as a unit, regardless of who is actually participating in therapy. An appreciative inquiry requires co-creation of a shared language to encompass the process of growth and change, in which cultural dilemmas and meanings are explored through dialogue, with the goal of generating a multidimensional understanding of love, intimacy, and autonomy across cultural differences. Carolina Vargas measured her migration success in light of Frankie's academic achievement and future chances. Although both mother and son spoke of their migration loss, therapy emphasized the resources available to them in multiple systems—resources for supporting positive developmental goals and redirecting their mutual expression of loving concern away from loss and toward growth. Although Clara was referred for depression, she understood her struggle as a pull home toward the family who needed her. Establishing goals for therapy that affirmed Clara's experience helped her identify practical resources in relationships and contexts that could assist her in rebalancing her culturally meaningful valuation of loyalty and interdependence. Her success in college was reframed as a desired resource for the entire family, and her responsibilities for caretaking and mediating were shifted to extended family and community.

3. *An exploration of past migrations emphasizes present and future goals for interdependent development and identifies existing and new cultural and relational resources in multiple systems that can support achievement of shared goals, even in the presence of trauma.* With a focus on the family's own goals at this moment in their shared passage, past migrations are explored to identify cultural resources of continuity and stability and to identify barriers to intimacy and mutuality that may be interfering with the process of change. Addressing traumatic histories will often form an important dimension of therapeutic work with immigrant women, and in this context it is especially important to use culturally based narratives and a strengths-based and multisystemic approach that fosters resilience and posttraumatic growth (Berger & Weiss, 2002; Rynearson, 2002; Shapiro, in press).

In closing, we would emphasize that clinical work with immigrant women launches a creative journey of transformation for all participants. As therapists, our attitude of appreciative inquiry and our stance of open-hearted listening help us abandon the certainties of diagnostic assessments, the comfort of ethnocentric judgments, and the reassurance of belonging to an authoritative school of psychotherapy. We travel together into unknown territories, discovering that love can be both lost and found in translation, finding new pathways by which loss and dislocation can be transformed through culturally meaningful reflections and practical actions that link the ancestral past to future strivings in the transcendent territory of the spirit.

Notes

1. In this and every case example in this chapter, names, nationality, and other identifying information have been changed to protect individual and family privacy. When modifying identifying information, which significantly changes family context, the case reports incorporate clinical experiences with other families to account for the impact of these contextual variations on clinical presentation and treatment.

2. Results from the 2000 census revealed significant growth in the number of people of all ages who were either immigrants or first-generation residents (Schmidley, 2001). This census reported 12.8 million women age 18 and older (total foreign born, 28.4 million) living in the United States who were born in other countries, 58% percent of whom were noncitizens. With an additional 14.8 million native born with both parents foreign born, and 12.7 million native born with one parent foreign born, 55.9 million, or one-fifth, of the U.S. population is of "foreign stock," to use the Census Bureau's revealing phrase. Earlier immigration patterns in which men arrived first and later sent for their families have been replaced by arrival of women in equal numbers as men (Hondagneu-Sotelo, 2003).

Twenty-one percent of the U.S. population under age 25 was found to be either foreign born or first generation (up from only 7% in 1970). The census also reported the presence of 2.8 million children born in other countries. About half of the foreign-born children were from Latin America, with close to 29% (8.8 million) from Mexico, and others from Cuba, the Dominican Republic, and El Salvador. Twenty-six percent of the foreign-born population is from Asia, totaling 7.2 million, with the majority from China, the Philippines, India, Vietnam, and Korea. Another 15% or 4.4 million of foreign-born residents were European born in the 2000 census, a significant decrease from 1970, when 62% of the foreign-born population reported a European country as their birthplace. Approximately 78% of the foreign-born residents from Mexico were not U.S. citizens, compared with half of those from Asia and 45% of native Europeans. Seven out of ten U.S. immigrants live in the six states of California (8.8 million), New York (3.6 million), Florida (2.8 million), Texas (2.4 million), New Jersey, and Illinois (1.2 million each), with more than 3 in 10 living in the Los Angeles and New York metropolitan areas (4.7 million each), followed by San Francisco (2.0 million), Miami (1.6 million), and Chicago (1.1 million).

Over 40% of immigrant women are heads of household, with 20% never married, 11% divorced or separated, 9% widowed, and 3% married with their spouse absent. The poverty rate for the foreign born overall is 17%, compared to 11% for the native population, with 22% for those from Latin America and 13% for those from Asia. Foreign-born women ages 25–54 had lower labor-force participation rates (67%) than U.S. born women (79%). Latin American women are the most likely to work in low-wage service, farm work, and manual labor. Fifty-five percent of foreign-born women workers earned less than $25,000, compared to 44.1% of native women, whereas 12% had earnings of $50,000 or more, compared to 13.2% of the native population; this difference in the upper range of women's earnings was not significantly different. Nearly 20% of immigrant women lack health insurance, and are more likely to seek health care for their family members than for themselves.

The U.S. census does not ask questions concerning legality of residency status, and U.S. immigrants who have entered the country illegally are reluctant to report that information, resulting in consistent underestimation and different totals depending on the method used. Estimates range from the Immigration and Naturalization Service (INS) number of 8.7 million, to a Northeastern University study that estimated workers to be as high as 11–12 million. Illegal status increases women's burdens of immigration, making it less likely that they will seek needed health and mental health services. Illegal status also appears to increase the vulnerability to risk of domestic violence.

References

American Psychiatric Association. (2000). *Diagnostic and statistical manual of mental disorders* (4th ed., text rev.). Washington, DC: Author.

Berger, R., & Weiss, T. (2002). Immigration and post-traumatic growth: A missing link. *Journal of Immigrant and Refugee Services, 1*(2), 21–39.

Bohart, A., & Tallman, K. (1999). *How clients make therapy work: The process of active self-healing.* Washington, DC: American Psychological Association.

Boyd-Franklin, N. (2003). *Black families in therapy: Understanding the African American experience* (2nd ed.). New York: Guilford Press.

Ballou, M., & Brown, L. S. (Eds.). (2002). *Rethinking mental health and disorder: Feminist perspectives.* New York: Guilford Press.

Comas-Díaz, L., & Greene, B. (Eds.). (1994). *Women of color: Integrating ethnic and gender identities in psychotherapy.* New York: Guilford Press.

Espin, O. (1997). *Latina realities: Essays on healing, migration and sexuality.* Boulder, CO: Westview Press.

Espin, O. (1999). *Women crossing boundaries: The psychology of immigration and the transformations of sexuality.* New York: Routldege.

Falicov, C. J. (1998). *Latino families in therapy: A guide to multicultural practice.* New York: Guilford Press.

Hondagneu-Sotelo, P. (2003). *Gender and U.S. immigration: Contemporary trends.* Berkeley: University of California Press.

Hubble, M., Duncan, B., & Miller, S. (1999). *The heart and soul of change.* Washington, DC: American Psychological Association.

Katz, A., & Shotter, J. (2004). On the way to "presence": Methods of a "social poetics." In D. Pare & G. Larner (Eds.), *Collaborative practice in psychology and therapy* (pp. 69–84). New York: Haworth Press.

Koenig, H., McCullough, M., & Larson, D. (2001). *Handbook of religion and health*. New York: Oxford University Press.

Leadbetter, B., & Way, N. (1996). *Urban girls: Resisting stereotypes, creating identities*. New York: New York University Press.

Luthar, S. (2003). *Resilience and vulnerability: Adaptation in the context of childhood adversities*. Cambridge, UK: Cambridge University Press.

Masten, A. (2001). Ordinary magic: Resilience processes in development. *American Psychologist, 56*, 227–238.

McHugh, E. (2001). *Love and honor in the Himalayas: Coming to know another culture*. Philadelphia: University of Pennsylvania Press.

Perez-Foster, R. (2001). When immigration is trauma: Guidelines for the individual and family clinician. *American Journal of Orthopsychiatry, 71*(2), 153–170.

Phinney, J., Horenczyk, G., Liebkind, K., & Vedder, P. (2001). Ethnic identity, immigration and well-being: An interactional perspective. *Journal of Social Issues, 57*(3), 493–510.

Rynearson, E. (2002). *Retelling violent death*. New York: Brunner/Routledge.

Sandler, I. (2001). Quality and ecology of adversity as common mediators of risk and resilience. *American Journal of Community Psychology, 29*, 19–63.

Schmidley, D. (2001). *U.S. Census Bureau current population reports: Profile of the foreign-born population in the United States: 2000*. Washington, DC: U.S. Government Printing Office.

Shapiro, E. (1999). From Byelorus to Bolondron: A daughter's dangerous passage. In M. Agogin (Ed.), *The house of memory* (pp. 230–240). New York: Feminist Press.

Shapiro, E. (Coord. Ed.). (2000). *Nuestros cuerpos, nuestras vidas [Our bodies, our lives]*. New York: Seven Stories Press.

Shapiro, E. (in press). *Grief as a family process: A cultural and developmental systems approach to integrative practice* (2nd ed.). New York: Guilford Press.

Torres, M., & Cernada, G. (2003). *Sexual and reproductive health promotion in Latino populations*. New York: Baywood.

Wyche, K. (2001). Sociocultural issues in counseling for women of color. In R. Unger (Ed.), *Handbook of the psychology of women and gender* (pp. 330–340). New York: Wiley.

CHAPTER 7

Class Tensions within Families
MAINTAINING RELATIONSHIPS
ACROSS DIFFERENCES

Sandra J. Jones

August 1992

On my way home from work at a computer company, driving by the ranch house where my ex-husband lives with his wife and step-daughter, I'm not surprised to see my brother Tommy's car in the driveway and the two guys sitting near the side deck. When he's working the day shift at the plastics company, Tommy likes to stop by Jimmy's after work to "shoot the breeze." Jimmy puts in a 10-hour day delivering automobile parts to garages in New England, but he's usually home by 4:00. I pull in behind Tommy's Honda and walk around to join them. Hearing them talking and laughing, I can imagine either of them saying, "Did you hear the one about the farmer and the three nuns . . ." They're like brothers, these two—on the same wavelength from the day they met.

They look up at me as I approach, and Jimmy says, "Hey, what's up?"

I respond, "Not much. We were away at Tanglewood this weekend."

He asks, "Oh, yeah? Who'd you see?"

I say, "We heard the Boston Symphony Orchestra."

With that, they burst into laughter, bending forward in their chairs. A sinking feeling comes over me, and I'm close to rage. "What's so funny?"

Jimmy sits up, looks me in the eye and says, "I thought you'd say Gordon Lightfoot or James Taylor!"

"What's the matter with the BSO?"

"Nothing," he replies with a grin, glancing at Tommy.

Tommy adds, "Just remember where you come from."

"How could I ever forget I come from Cli-en," I reply, stressing the local pronunciation of Clinton, which rhymes with linen, and is different from Cling-on, which is what Tommy calls Clinton because "you can never get away."

To these white Protestant working-class guys, going to the symphony rather than a pop concert seems ridiculous and out-of-character for people like us. "Remember where you come from" is a reminder of my class origins in a small town where members of our family, including Tommy and me, worked in factories. It is a rebuke and a charge to not "get uppity." In this interaction, Jimmy and Tommy used teasing as a way to critique class-related cultural differences and call me back home. I responded in kind, in a local dialect, participating in the tease and declaring our shared history. However, the social distance between us persists, leaving me to grapple with tenuous connections across contested terrain.

My experience is not unique. This chapter draws on research with women from working-class families who earned doctoral degrees, became college professors, and experience class-related tensions with adult siblings. Class is a relational concept: It is about relations of power between groups of people who occupy distinct social locations determined by a combination of factors that includes income, accumulated wealth, occupational prestige, educational credentials, associations and networks, and social identities (e.g., sex, race, ethnicity), whether or not individuals identify as members of a class (Bourdieu, 1998). Through participation in everyday life (e.g., home, school, work), individuals develop a sense of their class position and a consciousness and culture that is shared by group members and informed by material conditions and social relations of power (see, e.g., Bettie, 2003; Bourdieu, 1985; Rubin, 1976; Willis, 1981). The class into which we are born and raised influences our customs, attitudes, values, associations, networks, and understanding of the world. Therefore, it is not surprising that individuals tend to socialize with and marry people from the same class background, with its similar values and lifestyles, thereby reproducing class across generations.

However, a considerable number of individuals in the United States (about 40% in any given generation) move up in class status, a distance equivalent to the children of blue-collar fathers entering lower-white-collar occupations such as retail sales (Gilbert & Kahl, 1993). A smaller number (about 25%) move from blue-collar families into higher-status professions. Movement up the class hierarchy is associated with greater economic, social, and political power over one's own life and the lives of others. Individuals may change class status, but they can never escape class relations. We are all caught in a web of class relations—social and economic dependencies that maintain the class structure. Differences in economic, social, and political power between classes create tensions that are enacted in the workplace, school, neighborhood, and, in some cases, family of origin. Changes in class status by individual family members have consequences for the entire family system. Parents of children who move up in class status may be proud of their children's achievements but also feel estranged from them. Differences in class status between adult siblings can complicate and strain family ties, as described in the opening narrative.

Through a complex process of socialization, individuals appropriate ideas and values from the dominant culture, which positions people with higher class status as superior and those with lower class status as inferior (Freire, 1992). The internalization of dominant ideology by working class and poor people can result in "internalizing the enemy" and blaming oneself for failing to achieve higher status (Hertzberg, 1996, p. 133; Leeder, 1996; Russell, 1996). Individuals from poor and working-class backgrounds who move into the professions may report psychological distress, confusion about class identity, shame and guilt, estrangement from working-class family and friends, and disenchantment with class-privileged settings (Barker, 1995; Dews & Law, 1995; Jones, 1998b, 2004; Ross, 1995; Ryan & Sackrey, 1996; Tokarczyk & Fay, 1993). Women may experience greater psychological distress from estranged relationships than men because traditional gender roles assign women greater responsibility for maintaining relationships.

Although therapists use a variety of lenses through which to view family dynamics, there is a tendency to avoid a class lens. Therapists need to be attentive to class-related distress among clients, including class identity confusion and class conflicts in families. By attending to class issues, therapists can help clients identify and deal with the psychological and relational costs of mobility.

Exploring Class through Interviews

My interest in class is informed by my own experience of moving from the working class to the professions in my 30s. As a nontraditional, part-time college student working in the computer industry, I was keenly aware that becoming a professional required learning to act, dress, and talk like other professionals. However, doing so distanced me from working-class friends and family. I was caught in a double bind where "assimilation constitutes betrayal, while holding on to aspects of working-class identity marks out our unacceptability" (Reay, 1996, p. 445). Moving up from secretarial to professional status and remarrying a software engineer, who is also a first-generation college graduate, contributed to the class-related tension portrayed in my personal narrative at the beginning of this chapter.

I subsequently entered graduate school, where my experience of class took another turn. Between 1996 and 1998 I engaged in feminist interpretive research (Charmaz, 2000; Langellier & Hall, 1989; Levesque-Lopman, 2000; Reinharz, 1992) with 10 female academics to systematically explore women's subjectivity in the context of upward mobility from blue-collar families to academe. I conducted two tape-recorded interviews with each participant in her home or office that lasted approximately 2 hours each. The interviews were semistructured and focused on participants' experiences of social mobility.

I located participants through publications in which they wrote about their working-class backgrounds and through word of mouth. For the purpose of this research, I defined working class by a combination of self-definition and sociological indicators (parents' education and occupation). Six of the ten women I interviewed were white and identified as Polish, German Irish, Portuguese Italian, Italian, Eastern-European Jewish, and mixed ethnicity; two were African American, and two were Latina (Mexican, Mexican Salvadoran). Although not the explicit focus of this research, the women also differed in terms of region of origin, discipline, institution, family status, age, religion, and sexual orientation.

I analyzed interviews inductively to develop key concepts across participants while attending to case-specific particularities (Charmaz, 2000). I complemented cross-case analysis with a case-centered approach informed by sociolinguistic strategies to identify and analyze narratives, a storylike form of discourse found in interviews. When telling a narrative, interview participants verbally reconstruct a particular or habitual event. I parsed the narratives into lines and stanzas by attending to pauses, linguistic cues, and topic switches, noting unfinished expressions and words spoken with emphasis. Each line captures a single idea and each stanza an image. Words spoken with emphasis and stanza subheadings, which I added, are in italics. (For further information on narrative analysis, see Gee, 1991; Mishler, 1991, 2000; Riessman, 1993.) As a way to mitigate the inequality of power between researcher and participants, I engaged in a feminist reflexive process, disclosing my background as a woman from the working class and involving participants in interpretation. Participants gave feedback on both the transcripts and my analysis, and received a copy of the completed research report (Jones, 1998a).

This chapter examines an underside of upward mobility through higher education, namely, the ways in which class differences create or exacerbate interpersonal conflicts among family members. My analysis indicates that upwardly mobile women may experience a sense of estrangement from family members, guilt about socioeconomic privileges, working-class pride, and shame about their class background in elite circles. Upward mobility is a context for reconstructing identities and affiliations, which can lead to feeling "nowhere at home" (Overall, 1995). The narratives presented in this chapter reveal the ways in which these women negotiate their position as members of working-class families and their class subjectivities. These interactions reflect larger societal class relations and suggest ways that practitioners can help clients negotiate interpersonal and internalized classism.

Maintaining Relationships

Relationships among adult siblings are influenced by multiple factors, one of which is social class. Lifestyle differences due to economic resources, educational credentials, and occupational status situate adult siblings in relations of power within the family and larger society. In this section, I present analyses of four narratives that reveal class tensions between family members. The narrators are Nancy, Aurelia, Casey, and Maria (pseudonyms), all of whom are first-generation college graduates from blue-collar families. At the time of the interviews (1997–1998), they were 37–47 years of age and in tenured or tenure-track positions in the humanities or social sciences. Nancy and Maria have grandparents who immigrated to the United States from Italy and Mexico, respectively. Aurelia's mother immigrated from Central America, and her paternal grandparents from Mexico. Casey is an African American woman from the South. I chose these particular narratives because they reveal distinct aspects of class-related tensions in families, the ways in which these women negotiate these tensions, and the intersection of class, gender, race, and ethnicity.

A Gulf between Our Lives

Becoming a university professor with higher status and greater access to resources than working-class siblings can complicate relationships. Nancy, a third-generation Italian American, discussed problematic aspects of her relationships with two older brothers who did not graduate from college. Nancy went to college immediately after graduating from high school, and she taught for a year before entering graduate school. At the time of the interview, she had been a professor for 9 years. She told the following narrative in the context of talking about the importance of valuing working-class lifestyles in an academic world that devalues working-class lives. After discussing the importance of teaching her students, many of whom are first-generation college students, to be more critical of the social matrix, she talked about her relationships with her working-class brothers.

A gulf
I still definitely feel a gulf between my self and my family's lives,
my life and my family's lives,
and a sense of *loss*,
definitely.

Providing
And, you know, I sometimes wish that my brothers were in a place
    that was closer to where I am
so we could have—they could *help* me.
I feel a little bit like I'm the family member who does a lot of the
    providing,
so I don't really go to them for emotional support or intellectual
    support,
and I wish I could.

Grieving
How do I negotiate that?
I don't know.
I think, you know, it's an ongoing process of a kind of *grieving*.
I *definitely* work through this stuff in my writing,
when you say how do I negotiate that.
    Sandy: Do they still come to you?

Different worlds
    Nancy: Yes and no.
My middle brother—who I said, you know, is the one who I have
    most difficulty talking about
he really—no, he doesn't come to me at all.
Occasionally he'll write me a letter,
but there's really just a sense that we live in really different worlds.

Mother mediates
I see him at family gatherings,
but my *mother* kind of mediates so much of our relations that—
I only thought that *maybe* if—if my mother weren't with us anymore,
you know, if or when she dies,
and if she dies before we do,
then I imagine that our relationship will change.

Some kind of relationship

It will *have* to change.
I'll have to have some kind of relationship with my brother.
I mean, maybe that's a terrible way to think of it
I should be trying to have a relationship with him now (*laughter*)
but—
>   Sandy: Or it might become even more difficult.
>   Nancy: It might become more difficult *later*?
>   Sandy: To have a relationship without her there, mediating.
>   Nancy: Hmm, *well*, I don't know.

Not required now

I guess I kind of think that it would require us to have a relationship,
whereas we're not required to now
because now our relationship is with our mother.
She mediates between us, in a way.
yeah, his primary relationship is to my mother and his niece and
     nephew.
>   Sandy: I see.

He won't be vulnerable

And my other brother, he's turned me into some kind of perfect, I-
     can-do-no-wrong figure
whom he has to answer to,
so if he doesn't have good news he doesn't get in touch with me
     usually (*laughter*).
He just won't let himself be vulnerable really.

Miss Perfect

And—and he just sees himself as not making the right—not having
     made the right *choices*,
and I did.
and I'm Miss Perfect, you know,
so that's a kind of troubling position to be in,
because he doesn't see me as a human being, you know.
I symbolize something to him.

He does reach out

But he does call me when he needs things on a more profound
     level,
like that day when my father hit him.
He called me
and—so he does reach out in that sense.

Coming closer
And I feel, like I said, that I've gained him in some ways.
Since he's been getting an education
that something is coming closer.

The distance in Nancy's relationships with her brothers is large and accidental, not deliberate. Although they were raised in the same home, their lives diverged, leading them to "different worlds" separated by a "gulf." Through this metaphor, Nancy evoked the loss associated with upward mobility, which positions her far away from the everyday experiences of family members ("between . . . my life and my family's lives") and contributes to an internal sense of distance between herself and her family ("between my self and my family's lives"). She deals with this ongoing loss through writing. Upward mobility often requires geographic mobility, which may be a factor in relational distance; Nancy moved out of state, whereas her brothers remain in their hometown.

A key dimension of the loss Nancy experiences is a lack of support from her brothers. She represented herself as the one who does "a lot of the providing," and she expressed a wish that they were closer to her social location ("place") so that they could give her emotional and intellectual support. Her words suggest that they are unable to support her because of the social distance between them and because of her role as provider. Her role evokes stereotypical gender roles in which males rely on females for emotional support, and this may be part of the explanation. However, providing for them suggests some degree of close relationship, which seemed to contradict her earlier comments, prompting me to ask, "Do they still come to you?" Her initial reply was ambiguous ("yes and no"); the nature and extent of her providing remains unclear.

To some extent, Nancy's mother bridges the gulf, eliminating the need for direct contact with her brothers. As I listened to her, I thought about my relationship with my brother. Like Nancy's mother, my mother kept me informed about his life, and informed him about mine. However, her death did not result in a closer relationship with him. Nancy did not entertain the possibility, which I suggested, that having a relationship with her brother might be more difficult without her mother present. If or when her mother is no longer able to facilitate the relationship, Nancy will have "some kind of relationship" with her brother. However, "some kind of relationship" is not necessarily a satisfying relationship. Working-class families tend to place more emphasis on family ties than middle-class families and assign women primary responsibility for maintaining relationships (Rubin, 1976, 1994). Nancy's contention that she should initiate the relationship ("I should be trying to have a relationship with him now") reflects her internalization of gender roles and the importance of family ties in her Italian

American working-class family. Her connection to family is a central part of her identity and work, as reflected in her self-described role as the person who keeps the stories of her ancestors alive.

Nancy locates the strain in her sibling relationships with her educational and occupational achievements. Her success has been particularly difficult for her older brother, the first-born son, for whom she "symbolizes" something. He does not allow himself to be "vulnerable" with her, only calling when he has "good news." It is unclear whether a sense of working-class masculinity or pride associated with being the first-born brother inhibits him from disclosing his vulnerability, or whether her higher social status incites a defensive response from him. A belief that upward mobility is within the grasp of everyone can heighten a sense of inferiority among those who do not attain higher status. It is clear that Nancy's adult achievements shifted the gendered class relations within the family. The gulf separating her from her brothers is bidirectional: She moved away from their lifestyle and neighborhood, and they pulled back.

The shift of verb tense in her description of her older brother as "not making" to "not having made" the right choices reflects her sense that he is changing. Now that he is in college, their relationship has improved ("something is coming closer"), as evidenced by his ability to contact her when their father hit him. Why has college made a difference? It is clear that Nancy sees college as the "right choice," a choice that will decrease the social distance between them and increase their shared experience. The words attributed to her brother suggest that he sees education as the right choice ("he just sees himself as not having made the right *choices,* and I did"). From Nancy's perspective, it seems that improving her relationships with her brothers depends on the reduction or elimination of class differences, specifically, educational differences. This strategy privileges education. If education is the key to closeness, the relational strains will continue unless her brothers go to college. The idea that her brothers could identify alternative ways to conceive of their lives as successful is not engaged in this narrative.

The current roles taken up by Nancy and her brothers stand in contrast to their roles as children. She is their little sister. In another part of the interview, she described her middle brother as gifted in mathematics and science. He helped her with her high school studies and the transition into college, teaching her calculus. Her brothers have the potential to succeed academically, but other factors in their lives (e.g., depression, divorce, single parenting) hindered their college studies. Nancy's narrative suggests that a shift in roles occurred as a result of her adult achievements. She is the higher-status person, and the roles are reversed: Her brothers no longer mentor her, she mentors them—but the support she is able to provide them is limited.

Being perceived as someone who thinks she is better than less-educated family members is a difficult position from which to maintain relationships. As Miss Perfect, making all the right choices, it may be difficult for Nancy to be vulnerable with her brothers. How can she be vulnerable if her brothers do not see her as a "human being," capable of mistakes and wrong choices? On the other hand, her judgments of her brothers' choices and well-meaning advice may inhibit their expressions of vulnerability. As long as a power imbalance exists between them, Nancy's ability to repair the breach will remain limited. Her narrative evokes the question of whether intimate, reciprocal relationships can occur across differences in material conditions and social relations of power in a class-stratified society. Nancy's narrative suggests that the academic success of working-class women undermines working-class gender relations and conceptions of adult male and female success.

They Don't Understand

Aurelia, a second-generation Latina, talked about her relationships with family in the context of discussing how academics from the working class have a choice: They can (1) accept an academic identity and abandon their working-class identity; (2) claim a working-class identity and refuse an academic identity, walking around with a chip on their shoulder; or (3) straddle the fence between two worlds, claiming both identities. Aurelia identifies as a straddler, a position that has its own difficulties, as described in the following narrative.

Mom called

My mother called me last week
and she said, "What are you doing?"
and I said "Well, Mom, I'm gonna finish my dissertation."
She said, "Oh, how nice.

Did you hear?

"You know, Ruth was out of work the other day
she was sick
did you hear it?"
And she went on.
    Sandy: Right.

Taken aback

And I was like—I was taken aback for a second
and then I told [my partner],

and [my partner] said to me, you know, "She doesn't understand
    what it means to finish your dissertation."
[Sandy: Right] you know

She doesn't understand

She doesn't understand what it means
Sandy: Yeah.
She doesn't know how *important* it is.
She doesn't know how *hard* it is.
She doesn't know what sacrifice it took to do it.
    [Sandy: Right] you know

If she could

And it's like, "Well, that's nice," you know
"make you happy . . . I'm happy," you know.
Well, I'm glad she's happy for me,
but it would *really* mean something if she could say to me, "My
    God, that's been an enormous sacrifice," you know.

She never will

But my mother will never say it,
because she doesn't understand it, you know.
Sandy: It's learning to live with those kinds of pains. You know
    what I mean, that's a hurt to me, that people I care so much
    about don't really understand what I'm doing, or why I'm doing
    it, and my inability to convey that.

Closeness

Aurelia: Yeah, it is a pain, I mean—part of it, yeah,
but also—it also means that in terms of my own brothers and sisters
there's a—on one hand there's a certain type of closeness
but there's not an intimacy
    Sandy: Yes.

Loyalty

You know, we grew up together.
There's absolute loyalty.
If I needed something I could call my sister or my brother
and say "I need money. I need help. I need this,"
and they would *drop* everything and *help* me.
    Sandy: Right.

They don't understand

But they don't understand.
They don't understand my *life*.
They don't understand my choices.

[Sandy: Right] you know
They don't understand what makes me tick.

Why should they?
I don't understand what makes me tick—
why should they understand what makes me tick, you know *(laughter)*.

In this narrative, Aurelia conveyed the limitations in her family relationships, which she characterized as closeness without intimacy. The closeness is represented by a routine phone call from her mother and the "absolute loyalty" of her siblings, who live across the country in their region of origin. Her mother's nonchalant response to Aurelia's news about finishing her dissertation minimized her achievement, which stunned Aurelia ("I was taken aback"). Her partner provided emotional support, helping Aurelia understand her mother's indifference as a lack of understanding ("She doesn't understand what it means") and the significance of her accomplishment. She used repetition ("She doesn't know how *important; hard;* what sacrifice it took") to emphasize the experiential gap between herself and her mother. Her mother is "happy" for her, but she does not understand. Clearly, what was a culminating experience for Aurelia had little or no significance for her mother, who immediately shifted the conversation to Aurelia's sister's illness and loss of work, which may have been the purpose of the call (i.e., conveying information between siblings, like Nancy's mother did). Her mother's response may be influenced by an unclear association between completing the dissertation and occupational benefits. Aurelia had been in a tenure-track position for a few years at the time of this interaction, and she had a professional degree and occupation prior to her academic career. As such, there was no obvious career benefit to completing the dissertation.

Aurelia's description of the phone call evoked my own pain and frustration with family members who do not understand my choices. When I left the computer industry to go to graduate school, working-class family members were perplexed about why I would leave a well-paid position with good benefits. Inevitably, they asked the dreaded question, "Will you be able to get a better-paying job?" My reply, "Probably not, but I'm not doing it for that reason; I want to do work that's more satisfying," was met by a puzzled "Oh," at best. The privilege of being able to choose satisfying work over monetary gain is far removed from the lives of many working-class people. Women who pursue careers in higher education make what Valerie Miner (1993) has called an "irrevocable shift, moving beyond the family's imagination" (p. 77).

Aurelia elaborated my expression of pain by talking about the difference between loyalty and intimacy. She emphasized her siblings' willingness to "drop everything" and help her ("I need money; help; this"), and also their inability to comprehend her life ("they don't understand my life; choices; what makes me tick"), thereby conveying the depth of her disappointment about the lack of intimacy. However, she shifted the emotional tone of the narrative at the end, suggesting that she expects too much of them. Why should they understand her, when she doesn't understand herself? This movement away from any suggestion of blaming one's family is consistent with Lillian Rubin's (1976, p. 25) argument that working-class adults are keenly aware of the limitations associated with working-class lives and less eager to blame their parents than middle-class adults.

Writing dissertations, publishing research, and dealing with academic politics are foreign to the lives of working-class people. In addition to the stresses and strains in all family relationships, upward mobility through higher education contributes to an experiential and emotional gap between working-class women and their families. It is a class gap, influenced by gender and generation. Women of any class who choose a life that contradicts traditional gender roles may feel a gap between themselves and their families. Similarly, women and men of any class may develop interests and abilities that their parents do not understand. However, the experience of these women has a particular texture because of class: They have moved a great distance beyond their families' reach, resisting gender roles and class relations to pursue their interests. Although this movement has enriched their lives in multiple ways, it has positioned them in a different world and separated them, to some extent, from their families.

The connections between Aurelia and her siblings seem strong and supportive, a characteristic of Latin culture ("there's absolute loyalty"). It is important to note that her ability to ask and receive material support from them is influenced by the material and social conditions of their lives. Two of her three siblings are college educated, one of whom has a master's degree. Nonetheless, the quality of her relationships with family members has been compromised by her mobility. Lillian Rubin (1994) describes families as both a "haven in a heartless world" and a breeding ground for disappointment and discontent (p. 65). Disinterest and a lack of support due to not knowing the significance of events in academic lives may be understandable given limitations of life experiences, but it is still painful.

It's Hard to Balance Ideas of Success

Nancy's and Aurelia's narratives highlight the difficulties of negotiating significant relationships in which there is closeness without intimacy, and when loved ones see them in ways that contradict how they see themselves (e.g., as "Miss Perfect"). An issue touched upon in my comments on

Nancy's narrative is the danger of privileging education. This issue is brought into the foreground in a narrative told by Casey, an African American from a large Southern family. The context of the narrative was a discussion about success and how to value both higher education and working-class lives. Prior to the narrative, Casey described her sisters as having "standing in the community that I will never have" through their involvement with church activities and for rearing "good children." The setting of the narrative is a visit home in her second year of graduate school, during which Casey played Scrabble, a favorite family game, with her sisters. However, Casey usually won the game, which upset her sisters.

You're better

We were playing this game,
and all of a sudden this conversation started about being in graduate school
and thinking, "You're *better* because you have more education."
That time they said, "Because you've got more education, you just think you're better than us in that sense."

Go to school

And I said to my sister Cathy, "Well, you know, you could go to school."
And she was—she must have been about 40 at that time.
I said, "You can always go back to *school*—finish high school."
And then I said, "Since you are not working at this *time*,
why don't you enroll in a local community college and go there?"

I'm too old

She looks at me and said, "I'm too *old*."
Then I said, "Don't complain, don't complain,
just—you know, you can."
And she said, "No, but I'm too old, you can't."

Locked in

And I was supposed to *accept* that,
and I didn't understand how *she* could accept it,
how she could sit there and go on and on and on about *not* having an education,
her life being *locked in*, you know, and not have any outlets,
and not being able to accomplish some of the things she wanted to do in life because she wasn't *educated*.
Sandy: Right.

Opportunity

And so I said, "oh, here's an *opportunity*"
or hearing my sister Susan going *over* and over and over again
   about not finishing high school
"It's been *years*—you should have taken the GED."
And then she said, "Oh, I tried, but this happened and that happened."

Excuses

There was always a reason, *always* an excuse.
And I would try to urge them and *encourage* them to continue
and I just—they *never ever* wanted to hear it,
but they wanted to *complain*.

Success and discontent

And I just didn't understand that,
so I just think that's an example of how they would say "I am
   successful"
but yet they were not.
There was so much discontent
and so much unhappiness on their part about that *success* . . .
   Sandy: Yes.
. . . that I don't think it was acceptable for me.

Not acceptable

I tried to accept it
but it was not—in a sense it was *not* acceptable.
It's not something that I've been able to *balance* because—
and it's different—
and I think that if *I thought* that that was the best that they could
   do,
then I think it would be more acceptable.

The best she knew

Because with my *mother's* situation
and that was how I reconciled *many* many of my differences with her,
by coming to terms and saying "this is the best *she* knew how to
   do"
   Sandy: Right.
and "this is the best opportunity that was offered to *her* during her
   time,"
because those opportunities were *not* there for my mother.
   Sandy: Right.

They made choices
But for my *siblings,* the opportunity was there for *them,*
it's just they made *choices.*
They could have gone to college and just as I could have-
especially the second group—the second group of kids.

Enough is enough
I mean, I think one of the reasons was because of integration.
It really did do some things to them that I wasn't aware of.
But *still* I think there comes a point in your life where you make a
  decision to say enough is enough,
and this is what I'm going to do and you *do* it.

Don't complain
You don't continue to sit around and complain,
and that's what I saw many of them do
and *still* continue to do, over and over and over again.

The conflict
So that's why it's hard for me to balance that idea of success.
  Sandy: Yes.
I accept it because that's their *opinion* and I value that,
but at the same time, I guess the conflict that is there for me,
if I accept that as a standard, then what does that say about me
and my education or what I have?
what does that mean for *me?*
That is what is hard.
  Sandy: Right.

Encouraging children
And I don't think they really accept it,
simply because if they *did,* they would not push their children as far
  as they did
and *I* see them continuously encouraging their children to *do*
and be better at things than we were
  Sandy: Right.
all of them.
  Sandy: Right.

Never content
So that to me is an indication that they are not content
and they never will be.

Like the relationship between Nancy and her brothers, Casey's siblings critique her for thinking "you're better than us." In this narrative, Casey does not deny their charge. She responds by giving them advice ("urge them and *encourage* them") about how they can become better educated. She represents herself as active, involved in finding solutions to their dissatisfaction, in contrast to her passive sisters, whose complaints wear her down. In spite of her encouragement and suggestions, nothing changes. Her descriptions emphasize the monotony of these interactions through repetition: they "go on and on and on" covering the same ground "over and over and over again." The interaction Casey described is habitual, which raises some questions: Why do they cover the same ground over and again? Why do her sisters complain if their lives are successful? Do they complain about their lives as a regular occurrence, or are the complaints evoked as a defense with her? And why is it difficult for Casey to accept their lives as successful?

There is a pervasive sense in this narrative that mobility is largely due to personal choices. However, there is a larger sociohistoric context that frames these interactions, including a history of slavery, segregation, economic exploitation, and ongoing institutionalized racism. Casey refers to this larger frame, making an exception for her mother, who did "the best that she could do" at a time when educational opportunities for African Americans were rare. But she does not accept the limitations that her sisters give as reasons for not getting an education. While acknowledging systemic factors, such as the racial integration of schools that affected her siblings' experience of education, Casey attributes their limited educations to personal characteristics. She refused to accept age ("I'm too old") or life commitments ("locked in") as reasons for not pursuing a college education, which she sees as the solution to the disappointments in her sisters' lives. For Casey, success is related to contentment. Because her sisters complain, she is unable to accept their lives as successful or understand that her sisters may have some regrets but also some sense of accomplishment. She draws further evidence for their lack of success from the value her sisters place on their children's education as a way to improve their lives. In contrast to her siblings, Casey is the only one who does not have children, and the only one to move away, breaking community ties. As such, she may not fully appreciate the sacrifices her sisters have made and their pride in raising "good children" in a society that critiques the mothering practices of working-class women and blames them for social problems (e.g., delinquency, criminality; Walkerdine, 1996).

From her sisters' perspectives, Casey may seem out of touch with the reality of their lives, unable to see the real limitations they face and the ways in which their success as mothers required them to put their needs second. Her sisters pursued traditional working-class lifestyles for women: They married young and had children. They raised good children, with standing in the community. Not having children herself, Casey may be unaware of what it means to raise African American sons in a culture that imprisons so many of them and refuses jobs to so many others. Mothers whose lives have been limited by race and class boundaries may feel a sense of pride in preparing their own children for a different life, a life for which they are educated and have better economic and social chances than their parents had. Casey's sisters may also value their role as mothers and upstanding members of the community, which may be of higher priority to them than Casey's more individualistic road toward her definition of success.

The underlying tension in this narrative is the difficulty Casey has accepting contradictory values and standards of success. If the standards of success that her sisters live by are valid, "what does that mean for me . . . that is what is hard." Accepting her sisters' standards of success would cause Casey to question her choices and sacrifices. If higher education is the way to a better life, how can she value life choices that preclude education? If her sisters' lives are equally successful, what have her sacrifices gained her? Does Casey regret not having children? Does she miss the opportunity to be an active and appreciated member of their church and community? Have her gains outweighed her losses? This narrative engages the intersection of gender, class, and race, in particular, tensions between her sister's working-class family values and Casey's values as a professional single woman, and the contradictory feelings of both success and regret in all of their lives.

It is difficult to hold contradictory values and perspectives. There is a way in which valuing higher education precludes valuing less educated lifestyles. Privileging education obscures the fact that working-class people are often proud of the work they do and aspire to have better pay, better treatment at work, and more time with family rather than pursue a professional career (Zweig, 2000). On one level, Casey's dilemma represents an internalization of conflicts inherent in the class system (Ryan & Sackrey, 1996). The difficulty of valuing working-class lives and seeing them as successful reveals a deeply held contempt in a society that views the working class as something to escape. The lack of value placed on working-class lives by the dominant culture is part of the larger societal context within which Casey and Nancy experience strained relationships with their siblings. Being told by siblings that "you think you're better than us because you have more education" or being perceived as "Miss Perfect," an inhuman being who can do no wrong, are expressions of class relations, suggesting a sense of superiority (perceived or actual). These statements reflect a sense of estrangement and rebuke the educated person for snobby behavior. They also express resistance to a social system that privileges education and assigns higher social status to educated professionals.

Being Out in Left Field

Maria is a third generation Latina from a large family. Three of her six siblings have college degrees and professional jobs; her other siblings have high school educations or some college and blue-collar jobs. During the first interview, Maria talked about a lack of interest in her work by members of her extended family—including those who have a college education. I was reminded of similar situations in my life, and I asked her if she thought it was a gender issue. Although she acknowledged that gender played a role, she attributed their lack of interest in her work to a "difference in education." In the second interview, I asked if she thought differences in education were related to class differences. She responded by telling me the following story about her relationship with her brother-in-law, who has done quite well financially despite dropping out of high school.

Different interests

I think, of course, it is related to social class,
because you have people who have different educations and
    different lives that they live, different interests,
and that—that is—there's this overarching, you know, class
    structure there.

Little in common

For instance, when I'm at my sister Donna's house and her
    husband's there,
there's very little of interest that we have in common, maybe
    computer stuff
but he doesn't have much to say to me.

No interest

I always find that really interesting,
and I would *never* bring up any of my work with him, never
no interest to know.

At their level

And—*but* I would make a big effort to say, "Hey, what have you
    been up to?
how's the dirt bike?"
You know, to try and interact at their level,
and only if they ask me something would I say anything about my
    own work in those particular cases.
    Sandy: And what does he do for work?

Running equipment

Maria: He is, um, a mech—let's see, what would be his proper
term?
He works at the largest ice company in [the city],
which is very important when it's very hot,
and he maintains all of the equipment there
and running, you know, that they're running.
Sandy: Right, so equipment maintenance.

Not a lot in common

Maria: Yeah,
and he's very working class in all of his jobs that he's had,
and uh, he's a really nice guy.
I mean, we just don't have a lot of interests in common.
And a lot of times they think that I'm, like—I don't know
well, I'll give you an example.
Sandy: Okay.

Getting food

When they were—they were helping me move from—to my new
apartment in [a nearby city],
and I thought "Oh, okay, I'm gonna go run out and get some
food,"
and I bought everything that I think that they would like.
Instead of buying plain old French's mustard, I bought Grey
Poupon, okay?

For them

I don't eat *mustard*,
you know, I did *not* buy it for me,
I bought it for *them*.

I'm better

So my brother-in-law and my nephew made a really strong
comment about "Oh, yeah, Maria would buy this stuff," you
know,
"she just—" you know, kind of a comment that I think that I'm
better
or that it's, you know, *loftier* than, you know, basic French's.

It's for you

And I said, "Hey, you know, give me a break.
I bought it for *you*.

I don't even *eat* the stuff," you know.

Out in left field

Because—and because I try different foods,
or I eat what they think is exotic foods, you know, spicy things,
    Indian things.
I make different kinds of food than they're accustomed to
red meat and potatoes kinds of things
and so I think that they see me as being kind of, I don't know, out
    in left field sometimes.

I'm different

But I'm just *different*.
    Sandy: Right.
And so I *hear* comments about that
"oh, you would do something like that"
or, you know, whatever it happens to be that *separates* me as being
    different from them.

Normal

And to me it's normal
because my friends are like that
[my fiancé is] like that.

Experimental

They just are very experimental,
and we try different things,
and we've traveled.

Expanding

It's just different exposure
and a kind of expanding, you know, from how you grew up to
    something else
to trying different things.
    Sandy: Right.

Differences in experience

And food is just one issue,
one little issue there,
which is interesting
so in that way it kind of points out big differences in experience.

Maria organized this narrative around a seemingly small but consequential event that reveals a breach between her self-perception and how others see her. On one level, the dilemma Maria faces is to maintain connections with family members across "big differences." She portrayed herself as the one who tries to reach out and interact with her brother-in-law about his interests, whereas he makes no effort to reciprocate. On another level, the dilemma is related to Maria's sense of who she is and with whom she identifies. As such, the narrative is about how she makes sense of this interaction in an attempt to resolve a psychological tension between her working-class and academic subjectivities. Lastly, the narrative reflects class ideologies and conflicts between the working class and professional class, in particular, academia.

In this narrative, her brother-in-law and nephew were cast in working-class roles; they were the movers. Maria was in a traditional female role. She portrayed herself as appreciative and wanting to repay their kindness by providing something nice for them. As the action unfolded, Maria made two contradictory moves related to her sense of self and social positioning. First, she distanced herself from the mustard by claiming that she did not eat mustard. She added to this stance by belittling the idea that Grey Poupon was "loftier" than "plain old French's" mustard. Maria understood that the mustard symbolized putting on airs and being "out in left field," detached from their lives. Her strategy to reduce the distance between them by distancing herself from the mustard failed. The mustard signifies that she is removed from the real world, dwelling in an ivory tower. The conflict between Maria and her brother-in-law is about lifestyle; as such, it has some similarity to my personal narrative about Tanglewood.

In the narrative, Maria resolved the conflict by shifting to a different strategy: defending her lifestyle. She justified her purchase, arguing that she and her friends are more open, expansive, and experimental, in contrast to these "red meat and potatoes" kind of guys. This implies that Grey Poupon is better or more sophisticated than basic French's, as its name suggests. This strategy positions Maria as different, perhaps superior, to her male relatives and as such acknowledges the distance between them. Her earlier comment about trying to "interact at their level" may suggest a sense of superiority or awareness that she is perceived as such. Through this strategy, Maria positioned herself with her highly educated academic friends, claiming her identity and lifestyle as an academic, and acknowledging that she has changed from her working-class origins—how she "grew up to something else."

Maria's narrative relates class, occupation, education, interests, and taste, illustrating the signification of power relations in and through social roles and lifestyle. By purchasing Grey Poupon instead of French's mustard,

Maria invited her relatives to participate in her lifestyle. In a sense, she offered them the spoils of her sophisticated lifestyle in contrast to their more mundane tastes. Perhaps it was unconscious, or perhaps it was a small way to bring them into her world, to reduce the distance between them. Although her brother-in-law and nephew were willing to carry the artifacts of her research in Central America, they drew a line at adopting her consumption patterns. Or did they? We do not know whether or not they ate the mustard.

This narrative is about a "little issue" that points out "big differences" in lifestyle, revealing class relations in mixed-class families. The class conflict is covert: There is no direct talk about class relations or social status. The mustard (Grey Poupon vs. French's) symbolizes class interests. The contradictory moves that Maria makes in this narrative—distancing herself from the mustard and then defending her lifestyle—reveals a complex subjectivity that encompasses the contradictions inherent in the hierarchy of the class system. In/through the narrative, Maria shifted between class positions, resolving class tensions by asserting her lifestyle as "normal" and identifying with her highly educated, world-traveled friends.

Discussion

These narratives suggest that some family members view academic siblings as conceited or "out in left field," detached from the real world. Such critiques suggest that academics are a "class" apart from other professionals, a class of intellectuals (the intelligentsia). Women from the working class who become academics may be treated differently from those who become physicians or computer engineers. The latter are unambiguously useful in society, prosperous, and respected; in contrast, the world of academe is unimaginable to many people, particularly those who have not attended college or been exposed to the liberal arts. The academic family member is probably earning an unimpressive salary, and her motivation may puzzle her family. She was probably to the political left of her family and less engaged in relationships. Her choices in food, dress, entertainment, and other consumer goods may position her differently from both working-class and middle-class women (B. Greenberg, personal communication, March 26, 2004).

Upward mobility from working class to academe provokes internal conflicts related to class identity. Individuals may resolve conflicts between internalized working-class and upper-middle-class identities in different ways. Working-class academics might (1) fully assimilate into academic culture and reject their working-class background, (2) resist academic culture and wear their working-class identity like a badge, (3) claim an outsider status in both cultures, or (4) claim a border identity with a foot in both cultures. Although these resolutions may appear fixed, the social construction of self involved in such resolutions is a fluid, dynamic process that is always subject to change (Butler, 1993; Sampson, 1993). Insofar as identities are constructed in/through socially situated relationships within a moving field of existing power relations, individuals may construct context-specific resolutions to class-identity conflicts that are partial, temporal, and specific to a particular situation. It is also important to remember that the narratives in this chapter reflect the ways in which participants made meaning of events at a particular point in their lives. The meanings they make of past experiences will continue to evolve as they develop and encounter new situations.

Upward mobility is a progressive narrative that emphasizes the ways in which individuals have improved their lives and reproduces a belief in individualism. A consequence of progressive narratives is the tendency to represent the place of origin as inferior to the present location. This feature leads to the kind of dilemma Casey described: How can she perceive her sisters' lives as successful? There is a danger of depicting working-class family members as static, "locked in" individuals who are left behind, rather than as people who are also developing and who value aspects of their working-class lives. Working-class and poor people continue to develop, achieve, and make important contributions in their respective communities, such as Casey's sisters raising "good children" and contributing to their communities. It is also important to note that the career choices that these participants made limited and constrained them in particular ways. Like many professional women, Nancy, Casey, and Maria do not have children. The tension between career and family was particularly painful for Maria and Casey, both of whom expressed sadness when they compared themselves to their siblings in this area.

Implications for Clinicians

The analysis in this chapter demonstrates some of the ways in which upward mobility of one family member through higher education has consequences for that individual and his or her family. Bringing a class lens to therapeutic encounters can help practitioners identify class-related distress (which takes a variety of forms) and help clients develop healthy ways of dealing with class conflicts. For example, a clinician working with a young woman who is experiencing pain from distant relationships with her brothers (such as Nancy) might focus on helping the client process the loss associated with a relational "gap" and find ways to build relationships with her brothers.

Although these narratives are particular to the lives of these participants, some general implications for clinicians can be drawn from the analysis. First and foremost, it is important to identify class-related phenomena functioning at interpersonal and intrapersonal levels, including internalized classism. Explicitly discussing class issues is a crucial first step that enables people to externalize class conflicts, process painful emotions, and develop strategies to negotiate class differences. Second, whether working with an individual, a couple, or family, it is important to process emotions associated with class experiences, including loss, grief, anger, shame, inferiority, and superiority. Third, as an outcome of processing emotions, individuals need to develop understanding and insight into their experiences and healthy ways of processing class-related injuries. Fourth, in addition to helping clients identify ways to continue comfortable contact with family members (Ross, 1995), therapists can assist clients in identifying valuable aspects of working-class and academic lives, and finding ways to hold positive aspects of multiple class identities (Jones, 2001, 2003). To do so, therapists must examine their own class experiences and biases and the ways in which class attitudes are reflected in their relationships with clients (Leeder, 1996).

Critical self-reflection is an important part of this process for clients and therapists alike. People tend to be more comfortable talking about how they are marginalized than how they are privileged, and it is particularly difficult to examine our own feelings of superiority. It may be difficult to escape feeling superior when you are more highly educated than others in your family. Family members may assign a special status to a person with a doctorate, displacing birth order or gender statuses, and defer to your advice or resist it as utterances from "Miss Perfect." Class-conscious practice requires a critical examination of the ways in which we, as therapists and teachers, may give off vibes of superiority, contributing to social distances and estrangements.

By attending to class, therapists can help upwardly mobile clients identify and deal with the psychological and relational costs of mobility. However, class-related distress is a broad phenomenon affecting people at all levels of the class hierarchy, albeit in differing ways. From a psychodynamic perspective, self is constituted through a process of reflexive appropriation, occurring at the intersection of subjectivity (mind, moods, attitudes, opinions), the unconscious, and the social (Elliott, 1992). Dominant ideology about class relations is internalized at a deep unconscious level and is an active component in the negotiation of self (Elliott, 1992). Social status differences within families, regardless of an individual's class location, can cause psychological distress and interpersonal conflicts. Therefore, it is important for clinicians to listen for class-related distress when working with clients from a variety of class backgrounds.

References

Barker, J. (1995). White working-class men and women in academia. *Race, Gender and Class, 3*(1), 65–77.

Bettie, J. (2003). *Women without class: Girls, race and identity.* Berkeley: University of California Press.

Bourdieu, P. (1985). *Outline of a theory of practice.* New York: Cambridge University Press.

Bourdieu, P. (1998). *Practical reason: On the theory of action.* Palo Alto, CA: Stanford University Press.

Butler, J. (1993). *Bodies that matter: On the discursive limits of "sex."* New York: Routledge.

Charmaz, K. (2000). Grounded theory: Objectivist and constructivist methods. In N. K. Denzin & Y. S. Lincoln (Eds.), *Handbook of qualitative research* (2nd ed., pp. 509–535). Thousand Oaks, CA: Sage.

Dews, C. L. B., & Law, C. L. (Eds.). (1995). *This fine place so far from home: Voices of academics from the working class.* Philadelphia: Temple University Press.

Elliott, A. (1992). *Social theory and psychoanalysis in transition: Self and society from Freud to Kristeva.* Cambridge, MA: Blackwell.

Freire P. (1992). *Pedagogy of the oppressed.* New York: Continuum. (Original work published 1970)

Gee, J. P. (1991). A linguistic approach to narrative. *Journal of Narrative and Life History, 1*, 15–39.

Gilbert, D., & Kahl, J. A. (1993). *The American class structure: A new synthesis.* Belmont, CA: Wadsworth.

Hertzberg, J. F. (1996). Internalizing power dynamics: The wounds and the healing. *Women and Therapy, 18*(3–4), 129–148.

Jones, S. J. (1998a). Narrating multiple selves and embodying subjectivity: Female academics from the working class. *Dissertation Abstract International, 60*(015), 398.

Jones, S. J. (1998b). Subjectivity and class consciousness: The development of class identity. *Journal of Adult Development, 5*(3), 145–162.

Jones, S. J. (2001). Embodying working-class subjectivity and narrating self: "We were the hired help." In D. L. Tolman & M. Brydon-Miller (Eds.), *From subjects to subjectivities: A handbook of interpretive and participatory methods* (pp. 145–162). New York: New York University Press.

Jones, S. J. (2003). Complex subjectivities: Class, ethnicity, and race in women's narratives of upward mobility. *Journal of Social Issues, Special Issue on Psychological Meanings of Social Class in the Context of Education, 59*(4), 803–820.

Jones, S. J. (2004). A place where I belong: Working-class women's pursuit of higher education. *Race, Gender, and Class, 11*(3).

Langellier, K. M., & Hall, D. L. (1989). Interviewing women: A phenomenological approach to feminist communication research. In K. Carter & C. Spitzack (Eds.), *Doing research on women's communication: Perspectives on theory and method* (pp. 193–220). Norwood, NJ: Ablex.

Leeder, E. (1996). Speaking rich people's words: Implications for a feminist class analysis and psychotherapy. *Women and Therapy, 18*(3–4), 45–57.

Levesque-Lopman, L. (2000). Listen, and you will hear: Reflections on interviewing from a feminist phenomenological perspective. In L. Fisher & L. Embree (Eds.), *Feminist phenomenology* (pp. 103–132). New York: Klewer Academic/ Plenum Press.

Miner, V. (1993). Writing and teaching with class. In M. M. Tokarczyk & E. A. Fay (Eds.), *Working-class women in the academy: Laborers in the knowledge factory* (pp. 73–86). Amherst: University of Massachusetts Press.

Mishler, E. G. (1991). *Research interviewing: Context and narrative*. Cambridge, MA: Harvard University Press.

Mishler, E. G. (2000). *Storylives: Craftartists' narratives of identity*. Cambridge, MA: Harvard University Press.

Overall, C. (1995). Nowhere at home: Toward a phenomenology of working-class consciousness. In C. L. B. Dews & C. L. Law (Eds.), *This fine place so far from home: Voices of academics from the working class* (pp. 209–220). Philadelphia: Temple University Press.

Reay, D. (1996). Dealing with difficult differences: Reflexivity and social class in feminist research. *Feminism and Psychology, 6*(3), 443–456.

Reinharz, S. (1992). *Feminist methods in social research*. New York: Oxford University Press.

Riessman, C. K. (1993). *Narrative analysis*. Newbury Park, CA: Sage.

Ross, J. L. (1995). Social class tensions within families. *American Journal of Family Therapy, 23*(4), 338–350.

Rubin, L. B. (1976). *Worlds of pain: Life in the working-class family*. New York: Basic Books.

Rubin, L. B. (1994). *Families on the fault line: America's working class speaks about the family, the economy, race, and ethnicity*. New York: HarperCollins.

Russell, G. M. (1996). Internalized classism: The role of class in the development of self. *Women and Therapy, 18*(3–4), 59–71.

Ryan, J., & Sackrey, C. (1996). *Strangers in paradise: Academics from the working class* (2nd ed.). Boston: South End Press. (Original work published 1984)

Sampson, E. E. (1993). *Celebrating the other: A dialogic account of human nature*. Boulder, CO: Westview Press.

Tokarczyk, M. M., & Fay, E. A. (Eds.). (1993). *Working-class women in the academy: Laborers in the knowledge factory*. Amherst: University of Massachusetts Press.

Walkerdine, V. (1996). Working-class women: Psychological and social aspects of survival. In S. Wilkinson (Ed.), *Feminist social psychologies: International perspectives* (pp. 145–162). Buckingham, UK: Open University Press.

Willis, P. (1981). *Learning to labor: How working class kids get working class jobs* (2nd ed.). New York: Columbia University Press.

Zweig, M. (2000). *The working class majority: America's best kept secret*. Ithaca, NY: Cornell University Press.

PART III

Women and Paid Work

CHAPTER 8

The Impact of Culture on Women's Meanings and Experiences of Work

ASIAN AMERICAN AND ASIAN IMMIGRANT WOMEN

Mizuho Arai

Fourteen years ago, I came to Boston at the age of 21 to go to college. I had spent 3 weeks in Los Angeles when I was 17, visiting with an American family and learning English. But Boston was not the same as Los Angeles, and I was not the same as I had been at 17. I cried every day and lost my confidence because of the language barrier. Although I had studied English before I came to the United States, I was not able to speak and understand the everyday English I was actually hearing. I even had nightmares about failing exams and papers because of this language barrier. All of my confidence and pride were gone! But I was determined to learn and create my career.

When I was growing up, I never felt like I "fit in" to Japanese society because I wanted to be independent and free to do whatever I wanted to do. I wanted to be a career woman with a family. I wasn't sure I could have it all like that. I didn't expect to get married easily, because many Japanese men do not support women who desire both a career and a marriage.

As an Asian immigrant to America, I faced many challenges in the journey to my present place. I am now married to a white European American man, whom I met in a psychology master's program. At that time in my life, I was not expecting anything in my personal life because I was totally invested in my academic life and career. But I met this wonderful man. My husband had traveled extensively through Australia and many Asian countries, and he is culturally sensitive and respects Japanese culture and women. Thus he understood my culture and experiences (and I have not experienced some of the typical issues that many interracial and intercultural couples confront). We married soon after I completed a PhD program.

Currently I teach psychology, women's studies, and sociology university courses. My husband has recently started medical school, and we are planning to have children very soon. In the United States, as an immigrant woman from Japan, I have found a way to have career and family, to bring together these cultures and expectations to find success. My in-laws and my family, with the exception of my father, are very supportive. My father does not understand me and, clinging to traditional cultural values, he wishes to control my life. He has his own dilemma: He is proud of what I have achieved, but he feels threatened by my achievements. I don't "fit" his idea of an Asian woman.

My survival and success in my studies and my career depended upon the availability of many mentors—professors and friends who took the time to provide support and encouragement. For me, this support network has been essential, and I suspect it is for others too. Clinicians can and should be an important part of this network. But to do so, they must understand the impacts of culture and cultural differences on the lives of women.

This chapter discusses the impact of culture on women's meanings and experiences of work through exploring, in particular, the experiences of Asian American and Asian immigrant women as examples of the impact of cultural differences and expectations on women's experience of career and family.

Culture exerts a strong influence on people's attitudes toward, and their values about, family and work. People from a traditional society (e.g., Asian countries) frequently agree about traditionally gendered roles of men and women and adhere to traditional, frequently more conservative, morality and values. Although Asian people are moving toward an equal status for men and women, a gender gap still exists. The idea of combining career, marriage, and family is viewed as a much more remote and unrealistic thought for many Asian immigrant women. A major problem for Asian immigrant women (and Asian American women from traditional families) who wish to continue their careers after they marry, and particularly after they have children, is that so often they are expected to take on, almost single-handedly, the double burden of career plus housekeeping, child care, and care of the elderly. One aspect of this problem involves the attitudes, assumptions, and norms surrounding women's roles, which force women to bear a double burden, as illustrated by the voice of this Asian American woman:

"I don't think it's true that Asian women lack confidence. We know the reality of traditional Asian values and accept it and give up trying to change it. Actually, we do have hopes for our future, but women's success is prevented by the social system and its traditions. If Asian women want to keep working after marriage they then double their workload, because many husbands don't help with housework, and if they have a child, the women have to bring up the child, do housework, plus work. But it's very hard for us, so we choose either marriage or work."

Asian and Asian American men admit that women bear a double burden, but this is rarely questioned, as the voice of this male student demonstrates:

"It's fine for wives to work, as long as they continue to perform all of the necessary household chores and take care of children, so that husbands don't have to take on any of those responsibilities."

The prospect of having to confront cultural dilemmas and obstacles serves as a deterrent to planning for careers as part of their adult life paths for many young Asian immigrant and Asian American women from traditional families. Although there are many specific differences among Asian American women, those who are first generation from whichever culture seem to experience the most intense conflicts between their culture of origin and the Western culture to which they have immigrated. Many women who undertake the effort to have both career and family abandon their careers if they are economically able to do so, frustrated by the biases they encounter in the workplace and society, as well as the pressures from their families. Clinicians who come in contact with these women can help them confront and deal with the problems they are likely to face regarding career and family development.

Attending to Heterogeneity

Although there are differences between Asian immigrants and Asian Americans in comparison to European Americans, there is also great heterogeneity within people of Asian heritage in the United States. When empirical research on ethnic minority groups has been conducted, it has tended to follow a conventional model of race that subsumes numerous ethnic groups into one of four racial categories: Asian, black, Hispanic and white. For example, culturally distinct ethnic groups such as Cambodians, Chinese, Filipinos, Koreans, Japanese, Pakistanis, Taiwanese, and Vietnamese are lumped into one racial category: Asian. A conventional racialized model assumes that membership in a racial group is analogous with shared cultural values, beliefs, and attitudes.

However, each racial category has within-group ethnic cultural differences (Takeuchi, Uehara, & Maramba, 1999). For example, specific Asian American ethnic groups are distinguished from one another by characteristics such as language, cultural values and beliefs, history, religion, acculturation, place of birth, socioeconomic status, and age. Agbayani-Siewert (2004) indicated that the method of examining the values, beliefs, and attitudes shaped by culture, which includes social factors such as race, is well suited for studying the Asian American population, which is composed of 25 subgroups (Uba, 1993) and is the fastest growing racial population in the United States. Thus it is important to understand the existence of ethnic cultural differences within racial categories.

For example, there are significant ethnic differences between Korean and Vietnamese families as well as differences in the degree to which they conform to traditional family practices. Confucianism appears to have a stronger influence on the traditional family system in Korea than in Vietnam. In Vietnamese families there is a greater tendency for siblings to pool resources in providing filial care rather than relying on the elder son alone; this practice might be related to their poorer economic circumstances. In addition, Vietnamese women are permitted stronger kinship ties to their family of origin upon marriage than are Korean women, who are expected to live with their in-laws if they marry an elder son (Hurh, 1998).

Immigrant Asian groups (such as Koreans, Chinese, and Indians) also differ significantly from refugee Asian groups (such as Vietnamese and Cambodian) in relation to education and economic achievement related to career (2000 U.S. census data compiled by the Institute for Asian American Studies, 2004). For example, a higher proportion of Asian Indians, Chinese, and Japanese, as compared to the overall U.S. population, graduate from college and receive postgraduate education or training. However, 85.7% of Cambodian females and 71% of Vietnamese females have *less than a high school* education in Massachusetts. Data also suggest that Asian Americans as a group have the highest average family income in the United States, but Southeast Asians are among the poorest Americans. Those living below the poverty level include 24.6% of Cambodians and 21.2% of Vietnamese in Massachusetts (Institute for Asian American Studies, 2004). A substantially higher percentage of Vietnamese and Cambodians receive public assistance than do other Asian groups. Thus there are differences of education level and economics that are related to career and work issues among different Asian immigrant/refugee families. Clinicians must be aware of the great heterogeneity among Asian Americans when counseling about career issues.

Hap was a refugee who lost her family in a refugee camp and came to the United States 15 years ago from a farming background in rural Cambodia. She had received a junior high school equivalent education in Cambodia and worked as a sales person in a retail store and cleaned houses on evenings and weekends in order to support her family. She also took care of all household and child care responsibilities, because her husband believed in traditional family roles. Hap did not speak English well. Her limited language abilities made it difficult for her to obtain better-paying employment, but her husband had even greater challenges finding well-paying employment. Although he would have preferred to be the primary financial earner, Hap's income was necessary for the family's survival. Hap also had difficulties working with care systems because of the language barrier, so her daughter always went with her to doctor appointments to help her mother communicate with the doctor. This need for translation, as well as the financial demands on the family, affected the family roles and relationships.

Shivani was an Indian immigrant who came to the United States to study management. Her family was affluent and her father held the equivalent of a graduate degree. Shivani's education and background have contributed to her fluency in English and her associated educational and career success. After graduation with her bachelor's degree, Shivani worked as a bank manager and entered into an arranged marriage. Her husband supported her choice to have a career until she became pregnant. At that time, Shivani quit her job to take care of the baby. Her husband had a well-paying job that supported her family financially, so she could stay home and take care of her baby (and future children) with the help of a domestic servant.

Although more research is needed to examine specific Asian ethnic differences in family practices, existing literature (e.g., Agbayani-Siewert, 2004) does indicate patterns of similarities among the family systems of Koreans, Vietnamese, and other Asian ethnic groups that differentiate them from American family patterns—although, as Uba (1993) pointed out, most of the research has been descriptive rather than explanatory and has focused only on Chinese and Japanese Americans. The role prescriptions, family obligations, hierarchical relations, lack of emotional expressiveness, and collectivist values associated with the traditional family systems of China, Japan, Korea, Vietnam, and other Asian cultures contrast sharply with the emphasis on individualism, self-sufficiency, egalitarianism, expressiveness, and self-development in mainstream U.S. culture (e.g., Hurh, 1998; Min, 1998; Uba, 1993).

The Importance of Culture

Traditional Asian values emphasize solidarity, hierarchal relations, and filial piety (e.g., Min, 1998; Uba, 1993). Priority is placed on family interests over individual desires and needs in order to maintain stability and harmony. Status distinctions guide the way in which members are to interact with one another. For example, younger members are expected to display respect, deference, and obedience to elders, and wives are expected to show the same to their husbands and parents-in-law. Children, including adult offspring, are forbidden from expressing dissenting opinions or confronting parents, which is viewed as disrespectful (Min, 1998). Emotional expressiveness, including displays of affection, is discouraged, and self-control is emphasized (Hurh, 1998). Family ties and roles are central from birth until death, with a strong emphasis on family devotion. In general, parents are expected to rely on their children's support in later life. In Asian and Asian American families, the care and financial support of aging parents is a family matter, frequently the responsibility of the eldest son and his wife, who are expected to live under the same roof as the parents. Korean and Vietnamese cultures also derive from Confucianism a respect for the well educated, and education is considered the primary means for social mobility (Min, 1998).

These cultural values related to gender roles and family interactions have significant effects on Asian American women's careers. The emphasis within traditional Asian cultures of certain values may create challenges for Asian immigrant women who are seeking to prioritize careers or make nontraditional decisions related to balancing family and career. These Asian values, as noted above, include the importance of hierarchy according to generation, age, and gender; filial piety and family obligations; and the maintenance of solidarity and social harmony. Chuang and Lee (2003) found that Asian husbands' negative attitudes toward working wives would discourage the women from attaching to the labor market more value than to the presence of young children in the family. On the other hand, nonworking women's own attitudes toward working women did not show any significant effect on their work-related choices and commitments. This finding may imply that husbands' attitudes toward traditional gender roles might dominate women's career decisions. The implication is that in order to raise the rate of female labor participation among Asian American women, educating women to develop a perception of modern gender roles is not enough, by itself, perhaps particularly in collective cultures; it is even more critical to educate men to change their traditional attitudes toward gender roles.

Huong was a 22-year-old college student. Her Cambodian father and Vietnamese mother immigrated to the United States when Huong and her sisters were small children. Her parents held several jobs to support their family, which included Huong's uncles and aunts and their children. Huong performed well in school, and her parents were proud of her accomplishments and wanted to ensure that she would do well enough to enter a university. I met her when she took an undergraduate family and child psychology course that I taught. During the course of the term, Huong revealed that her father was pressuring her to marry a person whom she had never met. Her wish was to attend graduate school, but her father had arranged a marriage to take place upon the completion of her undergraduate program. Huong's mother knew she was very unhappy and did not want to push her daughter into an arranged marriage, but she felt she must follow her husband's decision. Huong's uncles had discouraged her from attending college, saying that it was a waste of her time; interestingly, her aunts have been supportive. Huong discussed her dilemmas with me. Her choice seemed to be whether (1) to pursue her educational goals or (2) to make her parents happy by entering into the arranged marriage.

Huong went to a counseling center and met with a clinician who was not culturally sensitive. The counselor interpreted Huong's desires to pursue her own dreams and goals, despite her family's hesitancy in allowing her to do so, as Huong being "oppressed" by her family. She perceived Huong's family as being "enmeshed" and Huong as too "dependent" on her family. The counselor contrasted Huong's personal desires versus her family's desires and could not see that Huong had multiple personal desires: to go graduate school but *also* to be a good daughter, as her family and culture defines it.

Huong came to talk to me after this disappointing session at the counseling center. She told me that her counselor did not understand her cultural background. She stated that she felt more comfortable talking to me because I am an Asian immigrant. I spoke with Huong about her multiple desires and those of her parents. I suggested that the support and understanding of her aunts might mean that they would be able and willing to speak on her behalf. Perhaps it would be possible to marry and pursue a graduate degree? Opening a conversation within the family would be the first step toward cultural understandings for Huong and her family. Thinking about Huong later, I also thought that it would be helpful for Huong to speak with other Asian immigrant women like herself, so that they could share their experiences and be supportive of each other. It would be helpful for clinicians to consider group therapy with Asian immigrant women such as Huong.

Decisions about work and family such as Huong faced may be complicated even more by the fact that Asian women's earnings are frequently necessary for a family's survival, as in the example of Hap. Immigrant men's wages decrease when they come to the United States, whereas the gender wage differentials are greater in Hong Kong (Glenn, 1996, p. 86). Even though Asian immigrant women's husbands have full-time jobs, it is not enough for their families. For example, Hap's husband earned about

$18,000 a year, a salary that was below the poverty level for a family of that size. Studying women in New York's Chinatown, Zhou (1992) found that the income earned by women in the labor market was necessary for the family's economic well-being because of the low-income jobs available to both immigrant men (who tended to work in the restaurant trade) and women (largely in garment work). Economic necessity is likely the chief reason that Asian immigrant women seek work or better-paying work (Grahame, 2003). The responses from the women in Grahame's study suggested that many immigrant Asian women defined their responsibilities to family to include their economic responsibility; they did not make a distinction between provisioning activities and nurturing ones. The job training they entered was seen as essential for their families' survival.

In Grahame's (2003) study it was not only the financial boost offered by the training that was attractive; the possibility that the job training would provide health care benefits was also important. In many Asian immigrant families, it was often the wife's job that provided benefits; many of the men worked in the restaurant industry, where jobs usually lacked such benefits. There were times in many families when obtaining these benefits was a matter of life or death.

For Asian immigrant families such as Hap's, the cultural transition of immigration can induce a particular type of stress for the husband, who is accustomed to fulfilling the role of breadwinner. Status inconsistency occurs after immigration, when skills, prior employment experiences, and educational backgrounds do not translate into jobs that are commensurate with actual experience and training. Due to racial discrimination and lack of proficiency in the English language, many immigrants experience unemployment or underemployment. Many rules and values that were once effective in immigrants' homelands are no longer relevant in their new host country. In many cases, unskilled jobs are more accessible to immigrant women than to men, thereby challenging family structure and roles. As a result, gender role reversals and immigrant women's improved social status produce family conflict and contribute to domestic violence in some families. Thus work experiences and choices have major implications for the well-being of Asian immigrant women and their families.

Individualism and Collectivism

The cultural value orientations of individualism and collectivism provide one useful construct with which to explore some of the cultural dimensions of values related to work and career for Asian American women (Arai, 2002; Leong, 1997). Triandis and his colleagues (1990) noted that *individualism* refers to cultural patterns that promote emotional detachment and independence from others, whereas *collectivism* represents cultural patterns that emphasize social integrity and regard for in-group (e.g., familial, community, or national) norms. The U.S. culture is typically described as more highly individualistic, fostering *idiocentric* personality traits such as self-reliance and self-realization (Leong, 1993). Cultural groups typically described as more highly collectivistic in orientation, such as Asian American cultures, advance *allocentric* personality traits or themes such as interdependence, loyalty, and family integrity (Triandis et al., 1990). Collectivist cultures place priority on group goals over individual goals. Therefore, collectivists' occupational choices reflect less on their own individual preferences and more on their perception of in-group expectations for an individual. Collectivists tend to accede to their families' wishes for them in life, including work and career choices; thus their families are likely to play a significant role on their career development.

Extended to the domain of career development, research findings (e.g., Leong, 1993) imply differences between individualists and collectivists in terms of their occupational choices and career plans. A key difference suggests that collectivists, living in individualist cultures, base their occupational plans and career choices more on the norms and expectations of their reference groups (e.g., family; Leong, 1993) as compared to individualists living in individualist cultures, who are likely to place greater emphasis on their own personal attitudes and goals in making their career plans and choices. Thus career counseling interventions for collectivists, such as Asian immigrants and Asian Americans in the United States, may need to incorporate the perspectives of the client's family and community rather than attend solely to his or her personal goals and values (Betz & Fitzgerald, 1993).

For Asian and Asian American women, negotiating the different cultural demands related to collectivistic versus individualistic cultures may create particular challenges. Because traditional sex-role behavior is emphasized in Asian cultures, it seems likely that the career aspirations of Asian Americans would be influenced by traditional sex typing. For example, Leung, Ivey, and Suzuki (1994) found that Asian American male students were more likely than European American male students to consider traditionally male occupations. However, Asian female students were more likely than their European American counterparts to consider nontraditional occupations for themselves.

The case of Huong earlier in this chapter is an example. Huong not only had difficulties because she wanted to go to graduate school rather than get married, but she also had difficulties related to her choice of major and career. She wanted to study sociology, but her parents wanted her to study accounting, which offered more financial stability. A collectivistic

cultural value of high respect for, as well as obedience to, parents is a dominating influence in many Asian families. Like Huong's parents, Asian families often expect their children to comply with family wishes, even if it
means sacrificing their own dreams and goals. Asian parents consider occupational alternatives that could give them the greatest survival value in the
U.S. social structure and tend to avoid occupations that could bring them
into direct contact with racial and cultural discrimination. Moreover, Asian
collectivistic cultures often encourage the individual to behave within the
traditional sex-role boundaries. Therefore, Asian American women are
more likely to consider college majors and occupations in the sciences and
technical areas because their parents expect a high value in selecting high-
prestige career options. Because conforming to the expectations of parents
is the way of life, Asian immigrant women are faced with the challenge of
resolving primary issues related to the existence of two differing
worldviews: those of their own culture (collectivism) and those of the dominant culture (individualism).

Clinical Implications

Clinicians can help their Asian American and Asian immigrant female clients learn about civil, legal, and political systems as well as American methods of problem solving, so that they are prepared (i.e., have the needed attitudes and behaviors or interpersonal skills) to deal effectively with social
systems and organizations. Cultural sensitivity and empathy for changing
mores are two primary clinical requisites.

First clinicians can identify the resources an immigrant family
already knows about or has used or managed in other environments.
Knowledge about the background of Asian immigrant families is also
necessary, including (1) the overall history of Asian immigration; (2) environment of the country from which the family emigrated; (3) the traditional cultural values of the specific ethnicity and country, especially concerning the family; (4) help-seeking behaviors of the people in that
country; and (5) coping behaviors of the people in that country. Some
Asian American and Asian immigrant women may see counseling as
shameful and embarrassing because of a cultural stigma attached to emotional expression in their societies (Atkinson, Morten, & Sue, 1998). As
noted, interdependence and collectivism are highly valued in Asian cultures, along with maintaining harmony and respecting familial authority.
Moreover, an emphasis on privacy may prevent Asian American and
Asian immigrant women from seeking help from outsiders and nonfamily
members. Some of these women, too, may feel uncomfortable expressing

themselves in English, so they tend to keep problems to themselves or rely on friends, family, and professors for help (Abe, Talbo, & Geelhoed, 1998; Yeh, Inose, Kobori, & Chang, 2001).

Asian American and Asian immigrant women should be encouraged to explain the struggles they are experiencing in attempting to balance two cultures in a respectful way. They might share how they are trying to find connection with other Asian American or Asian immigrant women, stay connected with the families, and become comfortable with their identities as Asian American or Asian immigrant women. Goals of culturally sensitive counseling include easing adjustment to U.S. culture, normalizing clients' experiences, and increasing coping skills in a safe, supportive environment. Social support validates the experiences of immigrant women and provides a powerful coping resource. It is helpful to provide opportunities for Asian American and Asian immigrant women to network with other Asian women in order to build a multicultural supportive community. This group can be a setting for socializing, practicing English, addressing academic/career, personal, and social concerns, and acculturation stressors. Empowering resources such as knowledge or information about where and how to obtain jobs, health care, education, and so on, are important for counselors to provide.

Intervention techniques such as family structural therapy, group therapy, and psychoeducational workshops may assist clients in (1) restoring orderly hierarchical family relationships, (2) teaching new roles and modifing family functions, (3) changing the family's perception of itself from incomplete extended family unit to altered but functional family system, and (4) building a new sense of belonging in the community. It is crucial that clinicians do not impose their own values but, rather, extend flexible, perceptive, and sensitive openness to the cultural values of the family. For example, clinicians may ask the family to articulate how families in their native country would deal with the particular problem with which the client is concerned. An important strategy to establish trust when clinicians are not Asian American is to honor the Asian tradition of respecting parental authority. Moreover, reframing the family dilemma in positive terms rather than blaming terms may promote changes in the feelings of anger, guilt, and confusion that are imposed by immigrant status and acculturation difficulties and then misattributed as negative feelings about the family. In conclusion, it is important for clinicians (1) to understand the strong impact of culture, particularly for immigrant women, (2) to consider the differences within a racial or ethnic minority group as well as the similarities in contrast to the dominant group, and (3) to adapt their pace and method of developing an effective helping relationship to the idiosyncratic and cultural variables of each client.

References

Abe, J., Talbo, D., & Geelhoed, R. (1998). Effects of a peer program on international student adjustment. *Journal of College Student Development, 29,* 539–547.

Agbayani-Siewert, P. (2004). Assumptions of Asian American similarity: The case of Filipino and Chinese American students. *Social Work, 49*(1), 39–51.

Arai, M. (2002). Career development: Comparisons between Japanese and American women college students (Doctoral dissertation, Boston University, 2002). *Dissertation Abstracts International, 63,* 02B.

Atkinson, D. R., Morten, G., & Sue, D. W. (1998). *Counseling American minorities* (5th ed.). New York: McGraw-Hill.

Betz, N. E., & Fitzgerald, L. F. (1993). Individuality and diversity: Theory and research in counseling psychology. *Annual Review of Psychology, 44,* 343–381.

Chuang, H. L., & Lee, H. Y. (2003). The return on women's human capital and the role of male attitudes toward working wives: Gender roles, work interruption, and women's earnings in Taiwan. *American Journal of Economics and Society, 62*(2), 383–406.

Glenn, E. N. (1996). Split household, small producer and dual wage-earner: An analysis of Chinese American family strategies. In S. Coontz, M. Parson, & G. Raley (Eds.), *American families: A multicultural reader* (pp. 74–93). New York: Routledge.

Grahame, K. M. (2003). "For the family": Asian immigrant women's triple day. *Journal of Sociology and Social Welfare, 30*(1), 65–90.

Hurh, W. M. (1998). *The Korean Americans.* Westport, CT: Greenwood Press.

Institute for Asian American Studies. (2004). 2000 U.S. Census Data. *Community profiles in Massachusetts.* Retrieved October 14, 2004 from Institute for Asian American Studies website: www.iaas.umb.edu/research/census/community_profiles/

Leong, F. T. D. (1993). The counseling process with racial-ethnic minorities: The case of Asian Americans. *Career Development Quarterly, 42,* 26–40

Leong, F. T. L. (1997). Cross-cultural career psychology: Comment on Fouad, Harmon, and Borgen (1997) and Tracey, Watanabe, and Schneider (1997). *Journal of Counseling Psychology, 44,* 355–359.

Leung, S. A., Ivey, D., & Suzuki, L. (1994). Factors affecting the career aspirations of Asian Americans. *Journal of Counseling and Development, 72*(4), 404–410.

Min, P. G. (1998). *Traditions and changes: Korean immigrant families in New York.* Needham Heights, MA: Allyn & Bacon.

Takeuchi, D., Uehara, E., & Maramba, G. (1999). Cultural diversity and mental health treatment. In A. Horwitz & T. Scheid (Eds.), *The sociology of mental health* (pp. 550–565). New York: Oxford University Press.

Traiandis, H. C., McCusker, C., & Hui, C. H. (1990). Multimethod probes of individualism and collectivism. *Journal of Personality and Social Psychology, 59*(5), 1006–1020.

Uba, L. (1993). *Asian-Americans: Personality patterns, identity, and mental health*. New York: Guilford Press.

Yeh, C., Inose, M., Kobori, A., & Chang, T. (2001). Self and coping among college students in Japan. *Journal of College Student Development, 42,* 242–256.

Zhou, M. (1992). *Chinatown: The socioeconomic potential of an urban enclave*. Philadelphia: Temple University Press.

CHAPTER 9

Women in the Workplace
AN APPLICATION OF RELATIONAL–CULTURAL THEORY

Judith V. Jordan
Patricia Romney

In this chapter we present a workplace application of relational–cultural theory (RCT) to demonstrate some of the core principles of consulting about the issues of diversity, authenticity, mutual empowerment, and management of conflict and disconnection. The organization depicted in this case study is a large not-for-profit corporation that was experiencing increasing tensions around the racial diversity of the workforce and styles of management.

Diane, an organizational consultant, had been called in by a manager who was no longer with the organization at the time of the dilemma we are presenting. Diane was originally trained as a clinical psychologist but for many years has worked as an organization consultant, coach, and theory builder in the areas of leadership consultation, diversity issues, and relational–cultural understanding of organizational dynamics. She had worked with this organization for several years. The CEO who had called her in for this particular consultation about diversity was supportive but slightly remote. The original manager of the division for which Diane was consulting was highly passionate about working with the "differences" among her employees, but she had recently moved to another company. Diane's assessment was that the new manager, Mary, paid lip service to the diversity agenda but seemed lukewarm to the prospect of really examining the effects of difference and power differentials on the organization.

In this context Diane's job as consultant was complicated. She was officially hired to do some serious work on intense and potentially volatile group issues: The organization had shifted in the previous 2 years from a predominantly all-white management team to a more diverse group, and there had been visible tensions within the group about race as well as the style of management. Although Diane had been hired by one manager, she was currently carrying on her work with a new manager. On a personal level, she had a good relationship with Mary, the new manager; there seemed to be respect, and the two of them had worked hard to get through several anxious engagements, including one in which an employee had charged a superior with racial discrimination around a performance assessment. Diane, an African American, and Mary, a white woman, both recognized that race was a hot issue in this setting. Although the racial tensions were more obvious, if difficult, to address, the style of management with which Mary worked (a top-down, rather hard-line and formal way of doing things) was a less obvious source of tension in the organization.

This particular consultation dilemma arose when a Latina member of the organization, Nancy, asked to speak to Diane as she was leaving the building at the end of the day. Nancy felt that she had been slighted in a meeting and that her superior, a white woman, had been engaged in a racist exclusion of her. Diane helped this woman examine what had happened and what steps she could safely take in the organization to address her concern. As they were leaving, Mary, who was also the manager of Nancy's division, walked by, gazed intently at both of them, appeared upset, and then proceeded to the parking lot without speaking to them.

In this case we will see how an acute disconnection between Nancy and Mary and between Diane and Mary could have led to an impasse and breakdown of a productive work connection. Instead, through using RCT to guide the consultation, Diane and Mary worked to do "good conflict" (not a smooth, linear process) and to move back into a mutually empathic connection following their disconnection. The consultation thus led to movement in a positive direction for the organization and the individual people involved. In this example we emphasize the reworking of a connection between two people, a manager and the consultant; although this example could be trivialized as representing "an interpersonal crisis," it underscores the powerful but often unacknowledged impact of relationships on the overall functioning of organizations. When movement from personal disconnection and power manipulations to mutual listening and learning occurs, the impact goes beyond the individuals involved and is reflected in shifts in the organization. For instance, in this case, not only did Diane and Mary move from disconnection to reconnection but there was also a lessening of tension among the diverse groups that were struggling with the movement from a homogeneous white culture to a diverse culture.

This case also illustrates the complexity of such movement; not everyone experienced a "good" outcome, and there were moments when all felt at risk in some way. Relational practice does not promise warm, cozy, and immediately comfortable outcomes. Furthermore, the case touches on the highly sensitive issue of race and the complications that may occur when there are misfits between a dominant work culture and what might be called new, more relational values and styles of working. Informal alliances were as important here as formal lines of authority; it was only when those informal alliances were acknowledged that people could begin to experience a real sense of safety.

When Diane got home she had a message on her answering machine from Mary, reprimanding her for doing "extracurricular consultation," undermining Mary's authority, and going beyond the bounds of the consultation. Mary added that she had informed Nancy's superior of Nancy's "insubordination," thus jeopardizing Nancy's position as well. Although Diane recognized the emphasis on formal lines of authority that characterized Mary's style of management, she was shocked at the vehement tone and the impulsivity involved in her swift report to Nancy's supervisor. She also felt hurt and angry. Knowing that she was traveling early the next day to another city to do another consultation, she picked up the phone and left a message for Mary, saying that she wasn't sure she could continue the consultation in the light of this reprimand. Diane felt that her own authenticity was crucial to successful consultations and that she therefore had to speak authentically about her experience of being treated by Mary like a "bad child." She also knew she had some power in this situation, because Mary did not want to lose "points" with her superiors for not taking diversity seriously and being unable to work with Diane. Diane also felt the importance of honoring the trust that Nancy had placed in her by going outside the formal pathways of naming a grievance. Nancy, a member of a marginalized group in this organization, had wisely sought allies and strategic input. Mary's failure to appreciate the vulnerability of those at the margin (Nancy) as well as her traditional management style had led her to respond in a closed-down, authoritarian manner that jeopardized the goals of the consultation.

When Diane returned from her trip, she received an anxious phone call from Mary, saying that she couldn't sleep, was terribly upset, and wanted to talk to Diane. At that moment something changed for Diane. Hearing the authentically distressed message and the vulnerability of Mary helped her remember the history of good work that they had done together. Diane was able to find the human piece of their disconnection and begin to move back into a place of empathy. The conflict was real and needed to be acknowledged, and Diane needed to bring her understanding of the difficulty to Mary, even if Mary didn't like it. But she could only do this in the context of an appreciation of the ongoing connection they had. Race, gender, and power differentials all played a part in this series of interactions. Mary had moved out of her stuck position as "the boss," was willing to share her vulnerability with Diane, and could allow Diane to see that she had had an impact on her. Diane moved out of her distanced position and was therefore able to engage in an authentic conversation with Mary. Both women relinquished their entrenched "positions" and in doing so were more open to the other's experience. In this interaction, both women felt mutually empowered and better understood. This shift allowed the two of them to actually do some creative thinking about this particular dilemma (i.e., Nancy's experience of racism in the organization) and to expand that thinking into procedural and structural interventions that would address the relational dilemmas that inevitably arise around race, gender, and other areas of diversity. In this case, Diane and Mary decided to hold meetings with the managers and workers to talk about setting up a possible task force to work on these issues.

This case was presented to a small collaborative group of clinicians, consultants, and business academics who use the lens of RCT to try to better understand organizational dynamics. Both of us participated in this group. We are both psychologists interested in RCT, women's issues, antiracism work, and organizational dynamics. I (PR) am a black, multiracial/multicultural woman, an organizational coach who has consulted with many companies throughout the United States on leadership, hierarchy, race, and other organizational issues. I (JVJ) am a white woman, a practicing clinician, and a founding scholar at the Stone Center, who has been working on developing new models of women's psychological development and organizational functioning. The study group is interested in the creation of new models of organizational functioning and change. In particular, the group critiques existing dominant work cultures and the ways in which they invalidate the experience of marginalized people, specifically people of color and women.

The aims of this chapter are as follows:

1. To explore the need for new models of understanding women's experiences in organizations.

2. To suggest that RCT is a particularly useful lens through which to view the special strengths and ways of working that marginalized groups bring to the workplace. It is furthermore useful in working on the dilemmas that arise in an organization when diversity issues and differing values and styles of organizing cause clashes.

3. To examine issues of power and hierarchy, the valuing of authenticity, empathy, and good conflict, and making the invisible "visible" from the perspective of RCT.

4. To delineate how reworking disconnections is central at the individual level and how the personal/cultural disconnections must be reworked to preserve or foster the well-being of the organization. What has been called the "soft" stuff in organizations (the relational work) is actually at the core of organizational work but is rarely valued or acknowledged (Fletcher, 1999).

It is important for clinicians working with women involved in traditional organizations to examine the ways in which these organizations may invalidate the woman's experience and thus contribute to her depression, anxiety, and isolation. Alternatively, the workplace may become a place of empowerment and validation when real change in traditional, patriarchal organizational principles takes place. Along with other feminist and multi-cultural voices (e.g., Ault-Riche, 1986; Boyd-Franklin, 2003; Comas-Díaz & Greene, 1994; Gilligan, 1982; McGoldrick, Anderson, & Walsh, 1989; Miller, 1976; Mirkin, 1994), the RCT organizational model emphasizes the importance of context and empowering women to question invisible and implicit values and rules of conduct that may be at odds with their own. Increasingly, the world of work impacts women's well-being. We embrace a model that does not automatically privilege the existing rules and culture but emphasizes the importance of mutual change and growth. Rather than forcing square pegs into round holes or bemoaning the lack of fit, organizations must be responsive to the needs and values of their incoming workforce (no longer only white and male). Mutual change and responsiveness are at the core of the relational–cultural understanding of what creates growth and creativity both in therapy and at work.

Relational–Cultural Theory

RCT posits that people grow through and toward relationship throughout the lifespan (Jordan, Kaplan, Miller, Stiver, & Surrey, 1991; Miller & Stiver, 1997). Growth occurs through the movement of mutual empathy and mutual empowerment. The outcomes of good connections are what Miller called the five good things: zest, clarity, sense of worth, productivity/creativity, and desire for more connection (Miller & Stiver, 1997). *Zest* refers to an increased sense of energy as an outcome of the interaction. In *clarity*, both participants get to know themselves, the other person, and the relationship better. Both feel stronger, more competent, a greater *sense of worth*, and, as a result, engage in more creative action. Finally, good connection leads to a desire for more good connection; in this way, it is a model of ever-widening circles of connection and community building.

Relational practice, as outlined by RCT, stresses the value of mutual empowerment, authenticity, and mutual empathy. At a personal level, experiencing these qualities requires (1) an ability to allow mutual influence, (2) an openness to impact, and (3) the ability and willingness to bring oneself as fully as possible into the relationship, with an awareness of the possible impact on others.

RCT points out that the standards of development that emphasize the emergence of a "separate self," autonomy, independence, and competition create multiple pressures for individuals. Although the dominant culture of 21st-century United States celebrates the importance of these qualities, we are not—any of us—independent, autonomous beings. In the dominant system (white, male, middle class, heterosexual, Christian), safety is achieved by establishing power over others rather than through building mutual connection. "Power over" others, as part of an organized system of stratification, is exercised in a way that creates disconnection and isolation, diminishes one's sense of worth, and undermines creativity. This system of invalidation and disenfranchisement, of deadening disconnection, characterizes those categorizations of people (race, sex, sexual orientation, religion) that relegate some to less worthy or unacceptable places in the culture. People are shamed or denigrated by differences in the stratified systems. In a stratified culture cultural differences lead to major disconnection, whereas meeting at places of difference can facilitate enormous growth in an unstratified system.

RCT suggests that as individuals and groups we are most productive and creative when we can bring ourselves authentically and fully into relationships and interactions. In order to grow and learn, a certain amount of vulnerability (i.e., openness to influence) is necessary. Jean Baker Miller (1976) once commented that "authenticity and subordination are totally incompatible" (p. 98). She pointed to the importance of "good conflict" in relationships, suggesting that, without conflict, relationships and the people in them cannot really change or grow. Good conflict does not involve aggression (i.e., the intention to hurt or control the other) or dominance over another person (i.e., the intention to suppress the other's experience). RCT posits that disconnections occur in all relationships. Acute disconnections may occur through empathic failure, misunderstanding, or the nonresponsiveness of one person (particularly the person with more power), but do not necessarily lead to problems. In fact, if an acute disconnection occurs and the less powerful person can represent his or her experience of the disconnection to the more powerful person, and the more powerful person can respond in a way that makes it clear that the less powerful person has been heard and valued, then the connection is strengthened and both people experience an enhanced sense of relational competence. If, however, one cannot represent one's difference (of opinion, values, feelings), then one is forced to shift into inauthentic functioning—that is, keeping certain aspects of one's experience out of the relationship—which ultimately drains the relationship of its vitality and creativity. This dynamic occurs when the more powerful person either does not respond or responds in a rejecting, invalidating, or shaming way, resulting in the less powerful person feeling less safe and less engaged. At a macro level in an organization, this dynamic often leads to less creativity and a "dulling down" of the work exchange. It is the climate typical of organizations that are heavily stratified and hierarchical, where only certain kinds of feedback are heard by those in power. A power system characterized by rigidity and hierarchy often silences the less powerful groups.

RCT recognizes that at the organizational level, most people are not invited into full authenticity, that lines of power restrict the quality of authenticity that can exist. But within these bounds, organizations are seen to be healthier when individuals can expect mutual respect and influence, when managers listen to and take in the experiences of those they supervise, and when workers feel that they "matter" in the organization. Rigidity of power lines, intolerance of conflict, and failure to respond to the expression of conflict have adverse consequences for an organization. Nevertheless, many managers are taught to exercise power in a top-down manner, and many organizations fail to acknowledge the importance of relational skills.

Relational–Cultural Theory and Organizations

Although RCT has been developed primarily in the clinical/academic realm, it addresses the sociopolitical forces that undermine whole groups of people, and it challenges the primary psychological theories that privilege separation and hyperindividualism. The RCT group that explored this case is particularly interested in working with the issues of conflict and diversity to foster a workplace experience of the five good things and growth of connections as an outcome of relational practice. Goleman (1995) has pointed to the significant role of "emotional intelligence" in the workplace, providing considerable data for the importance of empathy, and Senge (1990) has addressed the importance of a two-way flow of information in what he calls the "learning organization." Neither of these models, however, fully addresses the issues of power, gender, and diversity. Fletcher (1996, 1999) outlines several crucial skills for transforming the workplace into a more relational environment: (1) empathic competence, (2) emotional competence, (3) authenticity, (4) fluid expertise, (5) vulnerability, (6) embedding outcome, (7) holistic thinking, and (8) response-ability.

The forces of mutual empathy and mutual empowerment are as important for an organization as for an individual, albeit often more complicated. There are structural differences in power that are real and supported by the organization; people in both the role of "more powerful" and "less powerful" are affected by the constraints of these arrangements. RCT points to the ideal goal of exercising power to empower others (e.g., as occurs in healthy childrearing practices, teaching, therapy, many friendships). However, it is acknowledged that in many organizations, a strong component of exercising power over others is either that of preserving the power differential or augmenting it. Some of this power is straightforward. For example, the supervisor has the power to evaluate, recommend pay changes and changes in status, write letters of recommendation, and fire people. The supervisor may also use shaming and humiliation, emphasizing the inferiority of the "down" person, as an extension of his or her power.

It is not that we expect to do away with all power dynamics in an organization or even suggest that hierarchy can be eliminated. However, in bringing a goal of mutuality to organizations, we are suggesting a way in which both people in a power imbalanced relationship can be open to being influenced by one another, can engage in mutual empathy, and can have profound respect for each other's position. This is not a top-down system in which there is a boss and a "yes man/woman." Although there is clear and necessary acknowledgment of the power structures and differences between people in the assigned power they hold in an organization, in individual interactions the possibility of mutual growth and change must exist. And those in a "power over" position must maintain an interest in the empowerment of the less powerful people.

Achieving mutual empowerment in the workplace involves taking actions to increase the collective productivity and sense of well-being at the same time that one's own productive involvement in the work is enhanced. It can involve "empathic teaching" (Fletcher, Jordan, & Miller, 2000), which takes into account the experience of the other as one conveys information or teaches skills. It involves giving help, receiving help without an element of shame, and recognizing the power of collaboration. A key feature of mutual empowerment is the practice of "fluid expertise," which is "the recognition that expertise does not remain statically in one person, but can shift with different people's abilities. . . . [It is about] an openness to learning from or being influenced by others and a willingness to let others experience this openness and know that they have influenced you" (Fletcher et al., 2000, p. 254). Being valued, knowing that we have an impact, that we matter, and being responded to empathically and with respect are essential to a sense of well-being, in or out of the workplace.

Responsiveness to one another's ideas, feelings, and values is one of the most powerful ways to demonstrate the respect and real openness to change that are at the core of growth-fostering relationships. Many impasses in organizations, as in dyadic relationships, arise around experiences of shame or feeling silenced. Both of these dangers existed in this consultation. Nancy was shamed for seeking "extra help" from Diane. Mary felt shamed by Diane's failure to "work through the prescribed channels." Diane felt shamed by Mary's authoritarian reprimand. In a way, Mary was explicitly silencing Nancy and the question she was raising: Had racial bias been exercised in a meeting that she attended? And Mary was using her power to silence and immobilize Diane by reprimanding her. Mary's first reaction, a stonewalling attempt to get people "in line," led to a major disconnection with Diane. But Mary did not simply stay in a positional place of "being right and indignant"; she sought out Diane and clearly demonstrated her vulnerability and need for this relationship to weather the disconnection. Diane, demonstrating her appreciation of the ongoing centrality of the relationship and trying to strengthen the connection through authentic responsiveness, was able to convey that she cared about the relationship, the work, the consultation, and Mary as well. Although the specific dynamics that had led to this impasse did not get fully addressed, the rupture in the relationship was noted and the healing of that became a way of strengthening the work they were doing together.

> As Diane and Mary found their way back into empathy and mutual respect, they both had to open to possible influence from the other. Initially they had taken "positions" that made it difficult to deal with the conflict that had arisen. Diane felt protective of the consultation and the company's issues of diversity, recognizing that for her to be effective in the organization, the employees needed to feel safe in letting her know what might really be going on. Mary, a "by-the-book" manager, felt she had to protect her lines of authority and was threatened by the possibility that people might feel more comfortable bringing their grievances to Diane than to the preordained supervisors. Both were speaking from a place of authenticity and genuine belief. Their ability to move back into a place of openness with one another depended on a history of having worked together through some tough issues and having witnessed each others' vulnerability. Over the years they had worked slowly and carefully, taking small risks in revealing uncertainties and vulnerabilities. Diane could also see the ways in which "oppressive sociopolitical systems wreak damage on relational functioning" (Walker & Miller, 2001). Mary's acceptance of top-down authority and her sense of being threatened by Diane's responsiveness and involvement in Nancy's complaint led to a disconnection and failure to see the relational consequences of her punitive and "power

over" response. She herself was caught in an oppressive system of management.

Although Diane and Mary could not transform the rules of the organization, and they may not even have had that as a common goal, they could bring an openness to being moved by one another. Although the initial interaction of exercising hierarchy was done in a shaming way, and Diane's response may have been experienced by Mary as a countershaming power play, it served to rebalance the power in some way. And although both Mary and Diane were caught in anger, they found a way to stay with the complexity of this contractual relationship and maintain their willingness to interact, rather than withdraw into inauthentic relating. RCT views anger as a useful signal that "something is wrong" and finding a way to use it constructively is an important part of learning to do "good conflict."

Developing empathy is crucial to the negotiation of conflict and difference. Diane could not only empathize with Mary's pain around the possible failed consultation but also could empathize with her position as a woman trying to "make it" in a man's world. The "white man's rules" that prevailed in the organization led Mary to exercise power in a way that was not entirely syntonic for her. These rules also led to difficulty in relation to the issues of "power over." This was an organization that asked its members to acculturate—that is, to take on the dominant, hierarchical culture of the group. There was little interest in alternative ways of managing. The dominant group and its hierarchical leadership showed little motivation to accommodate or change in response to those members of the organization who did not embrace the dominant values. Although Mary and many of her staff did not fully embrace these values, they were encouraged to act as if they did. And they felt they should be able to manage like the successful, top-down men they saw elsewhere in the organization.

Tensions within the nondominant groups around race and authority also impacted both women. For Diane there was the possibility that a part of this dilemma resulted from the racial undertones of a white person being dismissive of, or unattuned to, the real and insidious effects of racism. Despite the cultural and racial complexities that arose, both women were motivated by deep commitments to the work, although the nature of their commitments differed. Diane was passionately dedicated to social justice, whereas Mary was deeply devoted to the productive work of her division. Both goals were supported by the working through of this conflict.

Diane and Mary resolved their conflict and practiced "good conflict" in some ways. They moved beyond the reactivity of the moment, which had led them to resort to more "power over" strategies. Diane was able to find a way to speak authentically about her difficulty moving forward with the consultation. Although initially this self-disclosure may have come from a place of shame and disconnection, as the feelings settled, it moved into a necessary place of telling the truth to those in power. Diane was also moving to a place of mutual empathy, feeling for Mary and also letting Mary see her impact on her. Mary, too, was willing to risk having her vulnerabilty seen. Diane brought an appreciation of the value of the connection itself. In order to make this project work, they both had to actively remember the largely successful history of their relationship and the consultation. Diane, being the "outsider," had to hold an appreciation of the larger cultural issues, both in the organizational culture (white, male, hierarchical, unfriendly both to women and people of color) and the larger culture (also white, male, hierarchical, unfriendly both to women and people of color). In this case they also took action to create a task force to facilitate the authentic representation of experiences of bias, prejudice, and alternative work values and styles. Furthermore, both women communicated directly with Nancy to validate her need to have a safe place in which to speak about her experience of discrimination.

In terms of the relational dynamics of this consultation, power moves, challenges to empathy, and readiness to move into good conflict constituted the core issues. The history of good working connection and sense of respect also informed the decisions of the principle players. Furthermore, the larger context exerted an important influence on the ways in which this exchange played out. Although the current administration honored the diversity mandate of the organization by continuing it, signals of covert distrust or devaluing of this agenda were perceived by various employees. This covert devaluation mirrors the larger societal messages in which "lip service" is paid to the importance of diversity issues without any real investment in changing the patterns of the dominant group.

Relational systems involving women at work are frequently embedded in contexts that do not privilege collaboration and mutual influence. Therefore, for all of the participants to agree on a common goal or common process is difficult. Not only are there issues of racial and cultural differences in ways of connecting, resolving conflict, and dealing with power, there are also gender complications. What Patricia Hill Collins (1990) calls "intersecting matrices of power" were operating throughout the consultation. Diversity work that does not explicitly deal with power differentials and stratification cannot facilitate real understanding or change. Any consultation around diversity that seeks only to "celebrate difference" is not seriously addressing the major disconnections that occur around differences that signify "less than" or "more than." In undertaking real diversity work embedded in a social justice model, an organization must be prepared to undergo change. Some of that change may be welcomed and some of it may be resisted as threatening, especially to the group in power. Mary had adopted a somewhat alien, but she felt necessary, system of imposing strict lines of authority and power; to move out of that position felt threatening to her. She feared a loss of status and being seen as "too nice" or not "tough enough." The larger work-related cultural values would have to change in order for her to be respected and valued for a more relational or mutual exercise of authority.

RCT emphasizes the importance of context. Just as individual relationships can be either growth fostering or destructive, so too can relational contexts contribute to growth, creativity, and productivity or their opposites. Because most work cultures have been created by successful white men, there is often an issue of "difference" as women and people of color come into the workplace, particularly when they come into positions of power. Fletcher and colleagues (2000) notes that there are four primary responses to those at the "margin" (hooks, 1984)—in this case, women:

1. *Fix the women.* They are "deficient" men and need to learn how to be "real men." For instance, in one organization where a very effective team leader was attributing success in developing a particular product to her team ("*We* did this"), a supervisor pulled her aside and suggested that she was "undoing" her own success, that she needed to learn to "toot her own horn" and take appropriate credit ("*I* did this") if she wanted to "get ahead."

2. *Create equal opportunities.* This approach highlights the structural obstacles to women's progress and attempts to alter these obstacles. It often incurs anger from the "inside group" (men) who sees the outsiders (women) as being given "special advantages." For example, when special accommodations are made to family needs, such as allowing flexible schedules for mothers of young children, other workers often feel resentful.

3. *Celebrate differences.* This response assimilates women into the workplace in a way that takes advantage of their "unique" experience. Often this approach pushes women toward "support positions" or human resources, the "people" offices in an organization.

4. *Revision the work culture, or make bilateral change.* The last response mode might be reframed by RCT as mutual influence. An example from another organization sheds light on the way mutuality and empathic listening can bring about effective results:

> Laura, a new vice-president for marketing, was invited to attend a meeting on her first day at the job, in which a decision was being made about marketing a new product. She had hoped to quietly observe the meeting but realized when she entered the room that all eyes were on her, that her new "authority" was about to be tested. But she honestly did not "know" the product or the process. She felt internal and external pressure to "take charge," "to show her stuff" as the new "boss."

When the team leader turned to her and said "What do you think we should do?" she responded, "I will take the responsibility for this decision, but first I'd like to hear from each of you what you would do in my shoes and why."

Laura managed to step into the organizational shoes of "decision maker" without sacrificing her authentic need for input, and she respected the flow of information "coming up from below." In this "small step" the work culture is changed as Laura herself shifts to move into a position of responsive authority. Both the work culture and the incoming workers are changed in a process of mutual growth. With an influx of relational values, the privileging of separation, competition, suppression of conflict, and independent functioning might be lessened. Instead there might be a growth of collaboration, a valuing of teamwork, and appreciation of the real work of developing growth-fostering connections in an organization. Joyce Fletcher (1999) has outlined four behaviors that constitute relational practice in organizations:

1. "Preserving" includes activities intended to preserve the life and well-being of the project, doing "whatever it takes" and sometimes putting aside one's personal agenda.

2. "Mutual empowering" is behavior intended to enable others' achievements and contributions to the project. An example of mutual empowering is empathic teaching, putting oneself in the shoes of the other. Mutual empowering contributes to the self-confidence and competence of others.

3. "Self achieving" is about using relational skills to enhance one's own achievements.

4. "Creating team" includes actions that foster group life.

Fletcher states that "relational practice is a way of working that reflects a relational logic of effectiveness and requires a number of relational skills such as empathy, mutuality, reciprocity and a sensitivity to emotional contexts" (p. 84). She notes that much relational work "disappears"; it is seen as gender determined, the "work of women," rather than as competent work. The skills, therefore, get overlooked. Skills such as mutual empowerment are often seen as being "nice" or sometimes even as "deviant," because professional norms of self-promotion and "me first" are so entrenched in most hierarchical organizations. Fletcher notes further that the misinterpretation of intention underlying relational practice is a powerful way of devaluing it; personal idiosyncrasy rather than competence or desire to work more effectively is seen as driving the behavior. Relational behavior is also conflated with images of "ideal" womanhood or femininity.

However, there is increasing interest in the business community in the importance of mutual change, two-way influence systems, and a recognition that the capacity to develop good relationships in work settings dramatically influences work productivity (Senge, 1990; Goleman,1995. Fletcher optimistically notes that "there are strong forces for change in today's globally competitive, knowledge-intensive business environments. Increasingly organizations are being encouraged—even warned—to reinvent themselves, push decision making to lower levels, encourage teamwork and collaboration, flatten the hierarchy and think systemically. These new organizational forms will need new kinds of workers" (p. 113). But these changes involve radical value shifts and new definitions of competence and success in traditionally competitive, top-down organizations. Identifying the goal of relational practice and its intended outcomes is important. For instance, when representing a team effort in a management meeting, instead of following the tradition of saying "I" saw this and "I did that" (individual attribution), use "we" and note that it was the outcome of a team effort. Also point to the norms in the organization that push people in the direction of personal claiming rather than group attribution. RCT supports questioning those individualistic norms in small ways and practicing a program of what Fletcher calls "small wins," in which one does not envision huge transformation but multiple and continuous small shifts.

Using her understanding of "small wins," Diane considered how to rework the disconnection with Mary. In her follow-up discussion with Mary, Diane focused on the importance of helping the employees find the pathway to protest that felt safest to them. For example, in this case, belonging to a marginalized racial group was a more important determinant of safety than following the institutionalized prescriptive pathway for grievances. Diane noted, "Although it is important to respect the institutional guidelines for registering a grievance, it is also important for management to remain responsive to issues of what really feels "safe" to people, particularly if they come from marginalized groups." She had to be very sensitive to the possibility of shaming Mary around this issue but was also trying to gently introduce an increasing awareness of the subtler forms of racism and marginalization that exist in almost all organizations. Although seemingly an individual interaction, it was important for the organizational group dynamics for Mary to follow up with Nancy, to apologize for her overreaction, and to talk with her and others in a task force that was then set up about how to best manage questions of prejudice and racial insensitivity.

The creation of this task force is an example of the importance of networking, in which growth is fostered in groups whose goal is to support and encourage individuals in an organization, particularly around making changes in the organization. It was necessary for Mary and Diane to convey to the organization its inability to effectively provide safe access for those with less power to address their concerns about prejudice or racism. With no safe forum available, employees are left to seek allies in opposing the practices that are used to devalue or "disappear" the relational work that occurs in all organizations. This outreach work involves finding ways to speak authentically (and strategically), to find the allies who can support one's position, and challenge existing norms in careful ways. Nancy had to find her own way in this area; she followed her inclination to talk with Diane rather than Mary. But the responsiveness and relational work that Diane and Mary undertook actually transformed her personal courage into an organizational structure (new task force on marginality, race, culture).

This is, in fact, the work of political resistance about which Carol Gilligan (1982) and Janie Ward (Robinson & Ward, 1991) speak. It is also powerful anti-shame work. Rather than assuming that those who experience the pain are the source of their own pain, this approach suggests locating the source of the pain quite clearly (i.e., the misfit between organization and certain individuals) and facilitating mutual responsiveness and change.

Women and other marginalized groups often "twist themselves" to fit into organizations, to "make it" according to the existing rules. They work very hard, often at great cost to themselves and their families. Because of these costs, women who have the economic capability to leave often do leave. Unfortunately, the question that gets asked most often is "What's wrong with this woman? Why can't she hack it?" The organization blames the "outsider" and works to "assimilate" her, to make her more like the "insiders," or it tracks her to the "people" departments of human resources and other people-oriented areas. Women who do not have the privilege of leaving are left trying to stay afloat in organizations that may trample on every relational value they hold. They feel shamed and blamed for not "fitting in better," not being as successful as their male counterparts. Change in the work culture in many organizations is necessary if women and other marginalized people are to feel "at home" and bring their full creativity to work. What is needed is a response that emphasizes the necessity of change in the organization as well as some accommodation to existing work culture on the part of the "outsider."

Clinicians are used to working with individuals, small therapy groups, and families. Whereas there is often an implicit awareness of context, an explicit focus on the organizations, communities, and sociopolitical milieus in which people exist is essential to real understanding and change. Without a critical awareness of the "culture of work" and the power dynamics that impact all workers, major areas of stress will be overlooked. RCT provides guidelines to help individuals identify and resist some of the disempowering practices that silence, shame, and stifle individuals and groups who do not comfortably embrace the prevailing workplace values and practices.

RCT offers a new way to examine the impact of power differentials and contextual factors on individuals and organizations. It seeks to reveal hidden biases, offer pathways of resistance to traditional and unexamined practices. By studying the patterns of disconnection and the necessary work of building relational resilience and reconnection following disconnection, RCT points to the complexity and centrality of relationships in human and institutional change. In identifying and resisting traditional and unexamined practices, the possibility for new organizational energies emerges. The work world can no longer be designed and run by one group in society to the detriment of many of the workers in it. There must be a process of mutual learning and responsivity that offers the possibility of new structures that can empower more than just the existing dominant groups.

References

Ault-Riche, M. (Ed.). (1986). *Women and family therapy.* Rockville, MD: Aspen.

Boyd Franklin, N. (2003). *Black families in therapy: Understanding the African American experience* (2nd ed.). New York: Guilford Press.

Collins, P. (1990). *Black feminist thought: Knowledge, consciousness and the politics of empowerment.* Boston: Unwin Hyman.

Comas-Díaz, L., & Greene, B. (Eds.). (1994). *Women of color: Integrating ethnic and gender identities in psychotherapy.* New York: Guilford Press.

Fletcher, J. (1996). *Relational theory in the workplace* (Work in Progress, No. 77). Wellesley, MA: Stone center Working Paper Series.

Fletcher, J. (1999). *Disappearing acts: Gender, power and relational practice at work.* Cambridge, MA: MIT Press.

Fletcher, J., Jordan, J., & Miller, J. (2000). Women and the workplace: Application of the psychodynamic theory. *American Journal of Psychoanalysis, 60*(3) 243–262.

Gilligan, C. (1982). *In a different voice.* Cambridge, MA: Harvard University Press.

Goleman, D. (1995). *Emotional intelligence.* New York: Bantam Books.

hooks, b. (1984). *Feminist theory: From margin to center.* Boston: South End Press.

Jordan, J. V. (Ed.). (1997). *Women's' growth in diversity: More writings from the Stone Center.* New York: Guilford Press.

Jordan, J. V., Kaplan, A. G., Miller, J. B., Stiver, I. P., & Surrey, J. L. (1991). *Women's growth in connection: Writings from the Stone Center.* New York: Guilford Press.

McGoldrick, M., Anderson, C., & Walsh, F. (Eds.). (1989). *Women in families: A framework for family therapy.* New York: Norton.

Miller, J. (1976). *Toward a new psychology of women.* Boston: Beacon Press.

Miller, J., & Stiver, I. (1997). *The healing connection*. Boston: Beacon Press.

Mirkin, M. P. (Ed.). (1994). *Women in context: Toward a feminist construction of psychotherapy*. New York: Guilford Press.

Robinson, T., & Ward, J. (1991). A belief in self far greater than anyone's disbelief: Cultivating resistance among African American female adolescents. In C. Gilligan, A. Rogers, & D. Tollman (Eds.), *Women, girls and psychotherapy: Reframing resistance* (pp. 87–103). Binghamton, NY: Harrington Park Press.

Senge, P. (1990). *The fifth discipline*. New York: Doubleday.

Walker, M., & Miller, J. B. (2001). *Racial images and relational possibilities* (Talking Paper, No. 2). Wellesley, MA: Stone Center Working Paper Series.

CHAPTER 10

Redefining the Career Ladder
NEW VISIONS OF WOMEN AT WORK

Barbara F. Okun
Lauren Gallo Ziady

"You may be able to do it all, but you can't have it all—at least, not all at once!" The reality of this statement confronts women who work and have families today, even though many with privilege were socialized to believe that if they wanted it, they could do and have it all. Women are in the labor force in greater proportion than ever before and in occupations tradition-ally accessible only to men. They are more educated, earn more, and gener-ally enjoy more labor-market benefits than their counterparts 25 years ago (DiNatalie & Boraas, 2002; Monthly Labor Review, 2002). Despite these advances, there still remain gender inequities in the number of women in top positions (glass ceiling) and in hiring salaries and raises (glass escalator) that contradict the popular notion of the declining significance of race and gender in the workplace. Gender and racial social stereotyping still prevails. Furthermore, in addition to structural biases, there are inadequate day care opportunities and unfriendly family financial and workplace policies that make it difficult for all but the most affluent to pursue traditional career advancement while raising a family.

Traditional career development literature suggests that the external barriers to optimal vocational development of women include sexual harassment; lack of mentors and role models; socioeconomic disadvantage; educational and workplace discrimination; prejudice related to race, ethnic-ity, gender, sexual orientation, and disability; and occupational stereotyp-ing (Gottfredson, 2002). Internal barriers include multiple role conflicts,

skill deficits, underestimation of capabilities and poor self-efficacy expectations, low outcome expectations, and constrictive role socialization
(Fassinger, 2002; McLennan & Arthur, 1999; McWhirter, Torres, &
Rasheed, 1998). Many of these barriers have lessened in recent years due to
sociocultural changes. Although much progress has been achieved, some of
these internal and external barriers may still be pertinent for some women.

Every day, newspapers and magazines report new studies illustrating
the wide variety of women's career aspirations and choices. For example, a
recent study of the Simmons School of Management (Blanton, 2004) found
that over 70% of the 571 women surveyed aspire to the highest leadership
positions; however, these women also believe that they do not have an
equal chance to fulfill this aspiration, compared with men. According to an
MBACareers.com (2003) quick poll, men and women have contrasting reasons for obtaining an MBA. Although both pursue an MBA to increase
earning potential, the commonality ends there. Men obtain an MBA for
networking and preparation for entrepreneurship and advancement,
whereas women hope that an MBA will gain them additional career opportunities and credibility in the workplace. Additionally, the survey revealed
that the long-term career goals for male and female MBAs differ as well.
Men acquiring an MBA aspire to become president or CEO of both public
and private companies or to start their own businesses. Women MBAs,
however, ranked management consulting, executive level vice-president
positions, and nonprofit executive management high among their career
goals. This discrepancy is likely based on the fact that women expect to
have children and therefore value flexibility and adaptability in their chosen career.

Thus the core issue for today's women is balance: work/career and
family; work/career and relationships; work/career and self-care. Each
woman's goals and criteria for balance are influenced by personality, partner status, relationships, health, energy, etc. Social systemic influences such
as race, culture, sexual orientation, class, economic privilege, and ability/
disability also influence women's ideas about, and attainment of, balance.
Those with more systemic privilege usually have more options open to
them. Balance is a core struggle over the lifespan, as circumstances, needs,
and opportunities continuously emerge and change.

We authors are of different generations. I (BFO) am older; I worked,
married, and had three children prior to entering (at the urging of my husband) a part-time master's program. I was able to complete a doctoral program with the help of a doting mother-in-law and a supportive husband. I
chose an academic career in order to have a flexible schedule that would
allow me to be involved as much as possible with my children's activities.
When my children left home to attend college, I became more intensely
involved in my career. I (LGZ) am younger; I married as a doctoral student

and am currently trying to time my internship and dissertation in order to have children and achieve my idea of a satisfying balance between self, family, and career. I (BFO) had no role models or societal support for my choices; I lived in a world where women were recruited by doctoral programs and universities to meet the Department of Labor's determination for gender equality in organizations (such as universities, clinics) receiving federal funds. On the other hand, I (LGZ) live in a more competitive, pressured world where university funding is decreasing, positions are being cut, and health care services reduced. Both of us appreciate the privilege of choice available to us due to family support related to finances and child care.

Women without children may choose more easily to have a traditional, linear career advancement path that is more typical of men. Women who have children, in contrast, have different choices and struggles in regard to balancing work and family; they may take the winding route or veer off their chosen path, becoming part of the "Opt-Out Revolution," a phrase Lisa Belkin (2003) coined to describe women who use maternity as an escape from the demands of high-pressured careers. Other women with children attempt to "do it all" because of financial pressures or for pure love of work. They combine family and work demands, unfortunately leaving little room for personal time. Blagg and Young (2002) talk about the inventive, alternative work situations that MBA graduates are developing after motherhood, pointing out the multitasking skills and shifting priorities that shape new concepts of work and career advancement. These include changing schedules, creating more job autonomy, creative networking, emphasizing the positive reciprocal influences of work and family, and setting new boundaries (Smith, 2002). The goal of boundary setting is to create structure and a time line of work and family priorities. As clinicians, we are noting the increasing number of successful career women who come for psychotherapy after the birth of their first child. Many are stunned by the intensity of their emotional attachment to their baby and are suddenly unsure about their original plans for returning to work after 4 weeks and pursuing career advancement. The same surprise often occurs for men, as more and more professional couples, both heterosexual and homosexual, reassess their priorities about work and family, take up co-parenting, (which requires paternity leave), and adapt work schedules to shared family responsibilities. Both men and women are surprised by the power of their attachment to their children, and they promptly begin looking for work and scheduling options.

This chapter focuses on four main areas:

1. To consider how women under age 45, who have some degree of financial stability, are redefining notions of "career," "advancement," "leadership," and "success."

2. To help clinicians understand the importance of attending to career issues as an essential component of psychotherapy.

3. To foster therapists' understanding of the organizational and larger sociocultural contexts of today's working women so that this expanded understanding can inform the women's psychotherapy.

4. To pay special attention to often neglected issues in considering women's experience of work, such as the impact of chronic illness, with or without disability; sexual orientation; and the impact that individual and family crises may have on career advancement.

The Clinician's Personal Issues

Female therapists of an older generation who lived through the struggle of tokenism and active discrimination often do not understand why younger women are not more fervent about fighting power abuses and seeking power and privilege in the workplace for themselves. It may even seem as if these younger women are taking for granted what previous generations of women had to struggle to gain. Whereas some older female therapists may question the lack of career focus in today's women, others, however, may question the seeming lack of family commitment. As in any clinical situation, it is important for us, as clinicians, to monitor and take charge of the possible influence of our own attitudes and values. There have been many clinical situations in which we (BFO and LGZ) have struggled with our concerns about the children of parents who were choosing to prioritize their career advancement over the needs of their own children. Talking to peers, seeking clinical supervision, and keeping up with the literature are all helpful antidotes to clinical subjectivity. It is important for clinicians to recognize generational changes and how women's choices are impacted by these changes.

Although many of today's younger women appreciate the sacrifices and struggles of their predecessors, they want to move beyond those struggles to change not only those ubiquitous patriarchal work cultures that are based on traditional hierarchical beliefs, policies, leadership, and organizations, but also the social stereotypes of "family," "spouses," and parenting choices. The demographics of our society and family structures are changing (Hacker, 2003; Okun, 2004). For example, there are an increasing number of (1) women who choose to have children without a partner or spouse, (2) gay and lesbian families, and (3) cohabiting families. The number of traditional nuclear families continues to decrease proportionally, whereas the number of families without fathers increases.

Today, many professional women are choosing to work part time, job share, or find some other way of getting off the "fast track." They are satisfied with this choice and will decide after school-age childrearing whether or not they want to pursue advancement in their original career or create some other way of fulfilling those needs. For these women, career success means the flexibility of being able to focus on different priorities at different times in their lives. As women realize that the fast track requires more than full-time work, many who have the options to choose are redefining "success" in terms of achieving a balance between family and career, rather than as traditional career advancement. These women may choose to be as involved as possible with childrearing even if they have partners who are also actively parenting. Other women, who also have the support to enable their choices, choose to prioritize their career advancement, involving spouses or extended family in child care or choosing to use their income to provide for nannies and other family services. Women's choices and trajectories may change over time, depending on individual, family, and work and financial circumstances. More and more, clinicians are sought to help women identify and understand their own meanings of a fulfilling balance and come to terms with unexpected changing circumstances.

Marilyn, a biracial (European American and African American) woman of 42, was the chief counsel of a state agency. She had worked for the current director in a previous job and had been brought into her current position when he became director. Raised in both African American and European American middle-class cultures, she grew up with the message to achieve, transcend cultural stereotypes, and "be your own person and show everyone you can do it all." Because of her history with her mentor/director, as well as her proven competence and high energy level, Marilyn enjoyed power and privilege within her work setting. She described herself as a "control freak" and a "perfectionist." Her husband, Todd, was an attorney in private practice.

For several years, this couple had been trying to conceive a baby. After many disappointments, they adopted an infant from Korea. Even on the airplane home from Seoul, Marilyn reported that Todd was more relaxed and at ease with the baby than she, and that she was anxious about what the other mothers on the plane thought of her. During Todd's 3-month paternity leave, Marilyn continued to work 60-hour weeks; in addition, she spent two evenings per week coaching the swimming team with which she had been working for many years. She came to therapy because Todd was becoming more and more concerned that motherhood and marriage were low priorities for his wife. Marilyn was disturbed about Todd's reaction and acknowledged that his perception was true, even though she and Todd were looking into the adoption of a second child. She was very concerned about the contrast between her actual feelings and her "superwoman" self-image and seemed relieved to be able to discuss them with a third-party therapist.

Therapy revealed that Marilyn was feeling shame about her priorities as well as guilt stemming from her belief that her years of bulimia had affected her fertility. But she also expressed a strong desire to be a "good mother," and she felt that she would be able to help her son develop a healthy racial identity, given her biracial identity. She felt as if she was "unnatural" for wanting her husband to accept the primary caretaker role so that she could continue her own activities. We discussed the sociocultural influences on her shame and her resistance to developing an emotional bond with her son. Her husband wanted more of shared family/career roles. The therapist and Marilyn explored her meanings and possible choices. For some women in Marilyn's position, the healthiest "balance" may have been to continue her emphasis on work and career advancement and help her develop a positive relationship with her son, whose primary caretaker would be his father. Marilyn chose a different balance; a few weeks into therapy she began to develop a closer relationship with her son, spending more time with him and beginning to perform some of the daily routines. As we explored her history and her recognition that she did desire to work and also have family time, she realized that some of her career drive came from her biracial identity, wanting to prove that she could succeed as well as a white woman might.

As Marilyn began to invest more of her time and energy in parenting, her boss, the agency director, simultaneously decided to take a position at a larger, more highly visible agency. He offered Marilyn the opportunity to go with him at a higher status level and salary. At this point, Marilyn felt panic. She was just beginning to think more about family, when a "chance of a lifetime" arose. If she stayed in her current position with the new director, she likely would not enjoy the same access to power and autonomy that she currently had, and she might not even be retained under a new regime. If she went with her former director, she would have more pressure, responsibilities, and visibility—and less time and availability for her husband and son. And what about the new adoption? Marilyn was angry about this dilemma.

Todd had been extremely supportive of Marilyn's therapy and urged her to explore various options. An important part of exploring Marilyn's choices concerned considering a better fit between her career needs, her family needs, and her organizational culture. It was important to expand options beyond the two already being considered. Together, Marilyn, Todd, and I began to explore the types of organizational culture that might afford Marilyn greater flexibility with regard to role and responsibilities, given Todd's current desire to find a different balance. At the same time, we began to work through her ambivalence about the disconnections between her self-image and her life choices.

The point of this vignette is to demonstrate how psychotherapy involves exploring all overlapping aspects of the client's life and the varying contexts in which he or she lives. Marilyn was following a traditional, patriarchal model of career advancement, adhering to family and cultural prescriptions to achieve and transcend gender and racial stereotypes; at the same time, she was following a nontraditional model of mothering that went against cultural prescriptions. For some women, this exploration of contexts might free them of shame at not being the "ideal" (and stereotypical) mother. For others, such as Marilyn, this exploration enabled her to rethink her notions of success and career achievement, which were biased by traditional models of career success, and she thereby felt empowered to consider various alternatives. As of this writing, Marilyn is awaiting a second adopted child, continuing to work at her old agency under a new regime, while exploring some challenging consulting work in the profit sector.

Elsa, age 43, and Henry, age 44, came to therapy because of Elsa's concerns about their 7-year-old son, who had special needs, as well as her concern about wanting to turn down a promotion she was offered at work. Both from working-class African American families, Elsa was an office worker in a large urban medical practice, and Henry was a uniformed auxiliary policeman. As in many working-class families of color, Elsa had the opportunity to attain higher-paying work with benefits more easily than Henry, who was studying diligently to try to gain a permanent security position. Elsa had been working for several years in this office and felt confident and competent. At home, she had assumed the family role of primary parent and home manager, based on her culture's gender norms. Career wise, she was the primary wage earner and provided health benefits for the entire family. The presenting problems were her preoccupying concerns about "not being treated right" by the school staff in her efforts to obtain services for her son, the effects of these preoccupations on her attentiveness at work, and anger at her perception of her husband as pressuring her to take a recent offer for promotion to assistant office manager, in order to make more money.

When Elsa was offered this promotion, she was tempted by the increased salary but concerned about managerial responsibility and losing the flexibility to run to school or home, when necessary, for her school-age children. Elsa was sure that Henry would not come to a couple's session, but when asked, he was agreeable. The therapist explained their rights with regard to obtaining a core evaluation of their son and services within the school and suggested several advocacy strategies. To Elsa's surprise, Henry was more than willing to be involved, and it was decided that he would visit the school in uniform (a symbol of power) to advocate for this mandated evaluation. It also turned out that Henry was not pressuring Elsa to take the promotion unless she wanted it. Elsa was struggling between her thinking that she "should" take it and her realization that she did not really want to take it. She was satisfied with her current status and work, and rising in the ranks had never been her goal. To her, this job represented a satisfying way of working and attending to family needs as well as having close relationships with peers. By the end of the second session, both Elsa and Henry felt united in mutual understanding and appreciation of their respective notions about family, work, and success. Henry acknowledged that to him, success means moving up the ladder at any opportunity (he was studying for the exam that would allow him to become a regular member of the force), but that it needn't mean this to Elsa. At the end of four sessions, Henry had succeeded in arranging for an evaluation of their son, and Henry and Elsa felt close again, having agreed that it did not matter who was the major wage earner as long as they could talk about circumstances on an ongoing basis.

In both of these case examples, I (BFO) used educational, coaching, and empowerment interventions in addition to relational and other psychotherapy models to help these women consider their unique needs and desires about achieving what would be a gratifying balance to them and their families. Each situation differs, depending on the people, sociocultural, and systemic influences. Considering the interface of all aspects of the client's life, including historical and current contexts, can lead to effective treatment planning and intervention. Both Marilyn and Elsa had to reconsider their definitions of career advancement and success in order to meet the competing needs and demands of many constituencies—self, family, work, and community. Both had to acknowledge the influences of their racial identities and heritages on their ideas about family and work.

Whereas women today have more choices than previous generations, an ever-changing world creates constraints and unpredictability. In the last few years, layoffs and long-term unemployment have been rampant in many parts of the United States. Some women do not have a choice about working, particularly if they are single or their partners are unable to find employment. Some have to stay in jobs or organizations they do not like to obtain health benefits (the same applies to men). Still, over the past two decades, women have been able to make more choices than they were allowed in the past. Depending on their educational and financial status, women can choose to enter just about any occupation; to cut back hours or even leave the workforce; to postpone having children (although they face increased risk of infertility); and, finally, women now have the choice of when and how to retire. Perhaps the greatest choice many women have is to try to define for themselves, within their financial and practical constraints, as did Marilyn and Elsa, what work means to them, what their aspirations are, and how they choose to prioritize and balance different parts of their lives. Obviously, different women have different choices, depending on family responsibilities, health, financial status, class, and governmental provisions.

Organizational Cultures and Leadership

The context of organizational cultures and leadership is a significant factor for occupational gratification and advancement. The traditional patriarchal organization is based on conventional gender and race-based hierarchical structure. The "rules" for channels of authority, evaluation, and promotion come from the "old boys' network," and authority is usually structured in a top-down format. In the past, women were primarily employed in ancillary roles—as assistants, secretaries, human resources personnel, etc. More recently, women may achieve management status if they play by those old boys' rules—although, as Hacker (2003) points out, there are few female CEOs and few women in senior management positions in U.S. organizations. In more traditional, patriarchal organizations, men and women experience very different career environments and career challenges. Barriers are built into the fabric of the organizational system with regard to process and policies of career advancement. For example, there is the hidden power of an informal communications network in which female managers are likely to receive more negative evaluations than men when using direct influence behaviors (Kanter, 1997). There is intense pressure for women to conform to stereotypical roles, and women are held to very different standards than are males. With the increasing number of women in professional graduate schools, women have greater opportunities for career advancement than they ever had before, but they still have to abide by the cultural patriarchal "rules" until they can create changes from their own power base. A study by Boyce and Herd (2003) suggests that white male-dominated traditional organizations attract leadership-aspiring women who score high on scales that measure masculinity; such scales assess degree of leadership traits of dominance, responsibility, achievement, and self-assurance. It may be that women who have worked in these traditional organizational cultures choose among multiple options, depending on their varying degrees of choice, whether (1) to remain in the environment, (2) to seek an alternative organizational culture after they have families, (3) to stop working, (4) to work from home part time, and so on. Some women claim to feel more secure in a traditional organization where the roles are governed by conventional operating rules that are well known.

Charlotte, a 53-year-old European American, middle-class woman, was the sole female senior consultant in a small, innovative public relations firm that describes itself as flexible and collegial. However, when push comes to shove, the firm is indeed patriarchal. Brought into the firm 12 years ago by her uncle, a founder and current board chairman, she consistently brought in more business than anyone else in the firm; she worked 7 days a week, stayed late every night, and was totally immersed in her job. Her only other interests were a series of on-and-off-again affairs with three married men. She is attractive, charming, and delightful, and clients want to work with her. She reported directly to a male president.

Charlotte came for therapy a year ago because her primary care physician suggested that the imbalance between her personal, social, and work lives was contributing to her low energy and symptoms of depression. Charlotte described herself as a "good girl" who needed to please people and work as hard as she could. She believed that males were authority figures whom she should please. As she described her background as one of two daughters of a domineering father and compliant mother, the connections between earlier relational patterns and current patterns emerged. Waiting for the "perfect" man to appear and fulfill her fantasies of love, marriage, and family had begun to be troubling, given that the years were passing, and she stayed involved with married men. She was exhausted when she was not working and had no time or space for anyone. At work, she was beginning to feel "undervalued" and "taken for granted." Charlotte and her therapist decided to tackle the work issues first, in order to alleviate stress and free up time, energy, and attention for other aspects of her personal life. The goal was for Charlotte to find a satisfactory balance in her life by developing a personal life away from work.

The first intervention, while establishing an empathic relationship, was to challenge Charlotte's thinking about males and females in the workplace, to teach her to understand that she was, in fact, describing a type of traditional organizational culture based on male norms; this psychoeducation allowed her to understand the constraints she was experiencing. Charlotte was very naive and had no idea of the covert operating rules and roles of the work environment to which she had devoted herself. She had a tendency to cling to her belief that only men are legitimate leaders. She was helped by an exploration of how leadership itself is gendered and enacted within a gendered context, so that she could understand how the board chairman and the president were in an alliance against her. She was asked to consider the impact of kinship and gender on this triangulation. She learned that, on a continuum from a patriarchal to a transformed leadership style, the male-dominated form is hierarchical, performance oriented and power based, whereas the transformed model stresses the empowerment of followers, collaboration, and more shared problem solving (Blustein, 2001). Charlotte could not transform the culture of her company, but she could learn to "take care of herself" within the organization, by insisting that she be evaluated on the same performance base as were the males at and above her level. With the help of therapeutic assertiveness training, Charlotte asked for a raise. She was coached every step of the way, but her boss was not willing to oblige at first. Finally, she did receive a token raise. Charlotte then learned that a younger man, who had not brought in any business his first year (and had even falsified his call records), received a higher bonus than she.

By this time, 1 year into therapy, Charlotte had shown great progress with her presenting problems: She had sold the home in which she was entrenched and moved into a larger home where she felt she could entertain; she networked and socialized with new friends; she took vacations and stopped working late; and on weekends she began to work with a dating service. Overall, she was less immobilized by depression when not working. For the first time, she allowed herself to feel anger at the inequities in her organization, and this anger enabled her to begin a serious negotiation with the president, who was thrown off balance by this new-found assertive behavior. It took months of steadfast persistence before Charlotte received a compensation package that she found acceptable. Coaching empowered her in all aspects of her life, and she felt stronger, more competent, and much more self-efficacious. Much of the therapy utilized cognitive restructuring (to challenge her ingrained stereotypic beliefs), bibliotherapy, role playing, and journal writing. Now she has moved on to differentiating between her ingrained fantasy beliefs and expectations and real-life opportunities. This transformation was slow and tedious but worthwhile: Being able to focus on concrete work difficulties enabled Charlotte to appraise her assumptions, to hold her head high, and to behave in an effectively assertive manner.

Charlotte is a good example of a single woman who needs balance between her work, her relationships, and her self-care activities. She also is an example of a woman caught between patriarchally socialized meanings of womanhood, work, success, and family and more current, postmodern models. By not attending to her personal relationships and self-care, she began to display somatic symptoms leading to anxiety, hypertension, and depression. Clinical work included exploration of organizational cultures and training in assertiveness skill development.

The rise of high technology and financial services has created alternative organizational cultures. Many of the high-tech and financial service organizations began with a diversified, mixed-gender network based more on competence than on traditional stereotypes (Agars, 2004; Hacker, 2003; Heilman, 2001; Ledet & Henley, 2000). The young developers in high technology have shared co-ed dormitories, become interested in more egalitarian family roles, and experienced a different gendered socialization than did their predecessors. The economy and state of technology enabled the emer-

gence of start-up high-technology organizations that required newer concepts of management to incorporate women's relational, collaborative, and
person-centered orientations. Typically, these newer companies have a
higher proportion of women managers than do traditional work organizations. There is higher gender equity, higher performance orientation, and
lower power distance. The family/work values of men and women in these
organizations tend to be more similar than dissimilar. These organizations
are not based on the old boys' network or on historical traditions. They are
more flexible and adaptive to societal changes and tend to appreciate and
value creative, original people who think "out of the box" (Carli & Eagly,
2001; Cotter, 2001; Heilman, 2001).

"Change-adept organizations cultivate the imagination to innovate,
the professionalism to perform and the openness to collaborate" (Kanter,
1997, p. 244). Newer styles of management are frequently based more on a
team principle. Team participation and management require high interpersonal skills, negotiation and consensus-building capacities, as well as
multitasking abilities. These organizational cultures attract women and
people of color, and there is a significant increase in senior-level female
employees. Women of color find these organizational cultures a "good fit"
because traditional race and gender stereotypes are less prevalent (Smith,
2002). The social stereotype that males are more competent and legitimate
leaders than females is not so ingrained in these newer organizations. Male
and female leaders are considered to have agency and communal capacities,
even if they are expressed and manifested differently. Performance and
competence are the major criteria for selecting managers.

Neglected Populations: Lesbians and Women with Disabilities in the Workplace

Lesbian Issues in the Workplace

At this time, it is unclear how attitudes toward lesbians have translated into
workplace behaviors. One study found, however, that 59% of lesbians in
their sample reported having experienced employment discrimination
(National Gay and Lesbian Task Force, 1991). Although overt displays of
discrimination seem to be less frequent (Dovidio & Gaertner, 2000), covert
ones are plentiful: A recent field study found that employers spoke fewer
words, terminated interactions, and engaged in more nonverbal forms of
discrimination (e.g., avoiding interaction) with lesbians compared to heterosexual employees (Hebl, Foster, Mannix, & Dovidio, 2002). A common
question asked in the workplace such as "Why aren't you married?" is an
example of a subtle form of heterosexism that can be quite painful. Dis-

crimination in the workplace still exists but typically manifests itself in subtler ways than in the past (Griffith & Hebl, 2002).

Katie, 41, and Chris, 31, came for couple therapy because of increasing conflict. Katie had been open about her lesbian sexual orientation since the age of 18 and was comfortable with her sexuality. Chris identified as bisexual and was not at all sure that she wanted to make the commitment Katie desired. She could not see herself in a permanent relationship with a woman. Chris was "out" to her family and a few close friends from childhood. Both women worked for the same governmental agency, but in different divisions. One of Chris's concerns was that no one at work should know about their relationship. Such subterfuge was difficult for Katie, because she was close to her colleagues and had been open about her personal life. Katie did not feel that the disclosure of her sexual orientation in the workplace had impaired her career advancement; Chris feared rejection and potential loss of advancement. Chris participated in the organization's sports teams but refrained from after-work social activities. She found herself edgy at work and brought this home as anger toward Katie. Katie, on the other hand, often became frustrated and resentful of what she experienced as Chris's "immaturity and withholding," related to Chris's uncertainty and need to remain closeted.

Self-disclosure of sexual orientation in the workplace has only recently received a portion of the attention it deserves, given that 10–14% of the United States workforce is composed of non-heterosexual workers (Powers, 1996). As with other minority groups, there is a recognized need to better understand the experiences of minorities who work in a majority context. Chris illustrates the lower levels of psychological well-being and life satisfaction associated with identity confusion and remaining in the closet. Closeted lesbian and bisexual women frequently experience health risks and focus an extraordinary amount of time on activities designed to cover up their stigmatized identity (Bepko & Johnson, 2000; Biaggio, Roades, Cardinale, & Duffy, 2000). For some lesbians, it may be healthier to be discrete about their sexual orientation at work than for others; however, a woman who is unable to be open about her sexual orientation in any realm of her life is likely to suffer more distress than those women who are out with family, friends, or coworkers.

In therapy, Chris gradually acknowledged that her gay supervisor had not experienced any stigmatization, at least to her knowledge. She began to realize that her discomfort stemmed more from her personal conflict about her sexuality than from the organizational culture. Research supports Katie's experience that lesbians who receive favorable and supportive reactions from others feel happier and less stressed in the workplace (Smith &

Ingram, 2004). The therapeutic work with this couple continued to focus on bridging the gaps in their "outness" and respecting their differing experiences at work and in their relationship expectations.

The process of "coming out" seems to affect men and women similarly (Griffith & Hebl, 2002); however, issues such as economic discrimination against women contribute to the unique challenges that confront women. Economic discrimination against women prevents the average working lesbian couple from earning as much as the average heterosexual or gay working couple (Hacker, 2003). This financial disparity is a considerable hardship for lesbian couples who choose to raise children while also juggling career and personal struggles. Career-focused counseling with lesbian clients may include an integrative approach to facilitate a more holistic understanding of the woman in context. It is important for clinicians to realize the uniqueness of each lesbian client. Individual differences, such as identity and comfort with sexual orientation and degree of "outness" to heterosexual friends, have been found to relate to disclosure behaviors at work (Griffith & Hebl, 2002) and should be explored in therapy.

Couple counseling and interventions designed to strengthen the interpersonal support system for women can aid in clients' ability to cope with homophobia in the workplace. Unsupportive social interactions in response to a lesbian's experience of heterosexism may result in additional distress for the woman who has been discriminated against (Smith & Ingram, 2004). For example, a family member might minimize the situation or blame the woman, causing her to internalize the discrimination, which often results in depression and/or anxiety. A clinician can help to remove the internalization of this subtle heterosexism, thereby externalizing the problem and relieving the client of the burden. Clinicians should understand the impact of heterosexism and continually work toward their own education of the issues that confront lesbians in the workplace.

Policies at the organizational level, such as domestic partner benefits and employment nondiscrimination clauses that include sexual orientation, diversity training that includes gay/lesbian issues, and over support of gay/lesbian activities show respect for gay and lesbian employees and help to protect them against overt forms of heterosexism (Griffith & Hebl, 2002; Smith & Ingram, 2004). Perceived organizational supportiveness, or lack thereof, should be explored in therapy as these types of organizational support typically factor into a woman's decision to disclose her sexual orientation. Analysis of these issues at the therapeutic level may help to decrease the level of stress created within the individual by the decision to "come out" in the workplace. Multilevel interventions aimed at equity for lesbian workers include advocating for nondiscrimination policies and providing diversity workshops. In order to work competently with lesbian women in regard to their career decisions, clinicians must be able to identify subtle bias and exclusionary behavior, of which the client herself may not be consciously aware. In addition, specifically asking clients whether they have encountered overt or subtle heterosexism conveys the clinician's knowledge of issues that homosexuals face and communicates her openness to discussing such issues (Smith & Ingram, 2004). Clinicians should also be aware of resources within the community, such as therapy or social groups, which can help the client, in an empathic environment, to develop her ability to seek support and foster coping strategies needed for dealing with heterosexism. Clinicians are encouraged to work in a proactive manner with their lesbian clients. Furthermore, they might work actively to combat heterosexism through teaching and advocacy. Enabling a lesbian client to assess the risks and benefits of "coming out" at work, while supporting her in mobilizing and strengthening her social support and self-acceptance, is key to effective therapy (Chung, 2003).

Career Development of Women with Disabilities

Researchers and clinicians are finally beginning to pay attention to the unique career development issues that challenge women with disabilities throughout the lifespan. We are just beginning to form a knowledge base about the variant normative family and organizational structures within which women with disabilities are encapsulated. The majority of individuals with disabilities are women (29 million, vs. 24 million men; Jans & Stoddard, 1999; McNeil, 2001). Research indicates that although more disabled women than men are considered to have achieved "successful" rehabilitation outcomes, the percentage of women achieving competitive employment is lower than the percentage of men (Jans & Stoddard); poverty is a common occurrence.

Women are doubly disadvantaged when gender interacts with disability, as both restrictive gender roles and low expectations based on disability lead to negative work outcomes (Noonan et al., 2004). Women with disabilities struggle with the same internal and external barriers in the world of work as do all women. These issues are compounded by realities directly related to their disabilities, such as chronic fatigue, lack of flexibility to travel, and absenteeism. Even more handicapping, women with disabilities are confronted with difficulties related to societal discomfort and ignorance and the resulting sterotype about people with disabilities, as well as practical/physical impediments (e.g., architectural barriers such as lack of ramps and technological barriers such as lack of TTY access).

In general, societal discomfort and lack of understanding leaves women with disabilities feeling less than valuable and wondering what they can contribute to the workplace. From early childhood even to old age, depending on the context in which they live, women with disabilities may be subjected to discrimination and made to feel as if they are really not as capable and as "good" as others. On average, women with physical disabilities report lower self-esteem than women without disabilities. Interestingly, for most women, this low self-esteem does not seem to be solely related to having a disability (Center for Research on Women with Disabilities, 1992). Often, women with disabilities become discouraged and struggle with depression and anxiety.

Frequently, people without disabilities are not sensitive to the manifestations of disability—for example, a slower walking pace or inability to use stairs—and therefore fail to notice that their colleague with the disability has been left behind. The importance of esteem-building activities and programs for girls and women with disabilities, be they within families, in schools, in churches, incorporated into medical and vocational rehabilitation services, or in the community, is indicated throughout the literature (Helmius, 2001; Taleporos, Dip, & McCabe, 2002), and clinicians should be aware of the importance of social support interventions. A 42-year-old woman with a neuromuscular degenerative disorder describes her thankfulness for the close relationships she experienced in the past, and currently experiences, with family members:

> "I was lucky as I was growing up to have a mother who loved me, no matter what. After she died, my younger sisters and I became even closer. Without their support and openness, I imagine I would have a difficult time waking in the morning."

Women with disabilities also confront specific challenges related to issues of body image. Society places enormous positive value and emphasis on having a perfect body, and this ubiquitous, impossible standard is often a further area of vulnerability for the self-esteem of all people who do not have perfect bodies, perhaps especially so for women with disabilities. Some women with disabilities state that they feel asexual, anonymous, or overlooked in the sexual spectrum of adult life (Cole & Cole, 1999). In addition, issues of behavioral autonomy, sexuality, reproductive capacity, motherhood, interpersonal relationships, and the onset of the aging process are all areas to be discussed when treating a woman with a disability. Very little research has been done on the life course of the individual human being with a physical disability, whether female or male, within the fields of medical sciences, social sciences, or the humanities. In addition, there is a lack of research contributing to the understanding of women within different cultural groups and the specific challenges these women may face in confronting both cultural issues as well as those related to their disability. All of these factors must be put into context as they impact career development in women with disabilities.

Katherine is a 42-year-old European American woman with multiple sclerosis who, along with her husband, is raising two young children. Over the course of her illness, it has been necessary for her to completely rearrange her work schedule. She has increasing difficulty with her speech as the day progresses, and is therefore only able to talk on the phone with clients in the morning. The rest of the day, she takes care of administrative work on the computer. Because she experiences numbness in her fingers, computer work presents an additional challenge. On several occasions, Katherine has been required to attend social events in the evening as part of her job. She must rest all day, sacrificing her other job responsibilities, in order to have the energy and cognitive capacity to engage in a social event. Despite all of this preparation, Katherine is still distressed and embarrassed at her word-finding difficulties and lowered verbal fluency at social occasions. Her employers have been supportive of her illness, yet Katherine constantly feels inadequate and frustrated by her inability to be as productive as she was before her diagnosis. The Americans with Disabilities Act (ADA) of 1990 requires her employer to make accommodations for her, and she is confused about whether her expectations (to be able to succeed and be productive) are feasible. In other areas of her life, as a mother and wife, Katherine often feels overwhelmed by the household pressures, resulting in additional feelings of inadequacy. She experiences increasing depression and despair as she attempts to live with a disability, while balancing work, family, and self-care.

In this case example, I (LGZ) initially used a humanistic approach to allow Katherine to begin the grieving process in order to ultimately facilitate her acceptance of her disability. Therapy revealed that Katherine felt trapped in a body that felt foreign to her. She was angry and frustrated and felt as if her life were spinning out of control. Not only did Katherine experience a loss of control over the changes in her body, but she also had lost control of her ability to work, effectively parent, and maintain a positive marital relationship. Throughout the process of exploration, understanding, and final acceptance of her disability under the framework of a combined narrative and cognitive approach, Katherine was able to externalize the problem and become empowered to accept herself while understanding her limitations.

It is important for clinicians to understand their female clients with disabilities in context, as career advancement cannot be examined without exploring development of the self over the lifespan. Development is unique for women confronted with lifelong disabilities. It is not only comprised of transitions and turning points, continuities and discontinuities, but the added dimension of possible barriers to independence (Rutter & Rutter, 1993). Women with disabilities confront many of the same challenges throughout development over the lifespan as women without disabilities, yet these challenges are tinged with possible discrimination and alienation, particularly in the workplace.

> Margaret is a 54-year-old European American woman with rheuma-toid arthritis who has been bound to a wheelchair for most of her life. After receiving her master's degree, she was politically active for many years in Washington, DC, advocating for equal rights for individuals with disabilities. She is currently the assistant director at a disability services center for college students in an urban area, a position she has held for almost 15 years. She is ready for a change in her workplace environment and therefore recently interviewed for a similar position at another more prestigious college. During her interview, she experi-enced what she considered to be the most egregious discrimination she had been confronted with in several years and was shocked that it came from the director of the Disability Services Center at an institu-tion that she revered. She was asked directly about her disability and what impact it would have on her ability to work. Not only did this individual display complete disregard for the federal laws set forth by the Americans with Disabilities Act of 1990, but he engaged in the type of subtle devaluation that is often experienced by individuals with disabilities. Margaret was left to wonder what impact her years of advocating for equal rights had had on society, and how a department created to assist individuals with disability could lack the knowledge to treat her as a respected equal. Margaret was offered the position in the end, but decided to reject the job in order to remain in an environ-ment that treated her with respect. She might have taken on this new job in an attempt to alter the culture and "educate" these college administrators; however, when asked why she decided against this challenge, Margaret replied, "I'm tired."

Recent research has shown that clinicians might best serve women with disabilities by working from an emergent theoretical model that con-ceptualizes a system of influences organized around a core dynamic self, which include identity constructs (disability, gender, racial/ethnic/cultural factors), personality characteristics, and belief in self (Noonan et al., 2004). Within this model, myriad contextual inputs are identified: developmental opportunities (education and peer influences), family influences (back-ground and current), disability impact (ableism, stress and coping levels, health issues), availability of social support (disabled and nondisabled com-munities, role models and mentors), career attitudes and behaviors (work attitudes, success strategies, leadership/pioneering behaviors), and sociopo-litical context (social movements, advocacy).

Career interventions for disabled women planning to enter the work world should include the development of their ability to build social sup-port as well as the development of strategies to cope with prejudice, to overcome internalized discouragement regarding gender and vocational success, and to understand the interactions among disability and other aspects of their salient identities (Noonan et al., 2004). In addition, current qualitative research findings suggest that the commonly used feminist therapy strategy of empowerment through "making the personal political," that is, engaging interested clients in proactive political and advocacy activities, may be a very effective approach for empowerment in the career arena through enhancing self-efficacy or even building professional networks (Noonan et al., 2004). Many women with disabilities appreciate when their community is supportive and therefore find solace in giving back through volunteer work activities.

Clinicians must consider the multivariate nature of the development of women with physical disabilities and the specific impact of the disability on career development. Women with physical disabilities confront many obstacles throughout the lifespan. An ecological perspective may help enable clinicians to work effectively in understanding and empowering the women within this population as they work toward career actualization.

Conclusions

The major themes of this chapter include recognition and understanding of the multiple contextual influences on women's work/career choices and advancement. The critical psychological issue for most women is achieving a satisfying balance between the work/career, family/relationships, and self-care components of healthy living over the lifespan. The types and degree of women's choices depend on their economic circumstances, individual abilities and disabilities, temperament and personality, family choices and opportunities as well as a degree of fit with their organizational culture and social systemic issues (e.g., gender, race, ethnicity, class, sexual orientation, health and political issues).

The meaning of positive balance changes throughout life. Some issues that we do not have space to address here include the impact of divorce, widowhood, elder care, and retirement on working women. It cannot be assumed that women are free to take responsibility for ailing parents and still care for other immediate family members. Women's situations differ, obviously, and some do not have the latitude to take off long periods from work. Many women entrepreneurs are attempting to address these concerns by developing consultation services that provide home care, elder care, and other human services across the country. The need for these innovative services will continue to increase, as will the challenge to make them available to all women and families, not only those with financial stability and privilege.

As clinicians, our goal is to consider all aspects of a woman's contextual issues and major role identifications as an essential component of any psychotherapy. Clinicians can use multiple theoretical orientations and clinical strategies to help women understand their roles and responsibilities in various contexts, so that they feel empowered to consider their options and develop an individual plan for achieving balance and prioritizing their goals and objectives. An empathic, supportive, collaborative, and encouraging therapeutic relationship is the bedrock of clinical intervention. We are all working women, and in order to help our working and nonworking women clients, we need to differentiate our own issues from our client's issues and serve as congruent role models.

References

Agars, M. D. (2004). Reconsidering the impact of gender stereotypes on the advancement of women in organizations. *Psychology of Women Quarterly, 28*, 103–111.

Belkin, L. (2003, October 16). The opt-out revolution. *New York Times Magazine,* pp. 5–22.

Bepko, C., & Johnson, T. (2000). Gay and lesbian couples in therapy: Perspectives for the contemporary family therapist. *Journal of Marital and Family Therapy, 6*(4), 409–421.

Biaggio, L., Roades, D. S., Cardinale, J., & Duffy, R. (2000). Clinical evaluations: Impact of sexual orientation, gender and gender roles. *Journal of Applied Psychology, 30*(18), 1657–1666.

Blagg, D., & Young, S. (2002). Women and work: Redefining success. *Harvard Business School Bulletin, 78*(1), 33–37.

Blanton, G. (2004, March 16). Women often eye top jobs. *Boston Globe*, p. D3.

Blustein, D. L. (2001). The interface of work and relationships: Critical knowledge for 21st century. *The Counseling Psychologist, 29*(2), 179–192.

Boyce, L. A., & Herd, A. M. (2003). The relationship between gender role stereotypes and requisite military leadership characteristics. *Journal of Research, 49*(7-8), 365–414.

Carli, L. L., & Eagly, A. H. (2001). Gender, hierarchy and leadership: An introduction. *Journal of Social Issues, 57*(14), 629–637.

Center for Research on Women with Disabilities. (1992). *National study of women with physical disabilities*. Retrieved July 8, 2003, from www.bcm.tmc.edu/crowd/national_study/national_study.html

Chung, Y. B. (2003). Career counseling with lesbian, gay, bisexual, and transgendered persons: The next decade. *Career Development Quarterly, 52*(1), 78–87.

Cole, S. S., & Cole, T. M. (1999). Sexuality, disability, and reproductive issues through the lifespan. In R. P. Marinelli & A. E. Dell Orto (Eds.), *The psychological and social impact of disability* (pp. 241–256). New York: Springer.

Cotter, D. A. (2001). The glass ceiling effects. *Social Forces, 80*(12), 655–681.

DiNatalie, M., & Boraas, D. (2002, March). The labor force experience of women from Generation "X." *Errata,* 3–15.

Dovidio, J. F., & Gaertner, S. L. (2000). Aversive racism and selection decisions: 1989 and 1999. *Psychological Science, 11,* 315–319.

Fassinger, R. E. (2002). Hitting the ceiling: Gendered barriers to occupational entry, advancement and achievement. In L. Diamant & J. Lee (Eds.), *The psychology of sex, gender and jobs: Issues and solutions* (pp. 21–46). Westport, CT: Greenwood.

Gottfredson, L. S. (2002). Gottfredson's theory of circumscription, compromise, and self-creation. In D. Brown (Ed.), *Career choice and development* (pp. 85–148). San Francisco: Jossey-Bass

Griffith, K. H. & Hebl, N. R. (2002). The disclosure dilemma for gay men and lesbians: "Coming out" at work. *Journal of Applied Psychology, 87*(6), 1191–1199.

Hacker, A. (2003). *Mismatch.* New York: Scribner's.

Hattery, A. (2001). *Work and family: Balancing and weaving.* Thousand Oaks, CA: Sage.

Hebl, M., Foster, J. M., Mannix, L. M., & Dovidio, J. F. (2002). Formal and interpersonal discrimination: A field study bias toward homosexual applicants. *Personality and Social Psychology Bulletin, 28,* 815–825.

Heilman, M. B. (2001). Description and prescription: How gender stereotypes prevent women's descent up the organization ladder. *Journal of Social Issues, 57*(14), 657–688.

Helmius, G. (2001). The paradox of discriminatory practices as a means of emancipatory strategies. *Community, Work and Family, 4*(3), 273–284.

Jans, L., & Stoddard, S. (1999). *Chartbook on women and disability in the United States: An InfoUse report* (Document No. H133D50017-96). Washington, DC: U.S. Department of Education, National Institute on Disability and Rehabilitation Research.

Kanter, R. M. (1997). *Frontiers of management.* Cambridge, MA: Harvard Business School Press.

Ledet, L. M., & Henley, T. B. (2000). Perceptions of women's power as a function of position within an organization. *Journal of Psychology, 134*(5), 515–526.

MBACareers.com. (2003). *MBACareers.com finds gender gap in male and female career aspirations.* Retrieved October 2, 2004, from JobBankUSA.com/careerarticles/career/ca72303a.html

McLennan, N. A., & Arthur, N. (1999). Applying the cognitive informal processing approach to career problem solving and decision making to women's career development. *Journal of Employment Counseling, 36*(2), 82–96.

McNeil, J. M. (2001). *Americans with disabilities: Household economic studies* (pp. 70–73). Washington, DC: U.S. Government Printing Office, U.S. Bureau of the Census, Current Population Reports.

McWhirter, F. H., Torres, D. M., & Rasheed, S. (1998). Assessing barriers to women's career adjustment. *Journal of Career Assessment, 6*(4), 449–479.

Monthly Labor Review. (2002, June). *125*(6). Washington, DC: Department of Labor.

National Gay and Lesbian Task Force. (1991). *National gay and lesbian task force survey*. National Gay and Lesbian Task Force Records, 1973–2000. Ithaca, NY: Cornell University, Division of Rare Book and Manuscript Collections.

Noonan, B. M., Gallor, S. M., Hensler-McGinnis, N. F., Fassinger, R. E., Wang, S., & Goodman, J. (2004). Challenge and success: A qualitative study of the career development of highly achieving women with physical and sensory disabilities. *Journal of Counseling Psychology, 51*(1), 68–80.

Okun, B. F. (2004). Human diversity. In R. H. Coombs (Ed.), *Family therapy review* (pp. 41–62). Mahwah, NJ: Erlbaum.

Powers, B. (1996). The impact of gay, lesbian, and bisexual workplace issues on productivity. In A. L. Ellis & E. D. B. Riggle (Eds.), *Sexual identity on the job: Issues and services* (pp. 79–90). New York: Haworth Press.

Rutter, M., & Rutter, M. (1993). *Developing minds: Challenge and continuity across the life span*. London: Penguin Books.

Smith, D. (2002). Making work your family's ally. *Monitor on Psychology, 33*(7), 58–60.

Smith, N. G., & Ingram, K. M. (2004). Workplace heterosexism and adjustment among lesbian, gay, and bisexual individuals: The role of unsupportive social interactions. *Journal of Counseling Psychology, 51*(1), 57–67.

Taleporos, G., Dip, G., & McCabe, M. P. (2002). The impact of sexual esteem, body esteem, and sexual satisfaction on psychological well-being in people with physical disability. *Sexuality and Disability, 20*(3), 177–183.

CHAPTER 11

Robbing Peter to Pay Paul

REFLECTIONS ON FEMINIST THERAPY
WITH LOW-WAGE-EARNING WOMEN

Vanessa Jackson

I grew up poor, hated, the victim of physical, emotional, and sexual violence, and I know that suffering does not ennoble. To resist destruction, self-hatred, or lifelong hopelessness, we have to throw off the conditioning of being despised, the fear of becoming the they that is talked about so dismissively, to refuse lying myths and easy moralities, to see ourselves as human, flawed, and extraordinary. All of us—extraordinary.

—DOROTHY ALLISON (1994, p. 36)

I am the daughter of Midwestern black working-class parents and grew up in the context of "enough"—enough food, adequate shelter, and access to medical and dental care. However, my parents repeatedly reminded my five siblings and me that "there was no money tree growing in our backyard." One of my earliest memories is sitting at our kitchen table pretending to write checks as my mother paid household bills. Although I was too young to understand it at the time, I remember my mother talking about "robbing Peter to pay Paul." As I grew older, I came to understand the anxiety, which she had hidden from me, created from ending up with too many bills and too few dollars at the end of the month. Unfortunately, I had not inherited my mother's skill in resource allocation, and a recent decision to self-fund a research project depleted my savings and left me wracked with anxiety when an unexpected bill showed up in my mailbox. As a therapist in private practice, I understand that I sit in a place of privilege, represented by my education and the power to label others through diagnosing them with a mental illness. However, in the past year, as I worked to rebuild my practice, I found myself among the ranks of the "professional poor," often sitting a few fee-paying clients away from financial disaster. This experience pushed me firmly into a place of "not enough." I realize that my experience was temporary and could be immediately solved by taking a position with an agency. That is my point of privilege—to remove myself from the economic margin when the fear and anxiety become overwhelming.

I start with my personal story of the day-to-day realities of living in the low-wage margins because I was amazed at how quickly I shifted into a space of panic and despair that narrowed my world and made me tense and less generous. The fear sucked up my energy and reached a level where it actually began to interfere with my ability to make a living. The most significant impact of my temporary poverty was that it put me in a place of shame. Politically meaningful work in domestic violence shelters, sexual assault programs, homeless shelters, and community mental health centers often leave feminist therapists barely clinging to middle-class status and can push us over the edge of poverty if we are the sole support of children or aging parents.

Millions of women struggle with the reality of poverty every day, with no relief in sight and no easily obtainable options with which to change their situation. The one thing that was clear to me in writing about a feminist perspective on therapy with women who live at or below the poverty level was the need to name the primary source of the pain these women experience. Women who live in poverty are the truest sisterhood because their ranks cut across lines of race, ethnicity, national origin, religion, age, sexual orientation, and geography. These are not "poor women"; these are low-wage-earning women. This distinction is important if, as feminist therapists, we are to engage in ethical and potentially healing relationships with our clients. The term "low-wage-earning women" helps us to always keep an eye trained on the economic conditions that create and/or maintain the challenges that lead many women and their families to seek our services. The phrase "robbing Peter to pay Paul" describes the shifting of limited dollars within the family budget to cover the most crucial household bills. However, the phrase also describes the shift in financial resources from the poor to the wealthiest 1% of the U.S. population.

The most insidious aspect of the classism in the United States is the vilification of families who live in poverty. Dorothy Allison's quote captures the emotional devastation that emerges out of the internalization of classism and the ongoing acts of invalidation that one experiences as part of a devalued group. Chester Pierce, a noted African American psychiatrist, described the impact of one manifestation of racism—"micro-aggressions"—daily acts of invalidation that left black people feeling "oppressed, defeated, demoralized and degraded in 100 ways each day of existence" (quoted in King, 1981). This same theory of micro-aggressions can be applied to low-wage-earning people in the United States. The effects of sexism that render women's daily lives a mind field of emotional and physical dangers compound these class-based micro-aggressions.

This chapter provides an overview of the economic conditions facing low-wage-earning women as a context for understanding the traumatic impact of being poor and female in the United States. I explore the impact of class on the clinical interface and common themes that emerged in my clinical work with low-wage-earning women. I conclude with feminist strategies for supporting healing for these women within the clinical setting and beyond.

Faces at the Bottom of the Well: Overview of Women's Economic Realities

Although some therapists continue to live working-class lives, the majority of us have moved into middle-class lifestyles. Within the warmth and safety of these lifestyles, it requires considerable conscious effort to stay connected with the day-to-day realities of low-wage-earning women. The U.S. Census Bureau recently released a report stating that the poverty rate for female-headed households had increased to 28% in 2003, and poverty among adult women had risen to 12.4%. In addition, 16 million women have no health insurance (Kaiser Family Foundation, 2004).

Gwen is a 37-year-old African American woman who was referred to the mental health center for treatment of crack cocaine addiction and parenting problems. Her two children, Antoine, age 12 and Shyniece, age 15, were also mandated into treatment as part of their probation through juvenile court. Gwen has been free of substance use for 6 months. The family had lived for nearly a year in an extended-stay hotel, The Lodge, with Gwen's 40-year-old boyfriend. The Lodge had long since ceased to be haven for tourist and business travelers and had settled into the business of serving as the closest thing to affordable housing in a large metropolitan area. Residents forked out $149 per week for a double room with cable (a necessity when you have children in a dangerous area with limited entertainment options). The family shared a cramped room, in which the adolescents shared a second bed; clearly, there was no privacy. Gwen used a hot plate to prepare any meals that were not eaten out at fast-food restaurants. She secured a job at a local factory, where she made $8 an hour, and she walked 2 miles along an access road to her second-shift position. Gwen and her boyfriend struggled to scrape together the $1,200 required for a deposit and first month's rent on an apartment. The family's life was reduced to work and the mental health center. Both adults were involved in a 12-step program and the children were involved in individual, family, and group therapy. There were four separate therapists and group facilitators involved with the family. Initially, little effort was made by mental health professionals to coordinate appointments. Fortunately, the child and adolescent program provided flexible funding that was used to assist the family with the rent deposit. This money would not have been available to a woman without children stranded in motel for nearly a year. Her life and her possibilities as a single childless woman would not have been viewed as worth the investment. Standing in their hotel room completely shifted my opinion of Gwen and her family. Their challenges in negotiating small conflicts looked completely different from the vantage point of a 15-by-15-foot room. The constant rubbing up against each other, physically and emotionally, set the stage for explosive conflicts. How do you create effective boundaries with your children when they sleep 4 feet away from you and your partner? Gwen's ability to maintain her recovery under her living conditions was nothing short of amazing, given the constant stream of dealers and customers who frequented the motel.

Once the family was settled in stable housing, the focus shifted to the reestablishment of parent–child boundaries. Gwen's therapist worked with her to express her frustration over her children's resistance to her attempts to set limits and her own history of having to fend for herself as a young adolescent. She was supported in her efforts to set clear limits with her children, even as she struggled with her limited experience at effective parenting. The therapeutic team consistently acknowledged Gwen's love for her children and her desire to create a stable, drug-free environment for them. Her children participated in a group for children affected by parental drug and alcohol addiction. Family sessions provided an opportunity for Gwen and her children to share their feelings and concerns about the chaos created during her years of substance abuse. Gwen's individual sessions open the door to her exploration of the connection between her drug use and her history of childhood sexual abuse. The family dropped out of service in the child and adolescent mental health program when the children completed their probation. However, Gwen continued in her substance abuse recovery program.

Low-wage workers are defined as persons who could not support a family of four on full-time wages beyond the government's official poverty level. In 2004 the Federal Register listed the Department of Health and Human Services poverty guidelines for a family of four as $18,850. An hourly wage of $9.06 is required to bring a single woman with three children to the poverty threshold (assuming she worked 40 hours per week for 52 weeks). But even an hourly wage of $10 per hour does not mean freedom from poverty. The poverty guidelines are not connected to reality in that they were established in the early 1960s and based on emergency food budgets and the assumption that 30% of a family's income was used for food. The current reality is that housing and medical care are the major expenditures in the majority of family budgets. Affordable housing has become an urban legend and out of reach for many low-wage-earning women. The National Low Income Housing Coalition (2004) reports that in 2003, an average national housing wage (hourly wage required to afford fair-market-rate housing that does not exceed 30% of monthly income) of $15.21 was required to secure a two-bedroom unit. In metropolitan Atlanta, the fair-market rate for a two-bedroom unit was $728 per month. For Gwen and millions of women like her, these equations lead to extended stay hotels, homeless shelters, and substandard housing in drug- and violence-plagued neighborhoods. Poor housing options open the door to "low-achieving" schools, inaccessible grocery stores, limited safe child care and entertainment options, and the simultaneous isolation from, and increased scrutiny by, middle-class society, which sets the standards for emotional health and productive living.

Low-wage-earning women are a diverse group, but women of color and immigrant women are overrepresented among the women in poverty. Racism, heterosexism, and ableism frequently intersect with gender to lock women into low-wage positions. Immigrant women may experience shifts in class status as part of the numerous losses inherent in the immigration experience. In addition, undocumented workers may be subjected to slavery-like economic exploitation as domestic, agricultural, and factory workers with virtually no legal recourse. Homophobia in the workplace may limit the employment options of lesbians/bisexual/transgendered women. Women frequently experience the double, and even triple, burden of multiple oppressions. According to the U.S. Census Bureau (2004) in 2003, the poverty rate was 24.4% for blacks, 23.2% for American Indians and Alaska natives, 22.5% for Hispanics, 11.8% for Asians, and 8.2% for non-Hispanic whites. In *The Working Poor: Invisible in America*, Shipler (2004), creates a bleak portrait of poverty among immigrant groups and notes that anti-globalization activists do not have to leave U.S. soil to protest sweatshops. The poverty-wage labor of undocumented workers provides for countless comforts and basic necessities that fuel the U.S. economy. Poverty is a feminist and a therapeutic issue. Feminist therapists pick up the poisoned fruits of poverty in battered women and homeless shelters, in psychiatric hospitals and outpatient clinics, in sexual assault centers, and increasingly in collaboration with welfare-related services. It is ironic that the mental health of women has become a public policy issue as welfare reform efforts drive more women into the low-wage labor market. Unfortunately, women overwhelmed by posttraumatic stress disorder, depression, or substance abuse are considered problem workers, in spite of the fact that many of these diagnoses are disabilities protected under the Americans with Disabilities Act. Temporary Aid to Needy Families (TANF), the nation's ultimate "safety net" for economically distressed families, has turned to social service agencies to patch up these emotional wounds, many caused by poverty, and get these women into the workforce. What is the feminist response to an invitation to serve as a tool of social control? How do we balance this mandate with the very real need of these low-wage-earning women to enter an emotional healing space in which they can address the myriad traumatic experiences and stressors related to the day-to-day terror of poverty? Although we may have limited control over how women access our services, what we do once they arrive can make all the difference between a health-promoting and empowering experience or a health-damaging acclimation to oppressive conditions.

Poverty in the Clinical Context

As clinicians, we have to understand that when low-wage-earning women show up in our offices, they have likely already negotiated an obstacle course of case managers, school officials, employers, child care providers, public transportation, empty gas tanks, and years of emotional pain. Even low-wage-earning women with insurance may be struggling to integrate the copayment into their bare-bones budget.

There is a slowly growing body of literature regarding the implications of class in feminist therapy. Hill and Rothblum (1996) assembled a crucial collection of articles that directly engage the issue of class and feminist therapy. Low-wage-earning women experience the same type of emotional problems that bring many women to therapy—sexual and physical trauma, depression, thought disorders, relationship and parenting conflicts. However, they arrive at the clinic doors with a distinct set of vulnerabilities that more economically privilege clients do not carry. Mickey de Valda, a white working-class man active in the Hearing Voices Network in England, notes that "working class people are more likely to accept their label and live it, act it out and become the schizophrenic [or borderline] they are told they are." McNair and Neville (1996) note the stereotype of low- and working-class black women as promiscuous and how this stereotype may dissuade these women from seeking help in the aftermath of sexual assault for fear that the responsibility for the assault will be placed on them.

The Wound of Meritocracy

Baker (1996) and Lerner (1986) address the myth of meritocracy in the United States that posits that where you end up economically is based on your merit. Therefore, if you are poor, it is due to your own failings, and if you are wealthy, it is through your hard work and intelligence. The insidious nature of meritocracy is that it operates essentially without acknowledging the existence of a class hierarchy. The historical amnesia of U.S. culture makes low-wage workers more vulnerable to the wounding influence of meritocracy. The challenges and accomplishments of the civil rights, women's, and gay/lesbian/bisexual/transgendered movements are recent enough to still be held in the cultural memories of most people. However, the challenges and successes of the labor movement, from the implementation of 40-hour work weeks to prohibition against child labor and the brutal union-busting efforts of business owners, are a distant memory. This historical memory of the triumph of collective action to improve working conditions and wages for working-class communities is complicated by the reality of ethnic, gender, and racial discrimination within trade unions (Tait, 1999).

The individualization of economic success or failure creates isolation and renders low-wage-earning women more vulnerable to internalizing a view of themselves as incompetent or undeserving. Clinical interventions that create an opportunity for exploring the context of economic exploitation of the working class can open the door for emotional healing *and* political action. This exploration can be achieved without ignoring the immediate emotional challenges of depression, anxiety, and other manifestations of trauma.

The dilemma of tackling the *oppression* versus the *depression* is familiar to people involved in the sexual assault and domestic violence movements. The challenge is how to render immediate aid while supporting an understanding of the systemic factors (e.g., sexism, racism, heterosexism) that target members of marginalized communities for oppression? Explicit discussion of class issues within the context of feminist therapy allows us to identify the "fiscal trauma" that emerges from society's willingness to create and maintain economic conditions that put marginalized individuals at risk of a variety of health and emotional problems.

Sue was working-class black woman in her mid-40s who had suffered a debilitating back injury and been unable to work for several years. Even without her injury, there were few employment options available in her rural town. Sue also suffered from severe clinical depression but had been erroneously assigned the diagnosis of schizophrenia, which resulted in her being placed on antipsychotic medications and in a day treatment program. In spite of her chronic physical problems and her psychiatric condition, Sue was repeatedly denied Social Security Disability income support. The lack of meaningful work and income fueled her depression and also required her to be dependent on an emotionally abusive family member for housing. Sue tried repeatedly to secure work that was not physically demanding. However, on the rare occasions when she was able to get a job, her explosive anger quickly resulted in her termination. In the day treatment program, Sue was able to connect with several other women who were involved in the mental health system and who had also been repeatedly denied Social Security income. During group discussions, staff explored the women's allegations of discriminatory treatment by the local Social Security agency and began to research strategies for securing new hearings. Although Sue was unable to get a new hearing for herself, she expressed a sense of relief at having her concerns validated by the other women and noted a reduction in her sense of isolation and helplessness. Sue stated that it was helpful to have staff and group members acknowledge the link between her depression, her feelings of rage, and her financial situation.

Chronic Stress and Poverty

In *Nickel and Dimed* (2001), writer Barbara Ehrenreich chronicles her journey through low-wage jobs in the United States. She describes the stress of unsuccessfully searching for affordable housing, engaging in physically and emotionally draining work, and the overwhelming anxiety of knowing that she did not have adequate resources to live. Ehrenreich, understands that she is playing at being poor, but she also introduces readers to the women who live this life, day in and out. It is a hard truth to witness.

Joan is a 40-year-old white woman who moved to a suburban community after leaving her husband when it was disclosed that he had sexually abused two of their four daughters. Joan left the relative economic security of her husband's salary and struggled to survive on child support and a low-wage job at a fast food restaurant. Joan brought her daughters in for counseling related to the sexual abuse and their increasingly out-of-control behavior. A petite, quiet, slightly depressed woman with a pleasant smile, Joan reported feeling under siege and out of control at home. She was invited to join the Mothers' Circle, a self-nurturing group for women who are parenting. Forming this group was my response to increasing complaints from my colleagues regarding "parents who will not comply with treatment." I did not know much, but I was clear that replicating the shame and abuse that these mother experience every day at jobs and in school, welfare, and juvenile probation offices was no answer to the attendance problems. After repeated invitations, Joan agreed to attend the five-session group.

During the first session, participants complete a self-care checklist. Joan's responses indicated that she was not current on medical and dental checkups; she was isolated, with no adult support network; and she did not get adequate sleep. Joan worked the opening shift at the restaurant and arrived at work by 5:00 A.M. She negotiated a schedule where she took an extended break around 7:00 A.M., which allowed her to return home and see her children off to school. Following her shift, she completed errands before picking up her children at school. Many afternoons were filled with therapy appointments. By the time Joan got all of her children to bed and settled down for the night, it was near midnight. She had operated for nearly a year on about 4 hours of sleep a night. Joan was depressed, but she also suffered from extreme exhaustion. In the Mothers' Circle she was able to tell the truth about her life and be witnessed by other women, many of whom had had similar experiences. It was a small step in breaking her out of a place of isolation. Joan stated that the most useful part of the group and the family sessions was to help reduce her guilt regarding the victimization of her children by their father. She was able to acknowledge that her ex-husband had also victimized her when he betrayed her trust and violated their children. She also was able to talk with other mothers and explore realistic mother–daughter boundaries. Joan noted that she had moved into more of peer role with her children and alternated between being afraid of the girls or acquiescing to their demands, which often put additional financial strain on her, in an attempt to secure their love.

Referring Joan to individual counseling was an option, but she has no time in her day for one more appointment. However, we compromised and I began to meet with Joan at the end of her daughter's session to check in on how she is doing, as a woman, not just as a mother. Although this level of support is less than what she truly needs, she had few alternatives that would not increase the stress in her life. The ultimate goal was for Joan to transfer more responsibility for some of the household chores to her children, which would allow her time to address some of her own personal needs.

Chronic stress can manifest in a range of physical ailments, including hypertension, migraines, back problems, and gastrointestinal complaints. A clinical assessment that includes a general question about medical concerns can be useful, in addition to providing information about low-cost clinics and offering to assist women in negotiating the frequently stress-inducing process of securing medical care. Because a fairly common response to chronic stress is self-medication with drugs and alcohol, it is important to explore the impact of the external conditions as one of many triggers for substance abuse.

Poverty as Trauma

I am wary of the risk of diluting the meaning of trauma as reflected in the experiences of physical and sexual assault, terrorist attacks, and war by adding to the list experiences of oppression that have become commonplace. I remember raising the issue of the traumatic impact of racism with a national expert on trauma, a middle-age, middle-class white male, who scoffed at the idea, stating, "an inability to catch a cab is hardly traumatic." However, numerous authors (Akinyela, 2002; McAdams-Mahmoud, 2002; Pinderhughes, 2004) have documented the traumatic impact of slavery, segregation, and racism on African American families and communities and the multigenerational transmission of that trauma.

The traumatic nature of poverty, reflected in malnutrition, premature death from preventable conditions, dislocation from housing, and prolonged periods of homelessness, may be harder to pin down due to the myth of meritocracy and the reality that individuals and families do shift social classes in America. According to the *Comprehensive Textbook of Psychiatry* (cited in Herman, 1992), the common denominator of psychological trauma is a feeling of "intense fear, helplessness, loss of control and threat of annihilation" (p. 33). In my conversations with no- or low-wage-earning women, especially at times of crisis such as an impending eviction, fear, helplessness, and despair are always present in the discussion. Although poverty may not be a trauma on par with physical abuse, it does create chronic levels of stress and exposure to a multitude of mental and physical health problems. House and Williams (2000) explain:

> What makes socioeconomic position such a powerful determinant of health is that it shapes people's experiences of, and exposure to, virtually all psychosocial and environmental risk factors for health—past, present and future—and these in turn operate through a very broad range of physiological mechanisms to influence the incidence and the course of virtually all major causes of death and health. (p. 90)

Whereas this concept of poverty as trauma requires further study, it is a useful categorization to utilize in dialogues with low-wage-earning women, because it implicitly (and appropriately) conveys the life-threatening and shame-inducing experiences that are beyond the view of middle-class America. In a recent conversation with a group of women that serves as a resource to mothers in a no- and low-wage-earning community, we talked about the stress and trauma created in their community by previous urban renewal and the current gentrification movement that transforms affordable housing for low-wage-earning families into what a protest sign described as "Yuppie Ghettos." The women noted that the recent placement of a sign announcing the development of $300,000 homes across the street from their community center was clear notice of their impending dislocation. They felt that this looming dislocation was a critical issue to discuss during a presentation on mental health in their community. Fullilove (2004) describes the multigenerational trauma and negative health consequences of "root shock," the destruction of communities and the massive dislocation of families and their support networks due to urban land-use policies.

Survivor Guilt and Fear

A common theme in therapeutic work with low-wage-earning women is that of "survivor guilt" or being a "class traitor." Upward mobility is the American dream, and there is a profound relief in reaching a space of economic security. However, many low-wage-earning women may experience a sense of guilt that they have pulled themselves above the poverty line but have economically left behind family and community members.

> Cara, a young black female client, recently spoke of her guilt over feeling depressed for "no reason" (she was in the process of escaping from an emotionally and physically abusive relationship) when she had been able to move from homelessness to homeownership. Cara reported that she looks for opportunities to help out young homeless people because she remembers the trauma of living in abandoned buildings after being kicked out of her mother's home at age 16. As we briefly sketched out a genogram, she noted a pattern in which daughters were put out of the house in mid-adolescence to fend for themselves. Cara is aware that her genuine commitment to giving back to her community has numerous safety risks (from taking in virtual strangers) and possible economic consequences, because maintaining her home for herself requires that she work two low-wage jobs. She struggles with the desire to provide assistance and the awareness that she still stands on economically shaky ground. For Cara, survivor's guilt manifests as an inability to enjoy her achievements. She is beginning to explore more appropriate boundaries that allow her to give back to her community while taking care of her own household as her first priority.

Another aspect of survivor guilt is the pattern of overspending to make up for deprivations. Often this generosity extends to family and friends.

> Susan was on the cusp of lower-middle-class status as a low-level manager at a company. She was able to purchase a home and provide a stable living environment for her daughter, which had always

been her dream after being raised in abject poverty as a child. Then Susan plunged into an "orgy of spending" that culminated in bank fraud and a failure to pay her mortgage for nearly a year before resulting in foreclosure on the property. Susan noted that her spending spree included buying numerous gifts for friends and family members. She has some awareness that her "generosity" is an attempt to balance the severe economic deprivation of her childhood. At the time of her consultation, Susan and her daughter were living in an extended stay hotel. She reported that she occasionally socialized with several other mothers at the hotel and frequently loaned small sums of money to neighbors and friends. Susan noted that the money she loaned was frequently needed for upcoming bills, including rent, but that she found it difficult to say no to others because she had often been the recipient of others' generosity. Susan's commitment to mutual aid, a long-standing and life-saving tradition in low-wage-earning communities, repeatedly pushed her into financial crisis. In therapy, we explored what Susan has begun to call her addiction to spending and the fact that her long-deprived "inner child" tends to go on spending binges on payday. She is able to understand the economic and social conditions that created the spending cravings, yet she still struggles daily to make decisions that honor her desire for security for herself and her daughter.

I have found it important to support individuals in finding ways to participate in mutual assistance that do not undermine their own fragile economic stability. Extending caring to others is a powerful affirmation of humanity and has a community-building impact. Long before government programs emerged, community sharing was the ultimate safety net. Quiet as it is kept, it still is today—and it represents a source of power and validation for low-wage-earning communities.

The Personal Is Political:
Therapy as a Tool for Liberation

Visibility and voice are powerful antidotes to poverty. As feminist therapists, we have been silent too long regarding issues of class and poverty. When we invite women to speak the unspoken aspects of their lives and bear witness to their pain and their triumphs, we are directly challenging for forces of oppression that say that their lives do not matter. The work of narrative therapists (Freedman & Combs, 1996; Morgan, 2000; Walgrave, Tamasese, Tuhaka, & Campbell, 2003; White, 2000) demonstrates the transformative power of engaging individuals in the retelling and reliving of their stories and the inclusion of the broader contexts of their lives.

All too often, low-wage-earning women lead fragmented lives as they encounter and attempt to negotiate various institutional systems. Shelters and hotlines see their physical and sexual abuse. Food pantries and homeless shelters see their hunger and lack of housing. Public clinics and emergency rooms see their poor health. Schools see the educational challenges that frequently bar them from living wage employment. Therapists see the emotional pain that results from carrying these multiple burdens. However, rarely are low-wage-earning women offered the time, support, and emotional space in which to connect the dots in their lives that maintain them in a place of poverty.

I have spent nearly 16 years involved in a self-help group based on the model developed by the National Black Women's Health Project (NBWHP; now known as the Black Women's Health Imperative). My training in the model occurred at Black and Female® retreats, and my primary trainers were low-wage-earning women who had integrated this model into their own lives and their community activism. NBWHP and the self-help model were based on four organizational goals (NBWHP, 1989):

1. To enable black women to understand the concepts and interrelationships of emotional, mental, physical, and spiritual health.
2. To provide black women with the information, skills, and access to resources to live healthfully.
3. To facilitate the empowerment of black women, both individually and collectively, to exercise control over their lives.
4. To ensure the survival of future generations of black people through the prevention of health maintenance and prevention.

The self-help groups provided women-controlled space, not dependent on government grants, third-party payments, or sliding-fee scales, in which we could talk about our lives. Women could bring all aspects of their lives into the healing space of the self-help groups under a broad definition of health that included, emotional, mental, physical, and spiritual aspects. As a self-help group developer, I routinely added a fifth aspect of health: financial stability. Although class tensions were a challenge for the NBWHP, as they are with many feminists, it was one of the few economically diverse spaces available to me as a feminist therapist from a working-class background.

I have integrated the goals of the NBWHP self-help model with feminist and narrative theory to create of principles that guide my clinical work with all women, but with special attention to the unique experiences of low-wage-earning women.

Guiding Principles for Feminist Therapists Working with Low-Wage-Earning Women

1. The therapist assumes responsibility for staying informed regarding the economic realities of low-wage-earning women. This responsibility involves staying current on information related to employment opportunities, wages, housing, child care, and transportation. Accurate information counters the myths regarding the poor that are pervasive in a capitalist, consumption-driven society. This information ensures an accurate understanding of factors that affect the behavior and emotional well-being of low-wage-earning women.

2. The therapist assumes responsibility for an active and ongoing exploration of her own attitudes and experiences related to class status. Specifically, the therapist should be cognizant of, and take responsibility for, changing negative attitudes regarding people who live in poverty.

3. The therapist respects the wisdom and strengths of low-wage-earning women and creates ongoing opportunities for women to articulate their unique stories regarding the impact of low-wage earning on their lives and possibilities. The therapist can invite stories of triumph, community, and love to assist clients in exploring stories that challenge the dominant narrative of low-wage earners as pathological and helpless.

4. The therapist assumes responsibility for demystifying the therapeutic process by clearly acknowledging and minimizing power imbalances. The therapist works collaboratively with women to create their plan for change, which is directed by the individual seeking consultation.

5. All engagements in the therapeutic process should be voluntary. However, if agency policies mandate involuntary treatment for low-wage-earning women (e.g., court-ordered treatment for addictions, child protective agency ordering family counseling following an abuse investigation), the therapist directly addresses the impact of the coercive intervention with the client. The therapist understands and communicates to the client that forced treatment is inherently shaming and that this system-generated shame must be addressed in the healing process. The therapist will support clients in identifying goals that meet their needs and will actively advocate true client/consumer-driven services.

6. The therapist is aware of the oppressive and potentially traumatizing impact of psychiatric labels on the identity and self-esteem of individuals. Low-wage-earning women are especially vulnerable to the shaming inherent in the diagnostic labeling process, because they often have limited education and knowledge that would enable them to resist the labels that could follow them for the rest of their lives.

7. The therapist values and assists low-wage women in identifying

healing experiences outside of the structured clinical hour. These resources include, but are not limited to, social action groups, spiritual/religious events, self-help groups, and self-development workshops.

8. The therapist understands that an apolitical stance in the therapeutic interface is a stand with the status quo. The personal is *still* political, and the therapist must function as an ally and advocate to support healing for low-wage-earning women in a capitalist society. This level of functioning involves helping the client to identify the external social, economic, and political factors that affect her ability to fully express herself in the world.

9. The therapist is committed to an economically diverse practice and utilizes a sliding-fee scale to ensure access to a broad range of clients. However, the provision of therapy is an income source, and a therapist has a right and responsibility to establish fee scales that allow her to secure a living wage. A therapist can engage in a range of creative practices, including groups, low-fee workshops, community presentations, and volunteer activities, to ensure that she is able to work in collaboration with low-wage-earning women.

10. The therapist is willing to accept leadership from low-wage-earning women and actively seeks out opportunities to participate in educational and political activities directed by low-wage-earning women. These actions are undertaken in the spirit of dismantling economic policies and practices that dehumanize people at all points in the class hierarchy.

Conclusion

Low-wage-earning women enter counseling with myriad internal and external challenges. In addition, these women are almost always embedded in the emotional and economic struggles of other immediate and extended family members. It is essential that feminist therapists take a position of honoring the multilayered stories of these women and actively encourage the telling of these stories in the therapeutic setting. However, it is equally important that we maintain a clear view of the pervasive social and economic challenges facing low-wage-earning women, who receive little comfort from the knowledge that they are victims of the "feminization of poverty." Feminist discourse on patriarchy rings a bit hollow in the face of the reality that the men in low-wage communities are equally limited in their economic opportunities. This does not mean that low-wage-earning women are free of other manifestations of patriarchal oppression. It does mean that issues of class have to be made more explicit in the discussion, just as women of color and lesbian/bisexual and transgendered feminists have demanded that issues of racism and heterosexism, respectively, be better integrated into feminist theory and clinical practice.

Feminist therapists must blend feminist theory with economic and political theories (Bracho & Latino Health Access, 2000; Brown, 1994; Friere, 1970; hooks, 1993; Lerner, 1986) that address the individual and community problems within a larger context. Unfortunately, much of the available literature on therapy with low-income women deals with black and Latina families, which creates the impression that the majority of these families are impoverished. At the same time it obscures the economic realities of Asian and Pacific Islander, Native American, and white families who struggle with poverty-induced or -aggravated emotional challenges. As Hill (1996) notes, "Class is complicated and difficult, but the first problem with class is that we don't talk about it. We can't afford that kind of silence" (p. 5).

References

Akinyela, M. (2002). Reparations: Repairing relationships and honouring ancestry. *International Journal of Narrative Therapy and Community Work, 2,* 46–49.

Albeda, R., & Tilly, C. (1997). *Glass ceilings and bottomless pits.* Boston: South End Press.

Allison, D. (1994). *Skin: Talking about sex, class and literature.* Ann Arbor, MI: Firebrand Books.

Baker, N. L. (1996). Class as a construct in a "classless" society. In M. Hill & E. D. Rothblum (Eds.), *Classism and feminist therapy: Counting costs* (pp. 1–23). Binghamton, NY: Harrington Press.

Bracho, A., & Latino Health Access. (2000). Towards a healthy community . . . even if we have to sell tamales: The work of Latino Health Access. *Dulwich Centre Journal, 3,* 3–20.

Brown, L. S. (1994). *Subversive dialogues: Theory in feminist therapy.* New York: Basic Books.

Ehrenreich, B. (2001). *Nickel and dimed: On not getting by in America.* New York: Metropolitan Books.

Federal Register. (2004). 69(30), pp. 7336–7338.

Freedman, J., & Combs, G. (1996). *Narrative therapy: The social construction of preferred meanings.* New York: Norton.

Friere, P. (1970). *Pedagogy of the oppressed.* New York: Continuum.

Fullilove, M. T. (2004). *Root shock.* New York: One World/Ballantine Books.

Herman, J. L. (1992). *Trauma and recovery: The aftermath of violence—from domestic abuse to political terror.* New York: Basic Books.

Hill, M. (1996). We can't afford it: Confusions and silences on the topic of class. In M. Hill & E. D. Rothblum (Eds.), *Classism and feminist therapy: Counting costs.* Binghamton, NY: Harrington Press.

Hill, M., & Kaschak, E. (Eds.). (1999). *For love or money: The fee in feminist therapy.* Binghamton, NY: Haworth Press.

Hill, M., & Rothblum, E. D. (Eds.). (1996). *Classism and feminist therapy: Counting costs.* Binghamton, NY: Harrington Press.

hooks, b. (1993). *Sisters of the yam: Black women and self-recovery.* Boston: South End Press.

House, J. S., & Williams, D. R. (2000). Understanding and reducing socioeconomic and racial/ethnic disparaties in health. In B. D. Smedley & L. S. Syme (Eds.), *Promoting health: Intervention strategies from social and behavioral research* (pp. 81–124). Washington, DC: National Academy Press.

Kaiser Family Foundation. (2004). *Women's health policy facts: Women's health insurance coverage.* Retrieved October 11, 2004, from www.kff.org/womenshealth/loader.cfm?url=/commonspot/security/getfile.cfm&PageID=37684

King, L. M. (1981). Missing links in the representation of mental health in the U.S. of A: Notes on the work of Chester M. Pierce, M.D. *Fanon Center Journal, 1*(2), 1–15.

Lerner, M. (1986). *Surplus powerlessness.* Oakland, CA: Institute for Labor and Mental Health.

McAdams-Mahmoud, V. (2002). We are making history now. *International Journal of Narrative Therapy and Community Work, 2,* 3–7.

McNair, L. D., & Neville, H.A. (1996). African American women survivors of sexual assault: The intersection of race and class. In M. Hill & E. D. Rothblum (Eds.), *Classism and feminist therapy: Counting costs.* Binghamton, NY: Harrington Press.

Morgan, A. (2000). *What is narrative therapy?: An easy-to-read guide.* Adelaide, Australia: Dulwich Centre.

National Black Women's Health Project. (1989). Organizational goals. *Vital Signs, 6*(1), 30.

National Low Income Housing Coalition. (2004). *Out of reach.* Retrieved August 20, 2004, from www.nlihc.org.oor2003/introduction.htm

Pinderhughes, E. (2004). The multi-generational transmission of loss and trauma: The African American experience. In F. Walsh & M. McGoldrick (Eds.), *Living beyond loss: Death in the family* (2nd ed.). New York: Norton.

Shipler, D. K. (2004). *The working poor: Invisible in America.* New York: Knopf.

Tait, V. (1999). "Workers just like anyone else": Organizing workfare unions in New York City. In K. Springer (Ed.), *Still lifting, still climbing: African American women's contemporary activism.* New York: New York University Press.

Twist, L. (2003). *The soul of money: Transforming your relationship with money and life.* New York: Norton.

U.S. Census Bureau. (2004). *Income stable, numbers of Americans with and without health insurance rise, Census Bureau reports.* U.S. Census Bureau News. Retrieved October 10, 2004, from www.census.gov/Press-Release/www/releases/archives/income_wealth/002484/html

Walgrave, C., Tamasese, K., Tuhaka, F., & Campbell, W. (2003). *Just therapy—a journey: A collection of papers from the Just Therapy Team, New Zealand.* Adelaide, South Australia: Dulwich Centre.

White, M. (2000). *Reflections on narrative practice: Essays and interviews.* Adelaide, South Australia: Dulwich Centre.

PART IV

Women, Self-Care, and Healthy Living

CHAPTER 12

Women, Psychotherapy, and the Experience of Play

Gretchen Schmelzer
Lise Motherwell

No Laughing Matter

A colleague and I (LM) are doing routine maintenance tasks in our office suite when a woman walks through the waiting room into another colleague's office and closes the door. Within seconds we hear laughter coming from behind the door. My colleague looks at me and says, "It's got to be supervision, they are having too much fun for it to be therapy."

Psychological inquiry is no laughing matter. After all, many of the issues with which clinical psychology grapples involve life and death. Dire issues require a certain solemnity, a mandate of seriousness, especially in relation to women's psychological issues, which include difficult topics such as domestic violence, rape, and discrimination. However, with all of the work still left to be done in women's psychology, we suggest that it is play which rejuvenates women for their work in therapy and their work in the world.

When we consider the dilemmas that our clients face in terms of setting both physical and emotional boundaries for play, it seems important to consider what we can do as clinicians to help women create more space for play in their lives. In working therapeutically with women, it is important to assess what they do to rejuvenate themselves, how they play, what interferes with play, and what increases the likelihood of play. Play is an often untapped source of strength for women. By helping them access this resource, we can bolster their capacity for the work they face in their lives and in treatment. In this chapter we explore the serious need for play as a catalyst to development and change in therapy and as a source of rejuvenation and connection in women's lives.

We believe that play may well be our first language in the world of psychology. Through our collaboration with one another, we have come to understand that play is often our default activity when we are feeling stuck in our work with clients or burned out as clinicians or as women. We both grew up in artistic households, where creativity was a valued and often used skill. This shared background element has influenced our thinking about, and use of, play in life and in treatment.

We come to the study of play as two white women who spent 10 years of our early training and clinical work with children and families—most of whom were from the diverse backgrounds typical of Boston neighborhoods— Irish American and Italian American families, African American and Latino families, and the recent Cambodian and Vietnamese immigrants. Our clients are all different from each other in culture and tradition, but most of them live at or below the poverty line. Both of us are products of parental divorce and experienced a range of economic circumstances during childhood. I (GS) went from working poor to upper middle class; I (LM) grew up in dichotomous households, with one parent uneducated and lower middle class, and the other with a graduate school education and upper-class status. These diverse circumstances have helped us empathize with our clients and understand the difficulties associated with poverty, such as poor access to education, health care, and child care and the privilege of choice that wealth affords.

The children from the families with whom we work have taught us much of what we know about play in therapy and play as a catalyst in development. Their parents, primarily single women, have illustrated for us how difficult it is to maintain play in one's life when there are so few resources, and what the cost to psychological health is when one is not able to play. Although many children are sent to us because they have not developed the capacity to play, there are at least an equal number who have taught us what we needed to learn or relearn about the necessity of play for development and rejuvenation. They taught us to trust in a world that is temporarily or temporally removed from reality; a world that is about sensation and not analysis, about present action and not outcome, wherein you get to choose and create, and re-create, when necessary.

Play is a means of helping a client connect to herself and her world, to harness her aggression in positive ways and to find her voice. It respects and works with her resistance and promotes her growth toward change and action. It encourages avenues of exploration that are often left ignored due to life pressures, difficult circumstances, and lack of time and attention. But play does not just benefit our clients. As therapists, it has the potential to energize us and reconnect us to ourselves and our passion in the work we are doing. It encourages us toward growth and change as well.

In contrast to more serious topics, play is not a subject that easily survives scientific rigor and psychological inquisitiveness without disintegrating into something that is no longer play. Whether intra- or interpersonal, play is interactional and thus a dynamic systemic process. Systems are difficult to understand through standard, quantitative, deductive inquiry. They have energetic and definitional properties that cannot be found in their parts (Kuhl, 2000), but instead are understood through the interaction among the various parts. A piano is a musical instrument that depends upon interacting systems. If you take a piano apart, you take away its "piano-ness"—it will no longer play music. It functions only as long as it is a whole system.

Likewise, play is best understood as a process rather than an end product. That is, what happens during the play is as, or more, important than the result of the play.

Work or Play?

Play has been difficult to define for anthropologists, zoologists, psychologists, and educators who have studied it across species and context. Play resists operationalizing (Schwartzmann, 1998) and is often defined from the negative, as in "not-work." Ellis (1973) defines play as an activity that is motivated solely by a desire for the reward inherent immediately in the activity itself (p. 14).

We interviewed a group of women across a range of ages and backgrounds to compile a sample of definitions of play:

"Fun . . . [it] could be work, could be recreational—what I like doing—I like thinking stuff that's creative. I like no distractions when I am playing." —Single white lesbian woman, age 44

"Play is any activity that someone enjoys—that they find relaxing or enjoyable. Play is getting in touch with your inner child and accepting your outer child." —Single African American heterosexual woman, age 37

"Play is not work, you are free to choose what you do—there is a lightness to it and you can decide if you want to do it." —Partnered heterosexual white Jewish woman, age 40

"I think of play as oftentimes being imaginative, different from work in that it's something that's done in leisure and it's also necessary and important in people's lives, in children's lives. In adult's lives too, but they often forget that. It's hard." —Partnered white lesbian woman, age 32

"Letting go, doing things with a sense of freedom and experimentation. Opposite of work, definitely freedom and experimentation is what comes to mind." —Married white heterosexual woman, age 51

"Play is when I am not stressed out—I am doing what I want to do and like to do—I don't think it is specific to one activity or another—I think it's more my attitude." —Single African American heterosexual woman, age 20

The view of play as an attitude rather than a specific activity is especially important and highlights the subjective nature of play. As Apter (1991) states, it is "not so much *what* is experienced in play . . . but rather the *way* of experiencing what one is doing in playing" (p. 14). Though we often know when someone is playing with us, it is hard to know whether someone is experiencing his or her activity as play. Imagine someone throwing a ball. Is that person playing, working, doing physical therapy, having fun? All of this is unknown from the behavioral description. Whereas some people garden for fun, for others it is drudgery—it is the same with writing, reading, exercising, cooking, and traveling. The activity does not tell the story, the subjective experience does. What may look like "real life" to the therapist may be play to the client:

> Louisa, a Haitian client, talked at length about the 3 days she spent preparing and cooking a traditional meal for a large extended family. For some people this would not sound like play at all. For her, however, the preparation and cooking of the meal were play. Her description of the activity had the typical elements of play: "I get to be creative, I get to enjoy my talents, and I lose myself in the process—all the smells and tastes and how everything looks—I can let the world fall away for a while." The stress she experienced was not about the task, but about being able to create the space in her life to allow those three days to happen.

How much we get to play and what we have available to us in terms of play are shaped by the context in which we live, our financial resources, our location, our culture and traditions, and our health and physical ability. In the larger cultural context, gender, race, ethnicity, and social class shape power and social relations, which impact and challenge individuals in their choices of, and opportunities for, play and leisure (Freysinger & Flannery, 1992). For most, the *choice* of when and how to play, or whether there is time for play, distinguishes "time off" from a "time out." If extra time were the only ingredient necessary for play, then surely the unemployed and the incarcerated would enjoy more play experiences than the employed or the free.

As stated above, play is often defined as "not-work." Yet this play–work dichotomy is a Western notion borne of the Christian teaching that play equals sin and the microeconomic measurement of work time versus leisure time as the prevailing way of understanding the allotment of time. Play is an activity that is freely chosen, but many adults do not choose the work that they do, and therefore they do not consider their work, play. The dichotomy has far less meaning for those who are fortunate enough to play and work in the same moments. This state of absorption in a work–play state, reported by athletes, artists, artisans and performers, has been called "flow" (Csikszentmihalyi, 1975). In nonindustrialized countries, the dichotomy has been less clear—for example, where adults only "work," but there is a distinction between profane and sacred work, in which, like play, the subjective experience is different. Some cultures have distinguished between play and rituals (Schwartzmann, 1978). In other cultures the difference between play and ritual is not as distinct. For example, in India during Diwali, the festival of lights, children light fireworks and small clay containers to welcome the goddess of wealth, Lakshmi. During Holi children sprinkle colors and water on their friends, which they do with much laughter and glee. In other celebrations, the children use puppets, songs, dance, and mime to portray important figures in Hindu religious philosophy (Roopnarine, Johnson, & Hoopers, 1994). Similarly, each New Year, Chinese children light firecrackers to drive out the old year, which is symbolized as a fierce monster and is believed to hurt people, which is why it must be driven away. One year the lighting of fireworks was considered to be a successful way of eradicating the monster, so it has become a yearly play form for Chinese children (Pan, 1994).

Can Jane Come Out to Play?:
The Meaning and Context of Play

Context—gender and culture, for example—has an impact on all human behavior and thought. Play is no exception. Though the "what" of play may change (the activity, the rules, the intended outcomes), the "fact" of play does not. All humans, in all cultures, and of all ages, play (Carlson, Taylor, & Levin, 1998; Farver & Howes, 1993; Osgoode & Howe, 1984;

Roopnarine et al., 1994). And though play has been considered so culture-specific that anthropologists have routinely studied play to infer the rules and norms of a culture, it is also true that play is one of the most dynamically changing aspects of a culture—because children, the guardians and architects of play, are the least conservative members of any culture and are more likely to adopt novel and foreign approaches to their play (Lancy, 1984).

We learn to play with "people like ourselves." This means that as children, across culture and context, we play first within family and kinship networks (Bloch, 1989), and then as we get older we are more likely to play with same-age peers in our neighborhoods and same-sex peers in our day care centers and schools (Maccoby, 1986)—which also means that we are more likely to learn to play with peers of similar socioeconomic status (given that neighborhoods and day care facilities often are comprised of children from families of similar economic status and race). These children typically remain playmates throughout the grammar school years, despite the integration of other students in the larger system of school (Ramsey, 1998).

Gender often determines the types of activities in which we initially engage—boys' play tends to be more active, aggressive, and object based, and girls' play tends to be more sedentary, constructive, and role and relationship based (Miller, 1987; Roopnarine et al., 1994). Thus the activities that we consider play, or our enactments of play, begin early and shape not only our future play but our future attitudes and behaviors in the workplace. Boys are more likely to be more inclusive of race, gender, and socioeconomic status in their play because their games tend to require more players and therefore they tend to be less exclusive. Girls' play tends to be more intimate and therefore more exclusive (Gilligan, 1989). The activities we choose as play are impacted by what we have available to us that match our internal and physical resources, as well as our financial and environmental resources. Context can have a big effect, and gender appears to impact choice of play activities from childhood to adulthood. Women from developed countries, for example, are more likely to choose "high end" cultural activities than are men (Katz-Gerro, 2002).

The research on whether the choice of leisure activities is determined more by race or by class has been equivocal. Some research indicates that race has an impact on choice of leisure (Stamps & Stamps, 1985), whereas other research indicates that class, not race, is the mediating factor (Floyd, Shinew, McGuire, & Noe, 1994). Hibbler and Shinew (2002) reported that racism acted as a constraint in interracial couples' leisure and play. They noted that for the couples in their study, it became "standard operating procedure to thoroughly investigate leisure offerings prior to participation in an attempt to not subject themselves or their families to overt racism" (p. 152).

Why Play?

Play is necessary for development. For all mammals, play serves an organizational and integrational role for emotional, sensorimotor, and social development (Haight & Black, 2001). Lack of play in animals is related to a decrease in brain development and lasting deficits in an animal's ability to learn from its environment (Black, Jones, Nelson, & Greenough, 1998). This loss of practice during play affects humans as well (Apter, 1991).

The capacity to play is not only crucial to the development of the core self and relationships; we maintain that it is the mechanism for change in psychotherapy. On her first visit to my (LM) office an 8-year-old white girl with difficult peer relationships picked up a metal "Slinky." She asked me to hold one end while she walked across the room with the other end. As she reached the end of the room, she let it go and it sprung back to the end I was holding with a stinging snap. I said, "Ow!"—but understood her action as a demonstration of her ambivalence about closeness and distance and how hurt she felt in her relationships. We created a diary/book in which she could write how she felt about each of her friends. After several months of treatment, she came in sobbing over an incident at school in which she had felt left out of a group of friends. As she cried, I talked to her about how painful her experience had been. We then wrote a story that created a more positive ending. When she told her mother that she had cried in my office, her mother asked if I had hugged her. She replied, "No, but her words felt like hugs." Clearly our play was transformative to my client, not only in her expression of feelings, but also in her experience of relationship. She could now accept my care and not feel the need to create distance.

Does Play = Fun?

When I (GS) worked in an elementary school as a counselor, the sign on my office door read "CFUN." This was an acronym for a community organization that loaned us their office during the school week to conduct therapy with the students. At the end of the year, one of my 7-year-old clients gave me a card addressed to Dr. Fun. "Isn't that your name?" he asked. For him it made perfect sense that the play therapy doctor's name was Fun.

Psychology has not focused much on fun, but there has been a recent push for study in the area of positive psychology. As Seligman and Csikzentmihalyi (2000) state, "psychology is not just the study of pathology, weakness and damage; it is also the study of fixing what is broken; it is nurturing what is best" (p. 7). They make an important distinction between pleasure and enjoyment, which may help us understand the forms of "fun" in play:

> Pleasure is the good feeling that comes from satisfying the homeostatic needs such as hunger, sex and bodily comfort. Enjoyment on the other hand refers to the good feelings people experience when they break thru [sic] the limits of homeostasis—when they do something that stretches them beyond what they were—in an athletic event, artistic performance, a good deed, a stimulating conversation. Enjoyment, rather than pleasure, is what leads to personal growth and long term happiness. (p. 12)

Although we discuss how play in therapy can be a useful way of exploring emotions that are difficult for women—anger, in particular—play is also a wonderful means of exploring positive emotions. Caldwell (2003) states: "Many modern therapies ignore this crucial phase, not realizing that most of us need help tolerating and basking in feelings of satisfaction and love. Most of us have been acculturated by groups such as family, society, or religion to limit our positive feelings" (p. 308).

Boundaries in Play

Play requires boundaries. In games and sports there are rules that delineate the boundaries of what is acceptable. Rules delineate the conditions of fairness and safety, identify expectations, and set time frames and physical boundaries (such as a field or board), creating structure for how the game will be played. Players agree on the rules before they begin to play. Imaginative play has fewer concrete boundaries and allows for more freedom (e.g., there are no explicit rules or limits to imagination), but there are implicit rules about what is play or playful. For example, mutual play includes a suspension of reality whereby each player understands that things can happen in play that would not happen in reality. Characters can have special powers, places can be built that do not exist, and the interactions between characters can include aggression and death. The most important implicit rules include those of emotional and physical safety. In child therapy it is common to tell children that anything can be said or done in the office, but that the child cannot hurt self, the therapist, or the toys.

Because play requires boundaries, it is an important activity in which one can learn about and practice boundaries. Huizinga (1994) notes that "all play has its being within a playground marked off beforehand, either materially or ideally, deliberately, or as a matter of course" (p. 10). The boundaries are both tangible (time/space) and intangible (imagination/

reverie). As Apter (1991) explains, "in the play state you experience a *protective* frame which stands between you and the real world and its problems" (p. 15). One woman artist we interviewed described this boundary between play and reality:

"I can see myself under a bush with a friend, creating a little world. And sand sculptures on the beach. . . . And there is a moment when you are in the play and then all of a sudden there is a moment [when you realize] that what you've created in play, others can see in reality. It's viewable from outside your imagination. I can remember standing on the beach and stepping back and laughing . . . almost separating from my play at that moment, because I am stand[ing] back in reality."

Boundaries become a crucial issue in the area of women's play. The intersection of the contextual demands on a woman and her ability to reasonably assert herself within this context will determine the scope of time/ space she may have for her play. In order to help our clients create space for play, we not only need to remind them to play more, but also show them how to protect their play time from the intrusions of real life.

Maria always showed up for her appointments an hour ahead of time. She had a busy schedule, working and raising three children, so she packed in as much as she could each day. Because she was so busy, she hated it when her friends were late and often felt self-righteous when they arrived 10 minutes past the agreed-upon time. Her anxiety and rigidity about being on time affected her relationships and left her little time for play or reflection. She was in a constant state of distress. I (LM) devised a plan to help her create time and play space for herself. She still came to the office waiting room an hour before her appointment, but, while there, agreed to spend her time playing with the Legos. Initially she felt that this time was "nonproductive," and she became anxious. Over time, however, she realized that the play space helped her to relax and gave her time to solve problems that had previously seemed overwhelming to her. One day she built a Lego bridge that she later realized represented how she wanted to work on her conflicted relationship with her husband. She suggested that he and she find a project to work on together. They decided to turn an unused room in their house into a "play room" for themselves.

We can teach our clients about creating physical boundaries by protecting the therapeutic frame: starting and ending on time, not taking phone calls or eating lunch during a session, creating consistent and reliable appointment times—and, just as important, protecting the play space the client creates for herself within the therapy session. In order to transfer this boundary to "real life," women need to say the word that it is often hardest for them to utter: "no." *No* is a word they can easily say to themselves, but not to others. Women's discomfort with conflict and anger, as well as the cultural demand that they care for others (Heilbrun, 1990), keep them from stating their needs and protecting their time to play. This fear of saying "no" leaves women with *no* time to play.

Another type of boundary is the more ambiguous mental boundary. Where is their attention during play? Is it on themselves, the experience, the sensations, or, as research indicates (Mattingly & Bianchi, 2003), is it on others and the dilemmas of daily life? How can we help women take what precious free time they do have, to experience the rejuvenation of play? One women client I (GS) had wrote her worries in a notebook before she went for a walk—she knew that they would be there when she returned, so she could focus on enjoying her walk. Another client who came to see me for overeating in the context of a medical disease had difficulty transitioning from work to home without eating. So we created a transition plan that involved her favorite form of play and rejuvenation—gardening. Upon arriving home, she would change her clothes and spend 30–45 minutes in the garden. Her family could still be around (and help if they wanted!), but she could reconnect with her home and herself in a playful and grounded way, and let some of the stress of her workday work itself out.

Therapy and Play

Traditional therapeutic practice is grounded in Western assumptions (Morris, 2001). If play outside of therapy is governed by the context in which women live—their ecological context of their culture, tradition, financial resources, family and work obligations, external support, and physical ability—then it is likely that play inside therapy also is governed by this ecological context. Therefore, it is important to take the client's context and what she considers to be play into account when facilitating play in therapy.

The most common forms of play in which we engage with our clients include humor, metaphor, the use of objects, toys, or drawings, teasing, jokes, and word play. For the purposes of this chapter, we focus on two—humor and metaphor—to explore play as a way to experience connection and as a way to express anger. Humor and metaphor are two aspects of adult play that often make their way into therapy—but, as Kegan (1994) notes, they are tools, not silver bullets.

Humor and Therapy

Like play, humor defies definition; however, it has been described in many ways over the years, including through a psychological lens. Harry Stack

Sullivan saw humor as a way of gaining perspective, and Victor Frankl saw it as a way of seeing oneself more objectively (Minden, 1994). From a psychoanalytic perspective, humor is viewed as a high-level defense and "one of a number of psychological processes which are functionally adaptive modes of withdrawing from reality into the world of imagination" (Minden, 1994, p. 126). Humor is also seen as a way of soothing oneself, a form of play, or a way to express difficult feelings.

As it turns out, laughter *is* the best medicine—especially for facilitating interconnections (Berk & Tan, 1989). In a recent study Marci, Moran, and Orr (2003) found that when patients laugh with their therapists, there is a greater increase in physiological arousal than when patients laughed by themselves. The benefits were noted for the therapists as well. Marci found that even when the patient laughs but the therapist does not laugh, the therapist experiences physiological benefits.

One caveat: Humor should be used judiciously in therapy. Humor can reveal, disguise, or express prejudice (e.g., ethnic jokes), gender bias (e.g., "dumb women" jokes), hurtful aggression (e.g., some types of teasing), and emphasize the power differential between therapist and client. For example, if I tease my client without her implicit or explicit permission, I may inadvertently shame her or subconsciously express my own aggressive feelings toward her. On the other hand, if the client initiates the teasing or indicates that she can tolerate teasing (e.g., by poking fun at herself or cracking a joke), the teasing can be an initial way of expressing difficult feelings about herself or the therapist.

Julia, a 25-year-old white client who had been hospitalized twice in 2 months, came to therapy after 6 weeks of day treatment. In our initial intake she presented as confused, anxious, and unable to say how she felt or to tell me (LM) a coherent story about her life. She would look down, cover her face with her hair, and look up at me shyly. Within a few sessions, however, she demonstrated an acute and quirky sense of humor. She teased me about my being a therapist always interested in the meaning behind things, but then said, "I know my humor is a defense," and shut down. I told her I enjoyed her sense of humor. She brightened, then told me that the hospital psychologist had told her that she used her humor to defend against her feelings. I believe that her humor showed her capacity for play, and that in playing together, she and I might find a way to connect. I began to banter in a playful way with her and neither interpreted her humor nor asked her how she was feeling. Several weeks later I was on vacation and, when I returned, I asked her how she felt about our missed session. She said, "You know, I missed last week. I surprised myself!"

This was her first verbal expression of a spontaneous feeling. She had begun to know herself and find her voice.

Metaphor and Therapy

Metaphor is a form of communicating in the language of *as if*, whereby a client can literally play with an idea through imagery or sensation to explore an experience.

> A colleague described a session with Jennifer, a white woman client, 35, who had never been in treatment, but who had a history of childhood trauma. Jennifer sat silently for many weeks, saying only a few sentences during each session. The therapist sat quietly and waited for her to find the space to talk. Several months into treatment Jennifer said that she was afraid to talk, that the act of talking felt dangerous, as if she were standing on a diving board about to jump into a pool, but there was no water in the pool. She was worried that if she leapt out, she would hurt herself. With an inviting smile her therapist said: "Maybe you can't see the water yet. But if I stood at the edge of the pool and threw in a pebble, you would see the ripple so you would be able to see the water in the pool. Maybe that's what I need to do." Once her therapist joined her in the metaphor (play space), Jennifer became more talkative because she had a found a common language and form of connection with the therapist.

When is metaphor play and when is it a form of communication? In the therapeutic context a metaphor can be thought of as an object, which is put "out there" by a therapist or a client to be considered. Like Winnicott's Squiggle Game (Winnicott, 1989/1964–1968), in which the therapist draws a squiggle and offers it to the child to turn it into something, a metaphor can become an object to mold, transform, or tell a story with. In this case the metaphor used by the client described her fear of talking: standing on a diving board with no water in the pool beneath her. Metaphor became play when the therapist joined her inside the image: standing at the edge, throwing pebbles into the water. The client created the metaphor, the play object, and the therapist picked it up and threw it back. If, instead, the therapist had directed herself to the feelings evoked by the metaphor—"It is really frightening for you to talk in here"—then the metaphor would not have been used as play; the metaphor would be a form of symbolic communication wherein the therapist articulates the explicit meaning, rather than meeting the client within the imaginary space of the metaphor.

In continuing with her work with Jennifer, our colleague found that the use of metaphor continued to be a tool for connection. Jennifer was extremely self-critical and had difficulty talking about her sadness and anger and trusting that the therapy relationship would stay together. Well into treatment, Jennifer came up with an image of a wolf. The wolf was strong and capable and not afraid of anger—she found that she could use the wolf image to talk about what she deemed her unacceptable feelings. For example, whereas she could not express anger about her therapist's vacations, Jennifer could use the wolf to voice her anger and disappointment. The image of the wolf then took on a heightened experience of play when Jennifer was distressed or went away on vacation—she asked her therapist to watch her wolf for her. They would plan an imaginary drop-off time and talk about what the wolf needed while Jennifer was away. Jennifer could articulate how she felt cared for when her therapist took care of this imaginary wolf. For the first time Jennifer understood and felt what it meant to be remembered—"not forgotten"—in a relationship.

Play as a Defense and as a Source of Connection

One question we have considered is when a therapist should add, include, or encourage play, and when a therapist should help her client move away from play. From our experience, play should be increased or encouraged when it serves the client as a connection to herself or the relationship, but shifted away from when it is used in a way that distances the client from herself or the relationship. That being said, there is no hard line about those distinctions—each therapy should be individualized based on the client's ability to tolerate closeness and distance, but in each case, the therapist and client need to talk about whether the play is helpful or is creating distance. One might ask oneself and the client:

> In what way does the play help the client to connect with a core aspect of herself?
> In what way does the play increase her capacity to engage in the therapeutic relationship?
> Is there any way that play impedes her connection to herself or to me?
> Am I engaging in the play only to protect myself from greater intimacy with my client?
> How does the play need to shift, or the work need to shift, in order to bring the client into greater, rather than lesser, connection to herself, her feelings, or me?

Talking about the *experience* of play does not, ironically, impede the play, at least in the work with adults. Instead, talking about a play experience can lead to further articulation of feelings, a deeper engagement with the therapist, and a strengthening of the client's coping skills (e.g., the ability to reflect, be flexible, imagine alternative possibilities, laugh at oneself, engage the other).

One way we assess how intimately a client is connected to herself is how well she is able to access her internal strengths and her external resources. If she is not engaging these two sources of support and strength, play is often way to reconnect her to them.

Dana, an African American woman, came to therapy because of anxiety related to a contentious divorce. Her ex-husband had arranged to move his items out of the house on her birthday. She was extremely distraught about her birthday coinciding with the anniversary of her loss. Dana had a successful career as a hospital administrator and a wide net of social support but felt that this loss and her feelings were too difficult to share with others on that day, especially since she was supposed "to be happy" on her birthday. This was a wonderful opportunity to use paradoxical play to reconnect her to her friends and the support they could provide. I (GS) suggested that she not fight having a "bad" birthday, but indeed invite her friends to a "really bad birthday party"—plan "bad" food—really play with it. Don't try to have fun, but instead—really just have a bad birthday, *with support*. When Dana returned the following week, she explained how much fun her friends had in creating the worst birthday ever—they all wore black, but put on costume jewelry—and they had written funny or loving poems for her and read them out loud. In the midst of a very difficult day, she was able to laugh and tap into a support network that she had worked hard to create and nurture. Play allowed her to connect both to her inner strength (the ability to laugh at her situation and create fun in the midst of tragedy) and her outer resources (her network of emotional support).

Play in Therapy as an Opportunity to Explore Anger

Feminist writers have argued that women's expression of anger is often censored, discouraged, or inhibited in Western culture (Bernardez, 1988; Miller & Surrey, 1990). Bernardez (1988) asserts that the suppression of anger in women is an attempt to keep them subordinate and in the role of the "feminine ideal"; that is, the all-giving, nurturing mother. Women's suppression of anger often leads to somatic complaints, feelings of helplessness, fear of losing control, fear of disconnection from others, withdrawal, numbness, depression, and anxiety (Munhall, 1992). Miller and Surrey (1990) assert that women's anger is relational and means something is amiss that needs to be addressed in order for the relationship to move forward. In other words, anger is energy that can be harnessed and transformed to deepen relationships. As we have seen in the above example, when women are able to express their anger constructively, they feel empowered, connected to themselves and others, and they develop self-esteem.

> A women's group that is meeting just before a month-long break for the therapists' vacation feels disconnected and scattered. The members leap from topic to topic and only superficially connect with each other. The leader believes the disconnection has to do with the summer break, but the group members ignore the therapist's inquiries and talk instead about the Lacey Peterson murder. In the last minute of the session, a client turns to the leader and says with intensity but also good humor, "I hope you have a really bad vacation." At first surprised by her bluntness but then delighted, the group members, including the leader, burst into laughter. The client has expressed, directly and playfully, the very feelings that the group members had been unable to express the previous weeks leading up to the break. The group now feels stronger and more connected as they disband for the summer.

The ability to author one's experience has been referred to as "voice" by the feminist theorists who note that women often silence their voices to remain in relationship (Belenky, Clinchy, Goldberger, & Tarule, 1986; Gilligan, 1982, 1989). When girls and women speak up, they encounter a dilemma: "Was it better to respond to others and abandon themselves or to respond to themselves and abandon others?" (Gilligan, 1989, p. 9). In the therapeutic relationship, *voice* is about the ability to communicate—to narrate, author, and speak one's experience. But as Brown and Gilligan (1992) note, voice is also about the listener: "We ask not only who is speaking, but also who is listening. . . . Instead of holding as an ideal a no-voice voice or an objective stance—a way of speaking or seeing that is disembodied, outside the relationship, in no particular time and place—we seek to ground our work empirically, in experience, and in the realities of relationship and difference, of time and place" (p. 23).

The act of speaking from one's own voice may be experienced by women and girls as an aggressive act within relationships that heightens their experience (and strengthens the dualistic paradigm) of being either connected or differentiated. Voice has power—"the capacity to produce change" (Miller, 2003). Women's discomfort with their own aggression and their lived experience with others' aggression (relational or societal) affect their ability to speak their voices and to risk that differentiation will end the relationship or their connection with another.

In its more traditional forms play can allow women the experience and expression of anger:

Rose, an African American woman in her 60s, had a long history of catering to the needs of her family. She had taken care of both of her parents through extended illnesses, and she had taken care of her grandchildren. She felt unable to speak on her own behalf, and she felt unheard during the instances when she attempted to speak. She was terrified by how angry she became at her spouse and her children, and she considered leaving home and moving. I (GS) wanted to let her have an experience of her anger to show her that it was manageable. I took an old phone book and had her rip out pages, ball them up, and throw them around my office. Her affect ranged from anger to excitement—she surprised herself in her ability to express her emotion without hurting anyone else. When Rose left, she asked if she could keep the rest of the phone book, in case she needed it. When she returned the following week she reported that she had calmly but firmly confronted her husband about his participation in household duties, and her daughter about moving out and finding a place of her own. Although initially surprised by her actions, neither the husband nor the daughter broke off the relationship, as she had feared they would, and my client got a chance to experience herself as a capable and effective communicator.

In this instance play served as catharsis and a form of exposure therapy for the affect: The object of anger was initially displaced onto something that could not break (balls of paper) and then transferred back to the actual objects (relationships) after the fear was tolerated successfully in therapy.

It is important to note that not all aggression is destructive. Positive aggression allows us to stand up in the face of negation, leave bad relationships, overcome obstacles to growth, push for new possibilities, and defend against harm (Jack, 1999). It is also a source of ambition, perseverance, courage, and creativity. The notion of a positive form of aggression could lead to a new paradigm of power (Miller, 2003; Walker, 2002). For example, Walker (2002) asks: "1) if power is a fundamental energy of relationship how does power look when used in the service of zest, clarity, mutuality, and affirmation of connection? and, 2) How might our relationship with power help us to more fully inhabit our lives?" (p. 4).

The societal expectation that women suppress their anger often leads women to withdraw from, rather than engage in, relationships and life. We believe that the use of play and humor in therapy can give women nonthreatening access to, and expression of, their anger, while also helping them get in touch with their creative selves. Furthermore, to give those clients who are unable to speak the room to play respects their silence and gives them another avenue through which to communicate.

When Jane Can't Come Out to Play

When we asked the women we interviewed what interfered with their ability to play, most cited lack of time as the primary mitigating factor. The research supports their experience (Eyler et al., 1998; Henderson, 2003). In the United States and Canada women get less leisure time than men, and women spend twice as much time doing housework and chores than men do (Bianchi, Robinson, Sayer, & Milkie, 2000). When men marry, their time spent on household chores decreases, the reverse is true for women (Gupta, 1999). Controlling for race, ethnicity, and socioeconomic status, women experience less free time than men (at least 30 minutes per day) (Mattingly & Bianchi, 2003). Women are responsible for creating and maintaining leisure time for others, especially children (Milkie, Bianchi, Mattingly, & Robinson, 2002), but do not prioritize creating this time for themselves. Barriers to play or recreation have been cited variously as lack of energy, job demands, physical illness, expectations and needs of the family, lack of facilities, and poor financial or environmental resources (Eyler et al., 1998; Henderson, 2003). The leisure literature describes barriers to play along two main dimensions: marginality (referring to social class and economic factors) and ethnicity (referring to subcultural values, languages, and traditions) (West, 1989, cited in Phillip, 1998, p. 215). For example, a Muslim immigrant woman may have the economic means to participate in an activity such as co-ed water polo, but may be forbidden to do so because of cultural or religious constraints.

For women of all ages, class is a predictor of the kinds of activities chosen for play and the playmates who participate. Women who have more financial means experience forms of play that are more diverse, involve participation in out-of-home activities, and include a wider range of social contacts. Within and across race, women from lower socioeconomic backgrounds engage in play that is less diverse, more home-centered, and includes playmates who are likely to be family members or other relatives (Shinew, Floyd, & McGuire, 1996). Other research has noted that for women, being poor, a member of an ethnic minority, and having less than high school education are associated with being less physically active during their leisure time (Ransdell & Wells, 1998). Given the widespread concern about women's health (particularly in regard to heart disease), physical activity as a component of play has become an important focus of attention.

In addition to the objective loss of available time for play in minutes and hours, research indicates that women have a different subjective experience of their leisure time (Mattingly & Bianchi, 2003). Men and women differ in their ability to maintain not only physical boundaries of leisure time ("This is my time"), but mental boundaries as well ("I will focus on the activity or myself during this time"). In contrast to men's ability to compartmentalize, women's mental boundaries tend to be more fluid. They are more likely to bring work problems home, home problems to work, and everyone else's problems into their leisure time (Mattingly & Bianchi, 2003).

Women who have trouble creating a play space for themselves in their lives may find it hard to create a play space in therapy—or maybe they do not even know how. Sanville (1991) has noted that some children who come into therapy are unable to play. They do not "send forth the usual affective signals that let the other person know what they are intending to do and what they are feeling; they seem unable to take into account the domain of relatedness" (p. 23). Their internal worlds are so chaotic that they cannot create a coherent story; they do not name characters, develop sequences, or express affect. She has found that these children do not respond to interpretation, but instead need the therapist to stay in the play with them. Slade (1994) adds:

> Choosing not to use interpretative or deductive language does not mean that therapy per se is not taking place. Serving as an organizing, enhancing or engaged play partner is hardly a simple task; in many instances, it is of enormous value clinically, and developmentally. With children who cannot play coherently or meaningfully, who cannot use the symbols of play and language to make sense of their emotional experiences, who cannot create narratives for their experiences, an essential and prior part of the work of treatment is to help them do so. (p. 81)

The same is true for our adult women.

Clients who cannot play report that they often feel confused and their minds go blank. They have no language for feelings, do not connect the past and present, and often have no story to tell about their lives. Abused women often feel ashamed, helpless, and overwhelmed. If we ask such clients to tell us what they are feeling or to tell us their story, we risk assaulting their sense of selves and leaving them feeling even more inadequate and alone. Winnicott (1989/1964–1968) reminds us that the child (or adult) plays if he or she can, and if not, "the treatment must be directed towards enabling the child [or adult] to become able to play" (p. 300).

When clients do not know how to play, we are more active, tend to initiate play rather than wait for the client to lead the therapy, use metaphor, interpret less, and look for "moments of meeting" (Stern, 2004) that often include playful bantering, humor, puns, or jokes.

Tina, an 18-year-old white woman who had been in residential treatment after she was emotionally and sexually abused by her father, came to see me for therapy. For 3 months she spoke not one word. I (LM) asked her questions, I told her stories, I sat with her, I read a book, I played with Play-Doh, hoping she might engage with me. Finally, about a month after Halloween she came into my office, sniffed, and said, "It stinks in here." She was right, a terrible odor had permeated my office (and although I also heard her comment as a metaphor, I chose to respond about the REAL smell in the office). I said, "Maybe we can explore together and find out what it is." In an adult version of hide and seek, she and I got down on our hands and knees, climbed up on the chair and desk, and looked in every nook and cranny. At one point I peered around a corner to find her almost nose to nose with me. I said, "Peek-a-boo!" She smiled and we continued our search. Eventually we found a rotting pumpkin that had been placed on a top shelf well out of sight. We both wrinkled our noses at the stench, while I removed it from the office. When I returned I pinched my nose closed and said, "You're right, it stinks in here!" She laughed and we began our work together.

Conclusion

Play is both primal and primary; that is, it hits the very core of who we are, and it is a fundamental source of healing and energy. Our primary recommendation for the area of play in psychology is research, but in an untraditional (and perhaps playful) sense. We suggest that each clinician increase the observation, awareness, and discussion of play in his or her professional and personal life. Ask yourself, your clients, your colleagues, your students, your friends and your family about their play: How do they define play? What kind of play did they most enjoy as a child or adolescent? What allows them to play? What interferes with their play? How do they play in their work life? How do they play in their relationships? Both therapists and clients should consider how play is used or not used in therapy. Who brings it in? What has been the impact?

As clinicians we view play not as much a technique (such as sand tray or role play) as we do a stance from which to work. How you choose to position yourself to the shared work in therapy will create an atmosphere wherein your clients feel invited to bring in their playful side—or not. One colleague shared a story that when she was in her 20s she sought therapy to help her cope with her father's illness. When she first arrived for her second session, the colleague said, "Hi, how are you?" The therapist responded, "That's not really why we're here now, is it?" Whereas most of us would agree that this response to a simple casual greeting is not likely to invite playfulness into therapy, it is also true that there are many subtler ways we communicate our commitment to play and playfulness within the realm of therapy.

Gender, culture, age, and economic status all have an impact on play. Who we play with, how we play, and our play activities are affected by the many contexts of our identity. It is true, however, that play simultaneously transcends those differentiators, connecting and integrating aspects of selves, relationships, and communities that need to be connected. It is in play that we connect our mind, body, and spirit, we connect to others in relationship, we connect to the natural world, and we have the possibility of connecting across difference.

References

Apter, M. (1991). A structural phenomenology of play. In J. Kerr & M. Apter (Eds.), *Adult play: A reversal theory approach* (pp. 13–29). Berwyn, PA: Swets & Zeitlinger.

Belenky, M., Clinchy, B., Goldberger, N., & Tarule, J. (1986). *Women's ways of knowing: The development of self, voice, and mind.* New York: Basic Books.

Berk, L., & Tan, S. (1989). Eustress of mirthful laughter modifies natural killer cell activity. *Clinical Research, 37,* 115.

Bernardez, T. (1988). *Women and anger: Cultural prohibitions and the feminine ideal.* Wellesley, MA: Stone Center, Wellesley College.

Bianchi, S. M., Robinson, J., Sayer, L., & Milkie, M. (2000). Is anyone doing the housework?: Trends in the gender division of household labor. *Social Forces, 79,* 191–228.

Black, J., Jones, T., Nelson, C., & Greenough, W. (1998). Neural plasticity. In N. Alessi (Ed.) & J. Coyle (Section Ed.), *The handbook of child and adolescent psychiatry: Vol. IV. Varieties of development. Section I. Developmental neuroscience* (pp. 31–53). New York: Wiley.

Bloch, M. (1989). Young boys' and girls' play at home and the community: A cultural–ethological framework. In M. Bloch & A. Pellegrini (Eds.), *The ecological context of children's play* (pp. 120–154). Norwood, NJ: Ablex.

Brown, L., & Gilligan, C. (1992). *Meeting at the crossroads: Women's psychology and girl's development.* New York: Ballantine.

Caldwell, C. (2003). Adult play group therapy. In C. Schaefer (Ed.), *Play therapy with adults* (pp. 301–316). New York: Wiley.

Carlson, S., Taylor, M., & Levin, G. (1998). The influence of culture on pretend play: The case of Mennonite children. *Merrill-Palmer Quarterly, 44*(4), 538–565.

Csikszentmihalyi, M. (1975). *Beyond boredom and anxiety.* San Francisco: Jossey-Bass.

Ellis, M. (1973). *Why people play.* Englewood Cliffs, NJ: Prentice-Hall.

Eyler, A., Baker, E., Cromer, L., King, A., Brownson, R., & Donatelle, R. (1998). Physical activity and minority women: A qualitative study. *Health Education and Behavior, 25,* 640–652.

Farver, J., & Howes, C. (1993). Cultural difference in American and Mexican-American mother–child pretend play. *Merrill-Palmer Quarterly, 39,* 344–358.

Floyd, M., Shinew, K., McGuire, F., & Noe, F. (1994). Race, class, and leisure activity preferences: Marginality and ethnicity revisited. *Journal of Leisure Research, 26,* 158.

Freysinger, V., & Flannery, D. (1992). Women's leisure: Affiliation, self-determination, empowerment and resistance. *Society and Leisure, 15,* 303–322.

Gilligan, C. (1982). *In a different voice.* Cambridge, MA: Harvard University Press.

Gilligan, C. (1989). Preface: Teaching Shakespeare's sister: Notes from the underground of female adolescence. In C. Gilligan, N. Lyons, & T. Hanmer (Eds.), *Making connections: The relational worlds of adolescent girls at Emma Willard School* (pp. 6–29). Cambridge, MA: Harvard University Press.

Gupta, S. (1999). The effects of transitions in marital status on men's performance of housework. *Journal of Marriage and the Family, 61,* 700–711.

Haight, W., & Black, J. (2001). A comparative approach to play: Cross species and cross cultural perspectives of play in development. *Human Development, 44,* 228–234.

Henderson, K. (2003). Women, physical activity and leisure: Jeopardy or wheel of fortune? *Women in Sport and Physical Activity Journal, 12,* 113.

Hibbler, D., & Shinew, K. (2002). Interracial couples' experience of leisure: A social network approach. *Journal of Leisure Research, 34,* 135–156.

Huizinga, L. (1949). *Homo ludens.* London: Routledge.

Jack, D. (1999). *Behind the mask.* Cambridge, MA: Harvard University Press.

Katz-Gerro, T. (2002). Highbrow cultural consumption and class distinction in Italy, Israel, West Germany, Sweden, and the United States. *Social Forces, 81,* 207–229.

Kegan, R. (1994). *In over our heads: The mental demands of modern life.* Cambridge, MA: Harvard University Press.

Kuhl, J. (2000). A functional design approach to motivation and self-regulation: The dynamics of personality systems interactions. In M. Boekarts, P. Pintrich, & M. Zeidner (Eds.), *Handbook of self-regulation* (pp. 111–169). Boston: Academic Press.

Lancy, D. (1984). Play in an anthropological perspective. In P. Smith (Ed.), *Play in humans and animals* (pp. 295–303). Oxford, UK: Blackwell.

Maccoby, E. (1986). Social groupings in childhood: Their relationship to prosocial and antisocial behaviors in boys and girls. In D. Olewus, J. Block, & M. Radke-Yarrow (Eds.), *Development of anti-social and prosocial behavior* (pp. 263–284). New York: Academic Press.

Marci, C., Moran, E., & Orr, S. (2003). Physiologic evidence for the interpersonal role of laughter during psychotherapy. *Bulletin for Psychotherapy of the World Psychiatric Association, 4,* 6.

Mattingly, M. J., & Bianchi, S. M. (2003). Gender differences in the quantity and quality of free time: The U.S. experience. *Social Forces, 81*(3), 999–1030.

Milkie, M., Bianchi, S., Mattingly, M., & Robinson, J. (2002). The gendered division of childrearing: Ideals, realities, and the relationship to parental well-being. *Sex Roles, 47*(1/2), 21–38.

Miller, C. (1987). Adult sex stereotyping of children's toys. *Sex Roles, 16*, 473–487.

Miller, J. (2003). *Telling the truth about power.* Wellesley, MA: Stone Center, Wellesley College.

Miller, J. & Surrey, J. (1990). *Revisioning women's anger: The personal and the global.* Wellesley, MA: Wellesley Centers for Women, Wellesley College.

Minden, P. (1994). Humor: A corrective emotional experience. In E. Buckman (Ed.), *The handbook of humor: Clinical applications in psychotherapy* (pp. 123–132). Malabar, FL: Krieger.

Munhall, P. (1992). Women's anger and its meanings: A phenomenological perspective. *Health Care for Women International, 14*, 481–491.

Osgood, N., & Howe, C. (1984). Psychological aspects of leisure: A lifecycle developmental perspective. *Society and Leisure, 7*, 175–195.

Pan, H. (1994). Children's play in Taiwan. In J. Roopnarine, J. Johnson, & F. Hoopers (Eds.), *Children's play in diverse cultures* (pp. 31–50). Albany: State University of New York Press.

Phillip, S. (1998). Race and gender differences in adolescent peer group approval of leisure activities. *Journal of Leisure Research, 30*, 214–232.

Ramsey, P. (1998). Diversity and play: Influences of race, culture, class and gender. In D. Fromberg & D. Bergen (Eds.), *Play from birth to twelve and beyond: Contexts, perspectives and meanings* (pp. 23–33). New York: Garland.

Ransdell, L., & Wells, C. (1998). Physical activity in urban white, African-American and Mexican-American women. *Medicine and Science in Sport and Exercise, 30*, 1608–1615.

Roopnarine, J., Johnson, J., & Hoopers, F. (1994). *Children's play in diverse cultures.* Albany: State University of New York Press.

Sanville, J. (1991). *The playground of psychoanalytic therapy.* Hillsdale, NJ: Analytic Press.

Schwartzmann, H. (1978). *Transformations.* New York: Plenum Press.

Seligman, M., & Csikszentmihalyi, M. (2000). Positive psychology: An introduction. *American Psychologist, 55*, 5–14.

Shinew, K., Floyd, M., & McGuire, F. (1996). Class polarization and leisure activity preferences of African Americans: Intragroup comparisons. *Journal of Leisure Research, 28*, 219–232.

Slade, A. (1994). Making meaning and making believe: Their role in clinical process. In A. Slade & D. Wolf (Eds.), *Children at play: Clinical and developmental approaches to meaning and representation* (pp. 81–107). New York: Oxford University Press.

Spangler, G., & Grossman, K. (1993). Biobehavioral organizations in securely and insecurely attached infants. *Child Development, 64*, 1439–1450.

Stamps, S., & Stamps, M. (1985). Race, class and leisure activities in urban residents. *Journal of Leisure Research, 17*, 40–56.

Stern, D. (2004). *The present moment in psychotherapy and everyday life*. New York: Norton.

Walker, M. (2002). *Power and effectiveness: Envisioning an alternate paradigm*. Wellesley, MA: Stone Center, Wellesley College.

Winnicott, D. (1989). The squiggle game. In C. Winnicott, R. Shephard, & M. Davis (Eds.), *D. W. Winnicott: Psycho-analytic explorations* (pp. 299–317). (Original work published 1964–1968). Cambridge, MA: Harvard University Press.

CHAPTER 13

Spirit Matters

WOMEN, SPIRITUALITY,
AND CLINICAL CONTEXTS

Tracy L. Robinson-Wood
Marilyn Braithwaite-Hall

This chapter focuses on spirituality in the lives of women within therapeutic contexts. The primary question that frames this work is, How can therapists successfully integrate spirituality into their work with women so that they see them as whole? Specific skills have been identified as helpful to clinicians in gaining insight when discussing spirituality: (1) the ability to examine their own prejudices and biases around spirituality and religion, both positive and negative; (2) becoming familiar with the literature on spiritual experiences; (3) exploring religion from a different culture than their own and being able to assess the relevance of the spiritual domain in the client's therapeutic issues; and (4) using a client's spiritual beliefs in the pursuit of the client's therapeutic goals (Cashwell & Young, 2004; West, 2000). In this chapter, we explore the enactment of these skills by way of a case study. First, we offer a glimpse of ourselves, in recognition that our multiple identities influence our perspectives and the positions we occupy.

We are women of African descent. We believe that to be healthy in the United States requires us to be aware of and nurture our spirit. What this means is that we know the importance of being quiet and listening to that still small voice that emanates from within, guides us, and allows us to make meaning out of our lived experiences, as they are profoundly influenced by the socially constructed and dominant discourses of gender and race. As adult women, we live in a world of which our mothers warned but equipped us with racial and gender socialization messages. Among their pearls of wisdom about excelling in the face of adversity and injustice was, "You will have to work twice as hard to get half as far, but hold on to God's unchanging hand."

Our upbringings coupled with our religious doctrines taught us to be dutiful, moral, caring, giving, helpful, productive, and loving to all others. Christianity is the religion in which we were raised and are now aligned. Both as girls and adult women, the association of God with whiteness and maleness was communicated through the media, classic art forms, church hymns—even from the images on the backs of fans used in many black churches. We have identified, critiqued, and challenged popular notions of God and power and have come to understand that messages such as "Don't question God" or "Just pray about it and let God take care of everything" can encourage a woman to behave with passivity and subordination. Yet we also know of the beauty and grace of "letting go and letting God" after we have done all that we know how to do.

We experience the dictates of patriarchy and androcentrism that encourage our, and other women's, economic and physical vulnerability. We bear witness to the factors that put most adult women across race, class, and ethnicity into therapy: child and adult sexual trauma, interpersonal violence within families that are supposed to be havens of rest and safety, and unrealistic caregiving burdens that render us selfless, exhausted, and resentful. As optimal resistors with a sociopolitical awareness of the genesis of hierarchy, we push back against subtle and blatant forms of race, gender, class, and religious oppression that press down upon our lives. Our spiritual lives call us to be aware of, and accountable to, our bodies and minds, insisting that we honor who we are. Our spirituality is strengthened by collaboration with communities of support that fortify our efforts to confront and overcome obstacles through the maintenance of life-affirming thinking patterns. Our resistance is achieved by nurturing our spiritual centers through prayer, which means both listening to and speaking with God. That others can listen and speak to God on our behalf makes prayer one of our most important coping responses.

Along our journeys, there were those who intended to help and those who meant to harm. We look back to all of these who, independent of their position, encouraged our spiritual evolution. This point is crucial in that it leads to three primary and guiding tenets of this work:

First, we believe that spiritual growth, as is the case with other dimensions of development, is most often a consequence of, and intricately linked to, suffering and crisis. Although we clearly acknowledge the place of spirituality in celebration, joy, meaning making, and transcendence, we also understand and accept that loss, pain, betrayal, and unwanted and unwelcome life events over which we have no control have beckoned the spirits of many to reach deeply within.

Another tenet of our work is that spirituality is a universal human experience. Whereas we acknowledge that our own religious and spiritual journeys influence our perspectives, we also emphasize the transcendence of spirituality in therapy for women across sources of difference, including (but not limited to) culture, age, race, class, and sexual orientation. *Spirit* comes from the Latin word *spiritus*, meaning "breath of life." This breath of life is a universal dimension. As a function of prayer, meditation, and other forms of spiritual cultivation, some people are more mindful of, and thus connected to, their spirit. Manifestations of this connection have been referred to as the "fruits of spirituality," which, according to West (2000), means that "being truly spiritual changes all aspects of who we are and how we live" (p. 10).

The third tenet pertains to the intersection of spirituality with other dimensions of identity, such as religion, class, gender, race, and sexual orientation. For example, it is rare to find black women who would not acknowledge God or a higher power as salient to their lives. Historically, the gendered and racial lives of black women have chronicled an active relationship with a creator who is regarded as loving and watchful. We believe that black women's dependence on and need for strength, justice, comfort, and support in a world often hostile to their racial and gender identities, have encouraged their relationship with Jesus, the suffering servant. For most black people in the United States, resisting oppression and striving for success are intricately linked to spiritual matters.

By way of a case study and with a focus on both the client and the therapist, we explore these tenets along with clinical skills supportive of spirituality as a topic within therapeutic contexts. Definitions and distinctions precede this case study.

Spirituality and Religion: Definitions and Distinctions

Religion and spirituality are interrelated, but they differ in important ways. *Religion* comes from the Latin root *religio,* which means a "bond between humanity and the gods" (Ingersoll, 1995, p. 11). Religion is the practice of beliefs about a higher being. Involved are behaviors, rituals, and routines related to the worship experience (Robinson & Watt, 2001). Religion is often associated with an institutionalized set of beliefs "by which groups and individuals relate to the ultimate" (Burke et al., 1999, p. 252). Expressions of religion tend to be associated with a denomination, are external, cognitive, behavioral, and occur in public contexts but can be intensely private as well. Religious aspects might also reflect a belief in a higher power.

Religion may encompass the supernatural, atheism, deism, and finite and nonfinite deities, as well as practices, beliefs, and behaviors that defy definition and circumscription (Spilka, Hood, Hunsberger, & Gorsuch, 2003). Religion has been described as having an extrinsic orientation where emphasis is placed outside of oneself, on institutions, religious leaders, and scriptures (Buchannan, Dzelme, Harris, & Hecker, 2001). Extremes in an external religious orientation can contribute to fundamentalism.

The human spirit is deep and mysterious. *Spirituality* is experientially defined, transcends the tangible, and connects one to the whole (Robinson & Watt, 2001). Experiences of the spirit tend to be universal, internal, and private, representing the essence of who people are. Although internal, spirituality has been regarded as the "outward expression of the inner workings of the human spirit" (Swinton, 2001, p. 20). Many people are aware of spirituality as having a transcendent and sacred dimension, wherein the experience is one of an altered state of being. Experiences with the divine are described as occurring within the person. Spirituality functions to provide hope, particularly in the face of distress and uncertainty, and gives one a sense of meaning and purpose in life while providing a sense of connection with others who are similarly minded (Ganje-Fling & McCarthy, 1996). As a contrast to the extrinsic orientation associated with religion, spirituality is viewed as having an intrinsic orientation. In this regard, "spirituality is seen as reliance on an internal authority, meaning that the expert is the individual, truth is derived from individual experience, and great value is placed on personal insight" (Buchannan et al., 2001, pp. 436–437). It can be said that a parallel exists between spirituality and a journey or movement along a path.

Church, synagogue, mosque attendance, and denominational affiliation neither correlate with nor dictate one's spiritual experiences. Persons who regard themselves as agnostic have spiritual experiences (West, 2000). For example, cultivating one's spirit and/or maintaining a strong connection with a church represents a foundation for the experience of most black people in the United States. Yet black people may not attend church regularly or even have a church home but may still regard themselves as religious and/or spiritual and "pray to the Lord" (Boyd-Franklin, 2003, p. 270) when needing comfort, particularly during difficulty times, such as illness, death, loss, and bereavement. It is possible to be spiritual and not religious, religious and not spiritual (Burke & Miranti, 2001), and both religious and spiritual. Wade-Gayles (1995) saw the distinction between religion and spirituality as follows:

> Religion and spirituality are like oil and water, insoluble. . . . Arguably there should be a line of demarcation between the two. Institutionalized religion requires us to be a congregation following an unchanging order of worship

and believing in a dogma, both of which have been linked to oppression throughout the history of human civilization. But spirituality frees us to worship wherever, however, and with whomever we so desire, each time anew and each time in celebration of the divine that is in us and in the entire universe. (p. 4)

Ingersoll (1995) identified seven dimensions of spirituality, many of which are seen in Wade-Gayles's (1995) description of spirituality: (1) one's conception of the divine or a force greater than oneself; (2) one's sense of meaning, or what is beautiful, worthwhile; (3) one's relationship with divinity and other beings; (4) one's tolerance of, or negative capability for, mystery; (5) the occurrence of peak and ordinary experiences that enhance spirituality (may include religious rituals or spiritual disciplines); (6) spirituality as play or the giving of oneself; and (7) and spirituality as a systemic force that acts to integrate all the dimensions of one's life (p. 11).

Cynthia was a 35-year-old, physically healthy African American woman living in a medium-sized city in Georgia with her husband, James, who was also African American. They were Christians and were heavily involved in their Church of God in Christ (COGIC). They have been married 10 years and have two school-age children. Cynthia sang in the church choir and spent several nights a week rehearsing as well as attending a variety of church meetings, including Bible study and women's auxiliary. Cynthia's time away from the home had increased, and she had become emotionally distant. Cynthia and James rarely made love. It was clear to James that something was very wrong with the relationship. Cynthia said, "I am doing God's work and serving the Lord and His church." In response to the growing tension in their marriage, James suggested that they speak with their minister for marital counseling. Cynthia told James that she could not speak to the minister. When James asked why, Cynthia confessed that she was having a sexual relationship with one of the women at church—and that she had been attracted to women for years before, during, and after college. In faith she prayed to God that He would heal (take away) these feelings, but they remained. What she felt during her times of prayer was a sense of God's peace and a steady but quiet internal voice that she should not marry. This was confusing to her, so she ignored this voice and attributed it to the devil "trying to steal her joy." After all, James was a God-fearing and handsome man who valued education and had the approval of her family. Although Cynthia was close to her minister, church, and biological families, she believed that she could not talk with any of them about this topic. She knew that they would judge her, and she already felt very ashamed, not only about her sexual behavior but also about her increased alcohol consumption, which took place mainly at night after her family had gone to bed.

Many nights, Cynthia retired to bed nearly intoxicated. Cynthia preferred to talk with someone she did not know. Cynthia's therapist was Alexa, a black, female, counseling psychologist. Alexa was Catholic.

Religious Discourses and Sexuality

Cynthia's religion was a crucial part of her life and a source of her strength. She had learned the importance of seeking God in prayer and trusting that, in time, with faith, things do change and get better. At the same time, her religion, as does her culture, contributed to her guilt feelings. According to both her religious and cultural training, homosexuality is an abomination before God and is not natural, particularly among black people. The African American community often reflects the attitude that homosexuality is inconsistent with being black (Riggs, 1994).

Clearly, Cynthia was wrestling with sexual identity issues; however, sexual identity is not determined by sexual behavior. For some, sexual orientation may be an evolving part of identity. The longevity of Cynthia's sexual feeling for, and attraction to, other women as well as the strength of her intrapsychic conflict is a strong indication that she may not be experimentally sexual with the woman from church but may be lesbian or bisexual. As a mother, wife, Christian, daughter, and African American woman, some of her identities conflicted with her new emotional and sexual experiences and behaviors. For Cynthia, the dominant discourses associated with her cultural, spiritual, and sexual identities were in conflict. For example, good Christian black women are heterosexual and are not prone to excessive drink; good mothers are not lesbians; earnest and faith-filled prayer can override or change ungodly same-sex feelings.

Cultural and religious messages have encouraged Cynthia to deny herself, particularly when doing so benefited others and glorified God. The dictates of gender socialization orient Cynthia and other women to meet the needs of others often at the expense of themselves. As a function of the centrality of men in the human experience, Cynthia was socialized to attend to the needs of others above her own and to function at all times, regardless of her own fatigue. As Singleton (2003) points out, Cynthia's mother taught her not to think about herself, otherwise she would wind up all alone. Both implicit and explicit messages about the superiority of males over women were central to Cynthia's religious training. Since Cynthia was a girl, she was socialized by her mother for economic independence, family responsibility, and daily accountability, yet she was taught to put others before herself.

Within the black community, women are culturally recognized as having fortitude, perseverance, and strength, particularly during adversity

(Boyd-Franklin, 1989). Women are generally more religious than men and function to bind the family into a church-centered support system, where particular roles and activities are assumed and performed. For Cynthia, being a good Christian black woman meant being compliant, cooperative, morally upright, chaste, and selfless.

Part of Cynthia's therapeutic journey requires an integration of spiritual issues that might help her to make meaning out of her religious indoctrination. The process of unpacking or deconstructing the meanings around Cynthia's religious teachings and spiritual insights and their influence on her current perceptions of sexuality, godly behavior, and right living are critical to Cynthia's reorientation. Therapy can help Cynthia understand the following areas: what her religion taught her about her sexual feelings and expressions toward the woman at church; what her spirit said to her prior to her marriage to James; if a difference exists between the voices of her religion and the spirit-led voice that gave her a sense of peace and told her not to marry. This act of deconstruction would be adversely affected if Alexa were also struggling with her sexuality, her spiritual affiliation, or had a wounding experience in her life due to infidelity. As human beings, therapists are at times vulnerable. Depending on the situation, they may be unable to explore certain themes or help certain clients with particular issues (Robinson & Watt, 2001).

Creating Safe Clinical Contexts for Discussions of Spirituality

Strong clinical skills are essential for good therapy but in themselves are not sufficient. The clinical encounter is an opportunity for spiritual healing—which means "moving from a place of brokenness, emptiness, and feelings of separation from oneself and others, to an awareness of one's infinite connection with a loving and caring Spirit or higher power, however the woman defines that power" (Robinson, 2000, p. 162). Therapy presents a tremendous opportunity for community and healing, along with friendship, love, work, and self-regulation (Witmer & Sweeney, 1992). Spirituality is a core dimension of life. However, some clinicians are uncomfortable with theirs as well as their clients' spiritual feelings and various expressions. The lack of training about spirituality in therapy, unfinished business with spiritual issues in their own lives, devaluation of the place of spirituality in existential and clinical concerns, fear of imposing their values onto clients, and discomfort with a topic often regarded as mysterious, controversial, and deep (or corny and passé) may contribute to therapists' discomfort with and dismissal of spiritual issues in therapy. Other reasons, such as lack of exposure to, and familiarity with, healthy forms of spirituality may also represent a barrier to an open discussion and inclusion of spirituality in the therapeutic event. Some people harbor anti-religious sentiment because religion is regarded as not scientific or logical. Others, therapists included, suffered from harsh and heavy-handed religious teachings that "lead us to regard all religion and all spirituality as harmful and unnecessary" (West, 2000, p. 17). Such negative experiences can contribute to clinicians' countertransference responses in therapy.

Just as clinicians have a responsibility to communicate to their clients that they (the clinicians) do not need to be protected from a discussion of race or related topics, there is a similar responsibility regarding spirituality. Multiculturally competent therapists understand that religion and spirituality can broaden the therapist's evaluation of the client's situation and provide different solutions (Kersting, 2003). Yet, out of fear of being perceived as ignorant, insensitive, or discriminatory, therapists will omit certain information or avoid asking particular questions. This fear can paralyze therapy and interfere with the client's growth. The clinician has a responsibility to communicate to the client that spirituality is a welcome topic in therapy.

To facilitate a discussion of spirituality, some skillful questions that therapists can ask their clients include:

1. Do you see religion and spirituality as similar or different?
2. How has spirituality helped you?
3. How has spirituality not helped you?
4. What has spirituality meant to you as a woman?
5. Has spirituality ever helped you to cope with a tragic or debilitating experience?
6. How have you experienced spirituality during moments of worship, celebration, and transcendence?
7. How does spirituality impact the way you look at problems or suffering?
8. What does it mean for you to attend or not to attend church, meeting, temple, synagogue, or mosque?
9. How has religion, compared to spirituality, supported and/or limited you?

How does Alexa use her clinical skills at diagnosis and insight to join Cynthia in a spirit of mutuality to help Cynthia to author her own life? Although it is true that Alexa exercises certain kinds of authority and Cynthia moves into a place of vulnerability in therapy, the therapeutic experience is one of empowerment rather than "power over" (Jordan, 1997, p. 143). A significant part of creating a holding environment in therapy requires Alexa to respect Cynthia and to honor her struggle. It is imperative that Alexa create a safe and nonjudgmental place for Cynthia to explore her concerns. Clearly good therapy does not rescue people, yet it does require Alexa to accompany Cynthia on her journey through her spiritual and sexual unrest and upheaval. In a safe space, Cynthia can give voice to her confusion and shame, and eventually her anger. In the safety of the therapeutic environment, Cynthia might gain insight into her abuse of alcohol until near intoxication as an attempt to medicate and anesthetize her depression. Because Cynthia has been drinking more, Alexa needs to ascertain how long this behavior has been occurring and if it is a suboptimal means of coping with her spiritual unrest, which is at the heart of her sexual conflict. Alexa needs to know and asks Cynthia how much her drinking has increased and what effect it is having on her life. Is Cynthia able to function without the alcohol? Is she able to get out of bed in the morning and attend to her normal activities and responsibilities? Alexa's response to Cynthia's answers to these questions is decisive and ethical.

Cynthia committed herself to a marriage relationship that she unconsciously knew was inappropriate for her. The energy expended to deny the truth about her sexuality is enormous, as is the conflict between her religion and her sexuality. With the help of therapy, Cynthia comes to understand that the weight of her guilt over satisfying her sexual and emotional needs and desires as well as her anger over having denied them contribute to her depression (Kersting, 2003). Cynthia's spirit spoke to her and she did not listen. Perhaps she could not. Her current crisis is a gift in that it offers her another opportunity to honestly listen to herself. Alexa presents Cynthia's situation from this perspective of hope in order to reframe it for Cynthia. With Alexa's support, Cynthia is more receptive to listening. Encouraging Cynthia to engage in bibliotherapy so that she can read the personal stories of other married women who started to question their heterosexuality helps her to listen. A spiritual time line or genogram serves to document critical events in Cynthia's religious and spiritual development. In time, depending on the evolution of Cynthia's therapeutic goals, marital therapy is also recommended.

Alexa assists Cynthia with the collision of crazy-making feelings around religion, spirituality, race, and sexuality. Helpful questions for Cynthia included: "How does your spirituality help you make sense out of your sexuality right now? What type of religious messages did you receive about your sexual practices? What did you think your spirit was communicating to you about your feelings for women prior to getting married? How do you think God regards the feelings you have for the woman you have been involved with at church? When you pray to God, what do you say? What are some of the critical points on your spiritual journey?" Responses to these and other inquiries are explored through spiritual journaling.

That Alexa views Cynthia from a place of strength and power, regardless of any powerlessness that Cynthia may feel as she presents for therapy, is an important therapeutic skill that reflects multicultural competence. Cynthia may question who she will be if she is not defined as a married woman within the context of a socially sanctioned heterosexual marriage to a man, with shared biological children. Some psychologists-in-training as well as professional therapists assume that having membership in groups traditionally marginalized (e.g., women, people of color, persons with disabilities, nonheterosexuals) render people powerless and oppressed. However, an automatic relationship between one's identity statuses and state of empowerment does not exist. This is not to say that people are not vulnerable as a consequence of racism, sexism, and homophobia. These very forces contribute to Cynthia's distress. Cynthia will experience ostracism and judgment from the black and Christian communities if she continues with her same-sex relationship. As a black woman, independent of her sexual orientation, she functions in a white-dominated society where her gender and race statuses are socially constructed from a place of marginalization. Despite these barriers, she—like many other people of color, poor people, and women—has relied on kinship networks to live her life with spiritual strength and integrity.

Because spirituality is intrinsically and individually defined, a woman's expression of it represents her evolution, freedom, and movement through life and signifies where development is taking place. Spiritual expressions may embrace externally imposed religious aspects learned at earlier stages of life. Examples of religious expression in a woman's spirituality could include partaking of communion, praying at particular times of the day, fasting, feasting, or refraining from particular foods during religious holy days, and reading scripture from religious texts. Nonetheless, a woman's spirituality occupies an internal space that allows her to critique the religiosity of her past and present. In doing so, she is in a better position to integrate the wisdom that is crucial to meaning making while letting go of doctrine and practices that may no longer be edifying. In the case of Cynthia, when she prayed that God would take away her desire for women, she experienced a sense of peace. Her inner voice—the voice of her spirit—told her not to proceed with the marriage. Alexa used this insight as a means of opening up other stories in which Cynthia's spirit spoke to her, but in a different voice from family and religious authorities, such as her minister and Bible Study leader. That she felt God's peace after asking God to remove her emotional and sexual desires for other women, feelings that she had been taught are reprehensible, is valuable information for Cynthia (i.e., it tells her that God can hear the unspeakable and that a voice she quickly attributes to the devil may instead be God's). The process of disentangling spiritual truths from religious doctrine is a process that Cynthia cannot negotiate alone. To do so is too cognitively distressing and dissonant pro-

voking. For example, Cynthia's religious convictions and cultural and gender messages eclipsed the message she heard in prayer. She married anyhow.
Alexa asks Cynthia to ponder and write down, "What have you been
taught about what constitutes an authentic spiritual message?"

Some people may be drawn to or use their spirituality for unhealthy
reasons. Spirituality motivated by fear, guilt, or shame is addictive and,
when used as a magic solution for life's problems, is best characterized as
unhealthy (West, 2000). Fukiyama and Sevig (1999) described unhealthy
spirituality as "growth blocking, resulting from rigidity, idolatry, authori-
tarianism, and practices that are life constricting or that deny reality" (p.
90). In therapy, it became clear that Cynthia buried herself in church work
in an attempt to resolve what must have felt like an unresolvable issue. Her
extramarital affair with another woman, increased use of alcohol, and lying
to her husband reflect overwhelming guilt and conflict. She sought to manage this conflict, constrict her life, and deny reality through frenetic activity
at church. Healthy spirituality is not a retreat into denial. Nor is it an abdi-
cation of responsibility and power to a higher authority, often regarded as
male. Instead, healthy spirituality supports personal freedom, honesty, and
interdependence while offering hope and providing meaning. Using Biblical
texts to reinforce healthy mental and emotional habits that change images
of God as punitive represents another spiritual tool that allows Alexa to
consider Cynthia's religion from a different perspective. Doing so assists
Cynthia in seeing her religion from a different perspective as well.

Spirituality and Therapy Intersections

Spirituality and therapy have many similarities. Both are oriented toward
helping individuals (1) learn to accept themselves within the context of
their environment and with others; (2) forgive themselves and others—
which allows them to release toxic and debilitating resentment and hurt;
(3) acknowledge their shortcomings and those of others as part of the
human experience; (4) confront corrective and destructive guilt; and (5)
modify patterns of thinking, behaving, and feeling that are self-destructive
and contribute to a lesser life (Burke & Miranti, 2001). Berliner (1995)
noted that "both psychological growth and spiritual conversion draw the
person out of old ways of being, through the deaths such letting go
requires, and into liberation forms of life consistent with one's true self"
(p. 113).

Another way in which spirituality and therapy are extremely similar is
their use of personal narrative: Both involve the telling and hearing of one
another's stories. Speaking within the context of teaching white students
about race and racism, Tatum (2000) said, "The sharing of stories has con-

sistently helped me to see another person's perspective. . . . Hearing each other's stories—'witnessing' to one another—seems very important" (p. 84). The experience of having another listen to one's story can be extremely therapeutic. The therapist's consideration and understanding of the client's personal, private, and powerful narrative supports the client in feeling heard and lessens the likelihood of the client leaving therapy feeling dismissed (Robinson, 2005). Good therapy should neither resemble nor reinforce the dominant discourses of society that perpetuate a woman's marginalization. Spirituality is narrative in that both spirituality and the narrative offer a different and alternative approach to understanding problems and the impact of problems on individuals and their communities. Through narrative therapy, dominant discourses that can silence a woman's lived experiences are explored (Buchannan et al., 2001). Women's lives become more powerful when they learn to listen to their intuitive voices. What is the life story that Cynthia wants to tell from her constructed meanings? Rooks (1995), in a chapter on women's spirituality, asks: "Could it be that an aspect of embracing spirit is the ability to access a space that allows our life-preserving voices to speak clearly, and with unchallenged authority?" (p. 106). Spirituality internalizes a woman's power in that she comes to know that the sacred, however defined, rests within her; it is not external, as she has been taught. This point is evident in Ntozake Shange's poem, "for colored girls who considered suicide/when the rainbow is enuf." Shange said that God was found within herself and the love she had for her (God) was intense and fierce. Alexa uses this and other poetry as a therapeutic tool of empowerment with Cynthia. The experience of empowerment reflects a woman's internal and intuitive "space" that, from struggle, she has learned to occupy peacefully.

Despite the similarities between spirituality and therapy, certain structural elements are unique to the therapeutic relationship. For instance, there is a formal beginning and ending of therapy. Clients or insurance companies pay money to therapists. Clients ask for help with areas of distress, and therapists provide help based on their training and expertise. Clients share more information about their lives than therapists share about theirs. Based on ethical guidelines, therapists agree to keep the session information confidential, whereas clients can share information from therapy with whomever they please. Finally, the therapeutic relationship is dedicated to the growth of clients (Mencher, 1997).

Clients require therapists' awareness and leadership to initiate conversation about difficult topics. Yet it is impossible to help clients explore gnarly and scary issues around religion, sexual orientation, gender, and race if therapists have not engaged in this very important work for themselves. Any unexamined biases that Alexa harbors toward nonheterosexuals constitute a barrier to a healthy therapeutic relationship. Alexa did not regard

Cynthia's sexual behavior to be objectionable or repulsive. However, if she did, she would not be an appropriate therapist for Cynthia and would need to refer her to someone who could be respectful.

To help empower clients, therapists need to ackowledge their clients' culture. In some cases, a client's culture includes religious practices and philosophies that not only differ significantly from that of the therapist but are perceived as unhealthy. In such a case, the clinician needs to rely on important clinical skills. These include the ability (1) to explore a religion that is different from one's own, (2) to assess the relevance of the spiritual domains in the client's therapeutic issues, and (3) to use a client's spiritual beliefs in the pursuit of the client's therapeutic goals. For example, Alexa is Catholic; Cynthia is Christian. Because Cynthia believes that her sexual behavior is largely due to the influence of Satan in her life; it is important that Alexa listen to Cynthia talk about what she experiences as a need to rebuke Satan and have people at church lay hands on her. Alexa could ascertain from Cynthia what type of meaning this belief has for her. Empowerment skills represent Alexa's ability to think flexibly about Cynthia's beliefs and determine how these beliefs can help or hinder Cynthia's therapeutic goals (Robinson, 2005). Alexa inquires into Cynthia's support system to determine if there is a "sister friend" in whom Cynthia can confide. Alexa understands the importance of community and recommends a prayer circle as a way for Cynthia to experience therapeutic support and acceptance.

Often when people conceptualize community, they think about being with people who are like themselves with respect to class, race, gender, and age. If the connective capacity is missing, being a therapist of color or a woman or both does not ensure that a female client of color will be able to work effectively on spiritual topics. Community is critical to the notion of the sacred and things spiritual and is at the heart of a "connective capacity" whereby people feel in relationship with one another (Palmer, 1999). hooks (1999) said that being guided by love means to be joined in community with all life. But a culture of domination, such as the U.S. culture, does not orient people to coexist in community. How do clients experience that connective capacity? In the presence of superb clinical skills, why does this connective capacity sometimes get suppressed or overlooked in the therapy room? As therapists, we seek to teach our clients new ways of being in the world. Hopefully, we are in the relationship based on our understanding of the sacred. The sincere regard for Cynthia's well-being that is conveyed through Alexa's eyes, the respect for Cynthia's courage to embrace struggle as she boldly puts one foot in front of the other, are sacred. Cynthia and Alexa alike have a mutual and human need for connectedness. It is this need that marks the therapeutic event as inherently spiritual. "If we recover a sense of the sacred, we will recover the humility that makes teaching and learning possible" (Palmer, 1999, p. 29). The process of Alexa and Cynthia learning from and with one another is sacred and therapeutic.

Pathways to Spirituality

A place of worship represents many different experiences for different women. For some, it is a space in which to receive validation—noticed and praised for one's hat, clothing, shoes, attended to, hugged, gazed upon, appreciated for volunteering, serving, and demonstrating a Godly spirit. Many women who attend some form of religious service during the week find that it is one of the only places where they experience peace and enjoy a sense of community with others who share their beliefs. It is a place where they can be real and accepted for their true self. Through religious affiliation, many celebrity vocal artists identified and refined their skills of singing in the choir. Others developed group facilitation and public speaking skills and learned to play an instrument. Others learned the value of community and being involved in a cause bigger than oneself.

Religious environments may also represent condemnation, judgment, fear, shame, and censor. For these women, their early religious training did not contribute to their empowerment. Instead, religion was experienced as oppressive and a source of bondage (Robinson & Watt, 2001). Due to a cultural climate of heterosexism that endorses heterosexuality as normal and superior, gay, lesbian, bisexual, and transgender people often do not find religion to be an affirming experience. In fact, many gay people "find themselves rejecting their religious faith in order to accept their sexual orientation" (Buchannan et al., 2001, p. 435). Their morality is questioned, as is their suitability as parents and married partners, in religious, church, and legal contexts. Such a negative climate has enormous implications for Cynthia and other spiritual women who are lesbian, bisexual, transgender, or simply questioning their sexuality. A perception of God as condemning of nonheterosexuals compounds a woman's culturally scripted powerlessness—the sense that she is not capable of directing or changing the course of her life in meaningful ways (McWhirter, 1991).

As a function of crisis or coping with, and/or suffering through, life's difficulty, a woman may find herself on a spiritual journey. As difficult as her journey is, spiritual growth is less likely without some dissonance and upheaval—feelings of pain, depression, hopelessness, and not being in control. "It is often, finally, a woman's own pain and sadness that make her change her life. Finally, it is impossible to deny her feelings any longer" (Duerk, 1994, p. 29). Loss and dissonance as a precursor to growth and change are consistent with most developmental theorists, who espouse a phase or stage of dissonance in their models of identity development.

Conclusion

This chapter sought to encourage dialogue within clinical contexts about the possible role of spirituality as a component of the client's issues seeking resolution. Therapy can assist people in their efforts to bring meaning, wisdom, and sanity into their lives. Many of us, as therapists, have offered help as well as benefited from the help we gave. Desperately needed are those of us willing and able to (1) foster a respect for spirituality as central to healing, (2) critique cultural patterns that are oppressive, and (3) encourage community between client and therapist. These aims ultimately require a crossing of borders that easily divide, such as race, gender, culture, religion, and position.

All persons independent of gender, race, class, sexual orientation, and religion who arrive at therapy for assistance need to be regarded as clients and treated respectfully. For therapy to be effective, clinicians need to learn the art of living in community as a core practice. In doing so, the therapeutic event is not seen as one of power over the client but as a joining with the clients in a connective way. Is it possible to give our best clinical practice to clients who we devalue or see as a problem? If therapists practiced the art of living in community, they might be less likely to assign ethnic-minority clients to junior professionals or provide low-cost, less-preferred treatment that consists of minimal contact and results in a much higher rate of premature termination among clients (Ridley, 1989). When therapists learn the art of living in community, women might receive fewer prescriptions for psychotropic medications and less frequent mental disorder diagnoses (Crose, Nicholas, Gobble, & Frank, 1992).

To explore this topic of spirituality in therapy, a case study of a client struggling with a collision between religious discourses and spiritual messages was presented. The intersection of religion and spirituality with other identities, such as race, sexual orientation, and gender, was discussed throughout. Specific skills were identified that are helpful to the clinician when approaching the area of spirituality in therapy.

References

Belenky, M. F., Clinchy, B. M., Goldberger, N. R., & Tarule, J. M. (1986). *Women's ways of knowing: The development of self, voice, and mind*. New York: Basic Books.

Berliner, P. M. (1995). Soul healing: A model of feminist therapy. In M. Burke & J. Mirant (Eds.), *Counseling: The spiritual dimension* (pp. 113–125). Thousand Oaks, CA: Sage.

Boyd-Franklin, N. (1989). *Black families in therapy: A multisystems approach*. New York: Guilford Press.

Boyd-Franklin, N. (2003). Race, class, and poverty. In F. Walsh (Ed.), *Normal family processes: Growing diversity and complexity* (3rd ed., pp. 260–279). New York: Guilford Press.

Buchanan, M., Dzelme, K., Harris, D., & Hecker, L. (2001). Challenges of being simultaneously gay or lesbian and spiritual and/or religious: A narrative perspective. *American Journal of Family Therapy, 29,* 435–449.

Burke, M. T., Hackney, H., Hudson, P., Miranti, J., Watts, G. A., & Epps, L. (1999). Spirituality, religion, and CACREP Curriculum Standards. *Journal of Counseling and Development, 77,* 251–257.

Burke, M. T., & Miranti, J. (2001). The spiritual and religious dimensions of counseling. In D. Locke, J. Myers, & E. Herr (Eds.), *Handbook of counseling* (pp. 601–612). Thousand Oaks, CA: Sage.

Cashwell, C. S., & Young, J. S. (2004). Spirituality in counselor training: A content analysis of syllabi from introductory spirituality courses. *Counseling and Values, 48,* 96–109.

Crose, R., Nicholas, D. R., Gobble, D. C., & Frank, B. (1992). Gender and wellness: A multidimensional systems model for counseling. *Journal of Counseling and Development, 71,* 149–156.

Duerk, J. (1994). *Circle of stones: Woman's journey to herself.* San Diego, CA: Lura Media.

Fukiyama, M. A., & Sevig, T. D. (1999). *Ingegrating spirituality into multicultural counseling.* Thousand Oaks, CA: Sage.

Ganje-Fling, M. A., & McCarthy, P. (1996). Impact of childhood sexual abuse on client spiritual development: Counseling implications. *Journal of Counseling and Development, 74,* 253–262.

hooks, b. (1999). Embracing freedom: Spirituality and liberation. In S. Glazer (Ed.), *The heart of learning: Spirituality in education* (pp. 113–129). New York: Putnam.

Ingersoll, R. E. (1995). Spirituality, religion, and counseling: Dimensions and relationship. In M. Burke & J. Mirant (Eds.), *Counseling: The spiritual dimension* (pp. 5–18). Thousand Oaks, CA: Sage.

Kersting, K. (2003). Religion and spirituality in the treatment rook. *Monitor on Psychology, 34,* 40–42.

McWhirter, E. H. (1991). Empowerment in counseling. *Journal of Counseling and Development, 69,* 222–227.

Mencher, J. (1997). Intimacy in lesbian relationships: A critical reexamination of fusion. In J. V. Jordan (Ed.), *Women's growth in diversity: More writings from the Stone Center* (pp. 311–330). New York: Guilford Press.

Palmer, P. J. (1999). A vision of education as transformation. In S. Glazer (Ed.), *The heart of learning: Spirituality in education* (pp. 15–32). New York: Putnam.

Ridley, C. R. (1989). Racism in counseling as an aversive behavioral process. In P. B. Pedersen, J. G. Draguns, W. J. Lonner, & J. E. Trimble (Eds.), *Counseling across cultures* (pp. 55–78). Honolulu: University of Hawaii Press.

Riggs, M. (1994). *Black is . . . black ain't* [Videotape]. San Francisco: California Newsreel.

Robinson, T. L. (2000). Making the hurt go away: Psychological and spiritual heal-ing for African American women survivors of childhood incest. *Journal of Multicultural Counseling and Development, 28,* 160–176.

Robinson, T. L. (2005). *The convergence of race, ethnicity, and gender: Multiple identities in counseling.* Upper Saddle River, NJ: Merrill Prentice Hall.

Robinson, T. L., & Watt, S. K. (2001). Where no one goes begging: Gender, sexual-ity, and religious diversity. In D. Locke, J. Myers, & E. Herr (Eds.), *Handbook of counseling* (pp. 589–599). Thousand Oaks, CA: Sage.

Rooks, B. (1995). Revelation by grace. In G. Wade-Gayles (Ed.), *My soul is a wit-ness* (pp. 105–108). Boston: Beacon Press.

Singleton, D. K. (2003). *Broken silence: Opening your heart and mind to therapy—a black woman's recovery guide.* New York: One World.

Spilka, B., Hood, R. W. Jr., Hunsberger, B., & Gorsuch, R. (2003). *The psychology of religion: An empirical approach* (3rd ed.). New York: Guilford Press.

Swinton, J. (2001). *Spirituality and mental health care: Rediscovering a "forgotten" dimension.* Philadelphia: Jessica Kingsley Publishers.

Tatum, B. D. (2002). Changing lives, changing communities: Building a capacity for connection in a pluralistic context. In V. Kazanjian & P. Laurence (Eds.), *Edu-cation as transformation: Religious, pluralism, spirituality, and a new vision for higher education in America* (pp. 79–88). New York: Peter Lang.

Wade-Gayles, G. (1995). *My soul is a witness: African American women's spiritual-ity.* Boston: Beacon Press.

West, W. (2000). *Psychotherapy and spirituality: Crossing the line between therapy and religion.* London: Sage.

Witmer, J. M., & Sweeney, T. J. (1992). A holistic model for wellness and preven-tion over the life span. *Journal of Counseling and Development, 71,* 140–143.

CHAPTER 14

Native American Women

FOSTERING RESILIENCY
THROUGH COMMUNITY

Nadine Tafoya

The sun shines brightly on the clear water running in the creek. The people known as Apaches have been preparing all year for the summer ceremonies and the special coming-of-age ceremony for girls to transition into womanhood. The girls' chaperones and medicine women are chosen and assume their roles and responsibilities for praying, preparing, and supporting each young girl through this life-changing event. They have harvested and prepared medicinal plants that are part of the process. They have prepared the buckskin hides for the young girls' dresses and moccasins. Special foods and other sacred things have been carefully collected and saved for the ceremony.

Four days before the ceremony is to begin the grounds and the encampment are made ready. All the family and their helpers work tirelessly as they make preparations for this momentous occasion. The long pine poles are tied together on one end. This is the framework for the big ceremonial teepee where the puberty ceremony will take place. The oak branches have been gathered and made ready to cover the teepee frame. Each of the girls has been prepared mentally and physically for the ceremony and the ordeal to begin. The grounds are consecrated and the energy of the tribe and the women has focused on getting ready for the dawn of this special day.

Each girl knows that she has been preparing for this moment. In fact, her family has been preparing her for this moment almost from the day of her birth. She is making the transformation from a girl to a woman at this time. She has strong medicine to impart to her people. She is carrying on a tradition that has taken place from one generation to the next for hundreds of years. Although there are many different bands of Apaches in the Southwest, all practicing different traditions and spiritual practices, this sacred ceremony is one of the most revered and important rituals that has endured even into the 21st century (Geronimo, 2001).

> In preparing for my first meeting with Charlotte and her daughter, I thought back over the days when I had been transformed from a girl to a woman in the eyes of my family and tribe. Charlotte had said on the phone that her 13-year-old daughter, Tamara, had adopted an urban culture that was at odds with her own. She was rebellious, failing in school, wanted to be independent, refused to help out around the house, and had been caught smoking in the house more than once. Charlotte thought that Tamara set a bad example to her younger brothers and sister. Charlotte had called after the most recent incident when her daughter sneaked away from school and lied about going to the mall instead.
>
> Charlotte was also concerned about Tamara's upcoming puberty ceremony. She worried that Tamara was not ready and, in fact, could not care less about all the fuss. The family had spent the past year in preparation for this event, while their daughter had grown more distant and urbanized. Tamara knew they were getting ready for her ceremony but had no desire to participate. She had a boyfriend and a life that did not include many of the old ways. Tamara had become more involved in town life and did not want to be dragged back to the old ways. She had begun to experiment with smoking and had started disobeying the rules. She claimed she wanted to "be her own person," "hanging" with her friends, away from her family.

> MOM: We're here today to talk to you about Tamara's behavior. The school said you might be able to help us. She's failing, she's not following our rules, and we don't know what to do. Can you do something?
>
> TAMARA: Looks down and mumbles something under her breath.
>
> THERAPIST: Tamara, it's good to meet you. I'm glad you're here. Why do you think you're here?

> The therapist noticed that Tamara had on black fingernail polish, several piercings, and her jeans were strategically ripped. Tamara, rolling her eyes, looked down again and made a small huffing sound.

> MOM: See!!! This is the way she behaves—we can't get her to talk to us either.

THERAPIST: (*smiling*) This reminds me of story about a young girl [Niethammer, 1977, p. 32]. This young girl was a Pueblo girl. She lived with her grandparents. Her grandparents had to work really hard. They lived on a farm and had animals, crops, and orchards to tend. Work on the farm was hard. They hauled water, chopped wood, and had to keep a fire burning in the kitchen constantly. Everyone in the family needed to pitch in when there was so much work to get done. This young girl had been away—she had been taken to boarding school and lived at the school most of the year. She was able to come home only on holidays. However, when she came home, she was lazy and wouldn't help with all the work and chores.

The grandparents were amazed at what had happened to their granddaughter while she was away at school. One time when the granddaughter came home and started behaving in the same indolent way she always did, the grandmother decided to teach her a lesson. The grandmother said to the granddaughter, "If you don't want to help here at home with the chores, go to the community field and pick us some *calabacitas* [squash] and chilies." So the girl thinks this is a fine idea. She takes her time getting to the community field, and along the way she meets some of her friends from the boarding school. They spend a great deal of time telling stories and gossiping about other girls at school. It is late in the afternoon when the girls finally get around to picking the *calabacitas* and chilies to take home. All of a sudden along came one of the *Tsabiyu* [masked figures from Christmas folklore] with some long whips made from the sharp-edged leaves of the yucca plant. "You do not mind your parent or grandparents," he said. Then he drew out his whips and beat the young girls.

Crying, the girls fled, but the masked figure ran after them, lashing them all the way. The girls tripped and fell, dropping all the chilies and squash they had picked. But still they kept running, trying to get away from the fearsome figure. Finally the *Tsabiyu* had used up all his yucca blades, so he called a warning to the girls, "This is what happens to girls who do not obey their mothers and fathers and grandparents. Now go home." The girls all went their separate ways but were never lazy or disobeyed their families again.

Mom and Tamara looked at each other and laughed.

MOM: We may have to go out and find that *Tsabiyu* too.

TAMARA: I'm not really that bad, am I?

What happened when the therapist told the story? Why did she tell a story rather than answering Charlotte's question? This chapter addresses working with female clients who are Native American. Particular attention is given to culture and community and how one can utilize these aspects in the therapeutic process. In order to explore this practice, examples derived from New Mexico's Apache and Pueblo tribes are used. I am Apache and live at Santa Clara Pueblo with my husband and family. However, these examples are helpful for clients from any Native American tribe. Native Americans in the United States have some shared history and experiences that have a direct impact on both individuals and the cultures and tribes within which they live.

The chapter is divided into four sections: (1) the initial historical context for Native women; (2) historical trauma and similarities among Native American clients; (3) differences among Native American clients related to tribe(s) of origin, acculturation, and other factors; and (4) cultural resiliency and adaptability: resurgence of community and cultural pride.

Each section provides the clinician with basic information and general guidelines about working with Native American women. Specific examples and scenarios are used to clarify how the more general information can be applied to the problems presented by individual clients.

Similarities within Native Women Clients Related to Historical Trauma

Before colonization, there were clear guidelines as to what women brought to the family and community. Depending upon the child's gender, everyone in the community knew what a child's destiny would be. As a child grew from one life stage to the next, he or she was prepared for his or her future role in the family and the tribe. Every individual had a strong sense of identity and belonging.

Female roles within the community encompassed not only mothering, nurturing, family, and child care, but also positions as spiritual leaders, tribal leaders, warriors, healers, and teachers/educators. Women were the keepers of the stories and stressed the importance of the traditional practices and beliefs. When a woman did not want to follow the traditional paths for women, she was still embraced by the community and she still carried a strong sense of pride and honor to be born into her tribe. Historically, just because a woman did not want to identify with the tribes' prescribed roles for women, it did not mean that her sense of identity or her sense of belonging to the community was eroded. Within the prescribed women's roles she strove to make a place for herself. She belonged to the community unless she transgressed in some way that resulted in ostracism.

Although women played important roles within the community, their contributions were not always accepted or encouraged by men. In the movie *Whale Rider*, the young girl had to fulfill a male role because there were no males in the modern-day tribe who could fulfill this role. Although her grandfather had impressed the importance of the role of the Whale Rider on her, he initially resisted the idea that a woman could fulfill that role. In her book *Daughters of the Earth*, Neithammer writes:

> Even in those Native American tribes in which women had a great deal of power and prestige, controlled the economic goods of the family and held sacred ceremonial offices, the line was always drawn at some point: The sacred bundle could not be handled by a women (who might be menstruating and thus defile it), certain offerings to very special supernaturals could only be made by men, or particular offices could be filled only by men. (1977, p. xii)

Throughout history, Native women have had to exhibit extreme versatility in order to keep the tribe thriving.

Furthermore, with colonization, the Western way of life was imposed on Native people. Women's roles were recreated using a European model. Spanish and English colonizers did not want to deal with women in leadership roles. Women were not treated or negotiated with; colonizers expected men to be leaders and wanted to deal only with the men. Native American women were relegated to the same position that European women held; they were considered chattel or property (Niethammer, 1977).

Later when Native children were unceremoniously forced into boarding schools, other more insidious effects of colonization occurred. The first major boarding school was Carlisle Indian School in Pennsylvania. In 1875, Colonel Richard Pratt, the founder of Carlisle Indian School, found himself with custody of a number of Indian prisoners. Rather than simple incarceration, Pratt decided that his prisoners should learn in a European school setting. The purpose of the school was "to civilize the Indian, put him in the midst of civilization. . . . To keep him civilized, keep him there" (Underhill, 1989, p. 207). With this philosophy or mission, Native children were ripped from their families and shipped over 1,000 miles away to schools on the East Coast. Their hair was shorn, their clothes taken from them, and they were forbidden to speak their languages or practice their religions. Not only was every vestige of their own culture stripped from them, but the smallest children were taken from their nurturing mothers, aunts, and grandmothers and remanded to Western caretakers who often abused them verbally, sexually, and physically (Tafoya & Del Vechhio, in press).

Results of Colonization

When Native American young adults returned to their homes and villages from the boarding schools, they understood little about the old ways of life.

They were strangers in their own communities. Youth incarcerated in boarding schools were without a family constellation and without role models to show them how to communicate, manage emotions, and set goals. Their exposure to positive parenting role models was extremely limited, and they did not learn how to parent as a result. As a consequence of this institutionalization, many generations of Native children have been raised without any kind of nurturing or positive parenting practices. The pain and suffering are a legacy that has been passed on from one generation to the next. Native American researcher Maria Yellow Horse Brave Heart (Brave Heart, 2003) and her colleagues have documented a variety of symptoms and issues related to historical trauma and unresolved grief. The dynamics of unresolved grief include symptoms and manifestations that affect every aspect of an individual's life include somatic conditions such as migraines, stomachaches, joint pain, dizziness, and chronic fatigue; physical stress and vulnerability to chronic health problems such as type II diabetes; depression; substance abuse; suicidal ideation and gestures; chronic, delayed, or impaired grief process (e.g., searching and pining behaviors that include thoughts, feelings, and behaviors aimed at reestablishing the presence of the deceased).

The trauma response, as documented among survivors of the Nazi Holocaust, Vietnam veterans, and the survivors of other wars, involves multiple psychological and physical components (Brave Heart, 2003). Duran and colleagues (2004) identified the prevalence and correlates of mental health disorders among Native American women in primary care. Although they did not find a direct link between boarding school experience and mental health disorders, they posited that the high prevalence of anxiety disorders in this group may be the product of a complex interaction of individual and community variables. Trauma response behaviors are also well documented in clinical treatment with regard to a variety of disorders, including posttraumatic stress disorder. The constellation of trauma response behaviors that is documented in the trauma literature applies to Native American women as well as to other populations, even though some of the initial trauma occurred many generations ago.

Trauma response behaviors include the following: psychic numbing; hypervigilance; disassociation; intense fear; survivor guilt; fixation on the trauma; victim identity, death identity, and identification with the dead; low self-esteem; anger; self-destructive behavior; weakened immune system and chronic diseases processes; depression; and substance abuse (Brave Heart, 2003). These processes, signs, and symptoms of both unresolved grief and the trauma response are endemic on reservations and among urban Native American populations in the United States. No family is untouched by these problems whose manifestations are evident communitywide.

Hopelessness and despair related to sociohistorical trauma are also common experiences among Native Americans. Women often present in therapy with persistent mood disorders, dysthymia, or anxiety. Although the client may not have internalized a negative self-image, she is confronted daily in her community with poverty, family violence, racism, and desolation. A recent health research study conducted by Duran and colleagues (2004) stated that mental illness, mental dysfunction, or self-destructive behavior affects approximately 21% of the total American Indian and Alaskan Native (AIAN) population. Their findings indicated that there was high comorbidity between substance-related disorders and mood and anxiety disorders. Among the women with any lifetime substance-related disorder, 74% had a lifetime anxiety disorder and 57% had a lifetime mood disorder. The authors explain another important finding in their study:

> The rate of lifetime substance abuse disorder found among the women in our study (62%; SE = 3.4) is considerably higher than any other reported rate in women. This finding should be put into context. Research on AIAN drinking indicates that (1) alcohol consumption and abuse levels vary widely by tribe and over time, (2) women have very high rates of alcohol abstention, (3) alcohol consumption is higher in urban areas than on the reservations and (4) alcohol consumption patterns are bimodal—there are large number of both abstainer and heavy binge drinkers in the population. (Duran et al., 2004, pp. 71–77)

The common history and shared colonization experience, including unresolved grief, trauma response, and internalized oppression, are part of the constellation of issues to explore. The following guidelines can be used to work with Native woman clients. It is not necessary to focus on specific tribal/cultural issues in the initial stages of therapy. The Native woman's "nativeness" comes first. One might conceptualize moving from working on the outside (shared Native history), toward the inside (exploration of more specific tribal affiliation issues and sense of belonging and identity shared with other members of the same tribe). When considering the more general, homogeneous Native experience, it is fine to suggest "pan-Native" healing traditions such as talking circles, vision quests, sweat lodge ceremonies, and the burning of sage to the client.

Guidelines for Initial Stages of Exploration, Discovery, and Assessment

Cathartic Release of Affect

During the initial process, treatment must provide for cathartic release of affect (Brave Heart, 1998). Women who experience this release come to understand the cumulative effect of generations of historical trauma. They become aware of and understand that their problems are not only specific to their individual history but are part of greater context that crosses generations and all tribes in the Americas. This experience of massive grief, loss, and change in culture and lifestyle has an impact on the individual that is greater than that individual woman's unique experience (the whole is greater than the sum of the parts). Some discussion of the history of genocide against Native Americans and the boarding school experience may be necessary to orient clients to the effect that trauma has had on the families and communities. Repression and racism should be identified as concomitant to the trauma process, and the impact that racist behavior has on daily life should be investigated.

Assessment of Family and Clan Affiliations

An assessment of the Native woman's connection to her "family" (i.e., of origin, extended, clan membership, and spiritual affiliations, both Native Ceremonial and Christian, e.g., godparents) should be explored. Sometimes a genogram is an effective tool to use. A genogram can be used to trace boarding school history, substance abuse history, strength of relationships between family members, conflicts between family members, and so on. Other ways of exploring family connectedness may be suggested by the client or the therapist. Visualization, role playing, and other typical counseling methods can be effective tools for this assessment. Identifying family and clan affiliations is particularly important for a Native American woman because her family connections, history, and degree of acculturation or traditionalism are essential information to use in making treatment decisions. You cannot put an acculturated woman into a traditional ceremony and expect her to reap the benefits of that ceremony. This Westernized woman would benefit the most from contemporary mainstream treatment modalities.

Assessing Acculturation and Tribal Identity

The therapist also needs to ascertain the client's levels of acculturation and tribal identity. Does the client live in the tribal community and, if not, how long has she lived apart from the tribal community? What are her existing ties to the tribal community? Does the family participate in cultural activities? Is the client and her family linked to, or tied in with, their tribal culture? Answers to these questions supply the therapist with insight into the woman's sense of self. Who does she think she is? Who are her people? The therapist also needs to assess the client's self-perception with regard to her identity within her tribe. Is her connection to the tribe strong or weak, positive or negative? Research indicates that strong tribal identity is a protective factor (protection from self-destructive behavior, such as substance abuse, promiscuity, etc; Brave Heart, 2003). Therefore it is important to explore tribal identity issues. Some individuals grow up without any known ties to the tribe. They may feel ashamed for not knowing customs, language, or even extended family members. On the other hand, some people do not miss what they have never experienced. In this case, their problems stem from other sources. Additionally, some Native women deal with internalized oppression. In these cases, they may be ashamed of any affiliation with their traditions and their tribal culture.

Assessment of Internalized Oppression

Internalized oppression—the incorporation of the belief that the oppressor's view of the Native person and culture as savage, uncivilized, and heathen is correct—is also an issue that has to be considered. Internalized oppression is often manifested as self-loathing, overidentification with the oppressive culture, and the scapegoating of others from their own tribe and culture. Native people experience a tremendous amount of racism and different forms of oppression from the non-Native society. Most of U.S. society has erroneous information and misunderstandings about Native Americans. Many people thinks Native Americans died out with the buffalo and that "Indian" describes all Native people. This is an example of stereotyping. It also puts Native people in the past rather than as a contemporary part of society today, a perspective that disenfranchises them as individuals and as a people and makes them an invisible, overlooked segment of U.S. society. Native communities contend with towns and cities that border the reservation, where more often than not, Native people are met with hostility when they go to town for daily business.

Native women are particularly vulnerable to insults both overt and subtle that target their gender and their ethnicity. "Squaw" is the mildest of the demeaning terminology that is still used to degrade and control Native women. "Squaw" was traditionally used to denote any Native woman as an object or a commodity to be used. Being called names contributes to identification with the oppressor and results in an internalized oppression that leads to self-hatred and an inability to function as a whole and healthy individual with a tribal or Native American identity. The Native woman then identifies with the oppressor. This identification causes an internal schism, because she is really Native and not the oppressor, and it results in ongoing internal conflict, shame, guilt, and insecurity.

Exploration of Connection to Traditional Ceremonies and Healing

Traditional ceremonies and healing processes provide grounding for Native clients, linking them to their culture and history. Clients should be encouraged to access the cultural ways that provide anchoring and emotional support, foster the cathartic release of unresolved grief and other suppressed or repressed feelings, and thereby facilitate healing. These traditions, as sources of protection and support, can also help to validate a woman's sense of self and confirm her identity and place within her tribal community and the greater society. Focusing on these traditional ceremonies as healing processes assumes that during the initial stages of therapy, the therapist has identified the woman's affiliation with her culture, family, and tribe. As noted, typical types of pan-Native treatments include talking circles, vision quests, and sweat lodge ceremonies. Traditional treatments that are tribally specific would have to be prescribed by a traditional healer (from that particular tribe) who would be consulted by the client.

Homogeneity among Native women clients has its roots in the systematic oppression that occurred as part of the colonization process. Native woman share a history of rape and slavery by colonizers that binds them together in shared suffering. The vestiges of this trauma continue today in intergenerational unresolved grief, decimation of language and culture, and the loss of identity. Assessment of these issues for any individual client is essential to moving the therapeutic relationship forward and to helping the client resolve her presenting problems. At the same time, knowledge of cultural differences related to tribal affiliation and an awareness of individual differences are also critical to facilitating the healing process. The next section explores how heterogeneity among Native women clients affects the progress of treatment.

Heterogeneity among Native American Women: Differences Related to Tribe(s) of Origin, Acculturation, and Other Factors

During the spring of 2004, elders from the Mescalero Apache tribe participated in a focus group as part of a traditional cultural night. Approximately a dozen elder men and women came together to answer questions about their history and culture. The Apaches lived a nomadic existence, and some of the elders in the group remembered when they still lived in tents and teepees and moved around. A woman's work involved gathering and harvesting food from the wild while the men hunted.

One of the elder women explained:

"We learned their beliefs in the Apache way—like not walking around in the house without shoes and other things we are not supposed to do. Also, that there were only certain times when we could cut our hair; and to look at the moon and stars to tell when bad weather is coming or when a death is coming. In the old days we had to carry water from the springs, gather wood and carry it to our camp. We were all poor, no hospital, no doctors or nurses. My grandmother helped my mother have me there at the camp. It's how we were brought up in the Indian way. We were brought up with the culture and the traditions."

An Apache woman who presents for therapy has a very different tribal history than a woman from another Southwestern tribal group, such as one of the Pueblos. At one time Apache people from many different bands were forced together on a small reservation in southeast New Mexico and were expected to live together and cooperate with each other, even though their languages, cultures, and traditions were very different. In addition, they were also expected to learn to farm and herd cattle—when they had no skills or desire to do so. They had always hunted and gathered for their livelihood. The Pueblo people, on the other hand, were never removed from their ancestral lands and already were farmers and herders. Spanish land grant rights accorded them their pueblos and they did not experience the same kind of forced removal history that the more nomadic Apaches did.

The different experiences of colonization and dislocation for tribes is not the only issue to be considered that shapes a Native woman's sense of self and community. The following case studies summarize some of the differences related to colonization that may shape a woman's sense of self and her position in the community, as well as some of the problems she brings to therapy.

Corinna was a 59-year-old grandmother of three. She came into therapy because she was severely depressed. She was diagnosed with diabetes, and her primary physician thought that Corinna needed some support to help her deal with this chronic disease. Corinna was a Pueblo woman who lived in a small community of less than 800 people. Her people have never been confined, treated as prisoners of war, or experienced forced abandonment of their pueblo, and homelands.

Corinna participated in annual Pueblo ceremonies that are linked to the cycle of the seasons as well as the Saints' Days celebrations of the Catholic Church. She spent a great deal of time shopping, cooking, baking, and cleaning for every feast day, which occurred with every season change. This preparation was an obligation that tied her to the family, the extended family, and the community. The women worked together to prepare for the elaborate feasts when they open the matriarch's house to the community and to friends who have been invited to watch the dances and to eat afterward. With her family and community responsibilities, Corinna had very little time left for herself. In the midst of all the seasonal activities and preparations, she still had to deal with family crises and care for elders and children within her extensive family system. In addition, she worked full time as an administrative assistant to the tribal court judge.

As Corinna enters therapy, she is feeling overwhelmed and unaccustomed to providing nurturing for herself. She is comfortable with her role as nurturer to her extended and immediate family, but there is no time left for herself, and she has never had any role models from whom to learn how to nurture herself. In the communal life of the Pueblo, the needs of others must come first, and each community member is expected to give back to the community. This custom is both a strength and a resource for Corinna to draw upon, while also causing ongoing stress in her life. The demands of the community offer the reward of drawing everyone together, but the amount of work that goes into preparation is extremely time consuming and exhausting. The complexities of diabetes and the stress that comes from a long history of oppression, which contributes to the development of somatic diseases such as diabetes, now require Corinna to pay attention to her own needs in a manner for which she has not been prepared. The ongoing and extensive work required of each individual to the community is an issue specific to the Pueblo tribe. The communal needs for support of the religious obligations to the church and traditional ceremonial activities, as well as day-to-day demands for help with births, weddings, and deaths, are not typical of the dominant culture or of many other tribes in the United States.

An intervention strategy for Corinna can utilize the healing practices that are available within her pueblo. She can be encouraged to utilize her strong family network to help her deal with her current medical condition, and traditional healing ceremonies prescribed by healers within her pueblo and not shared with outsiders can be utilized, if she so chooses. She can also be referred to other community health resources that will provide education and support to Corinna and her family.

Jennifer entered therapy through a local women's shelter for victims of domestic violence. She grew up on the Apache reservation and attended postsecondary schools in the region. She had an undergraduate degree in sociology and had worked for the tribe for a number of years. She married a European American outside the tribe, and they lived in the town adjacent to the reservation.

Jennifer's parents were the product of boarding schools and experiences of racism and oppression throughout their lives. They wanted better for Jennifer and their children and pushed the issue of European American education as the way out. Although her parents practiced their traditions, spoke the Native language, and were involved in the cultural traditions of their tribe, they never pressured Jennifer to be involved in these activities. Jennifer was aware of cultural ceremonies and practices but was never interested in participating in them.

Jennifer currently lived a daily existence of fear, pain, and depression. She never knew what would set off her husband's anger or when the next blows would come. She had three sons, who watched their father beat her. Jennifer was afraid to let her parents and family know what was going on, so she kept silent about the abuse. She finally chose to seek help and to leave her home when the oldest boy started to stand up for her and tried to protect her. Her husband severely beat him too, and that was when she gathered the children and left.

After being referred to a women's shelter for victims of domestic violence, Jennifer sought counseling to try to get back on her feet. Her treatment will take a different path from Corinna's. She has been isolated from her Native culture and community traditions, originally by her parents and then by her husband, who is an outsider. The dynamics of domestic violence cause the abuser to isolate the victim and to deny her access to any form of support or resources outside those that he might offer her. Throughout the course of treatment, the therapist will focus on educating Jennifer about the cycle of abuse and its effect on her and the children. Because Jennifer is so removed from her tribe at this initial stage of treatment, the community is not the logical place to go for support. She may benefit more from a women's self-help group that focuses on her needs and the needs of her children.

Jennifer's problems are specifically Apache in that her exposure to traditional tribal language and culture was limited by her parents. Although they participated, they did not teach their children. The Apache way of life does not require the same amount of communal contributions and involvement as that seen in the Pueblo way of life. Historically, Apache people lived in bands; they were spread out and nomadic. Today, involvement in traditional ceremonies is more an individual decision rather than an expectation of the community, as seen in Pueblo tribes. Jennifer can lead a more autonomous lifestyle and is less in a fish-bowl-like situation than Corinna was. Jennifer is an example of a contemporary Apache woman; she is more acculturated and less tied to traditional tribal practices.

The two clients, Apache and Pueblo, presented with issues and resources that are unique to their ages and stages of life as well as to the tribal communities from which they come. The therapist must first establish rapport and then elicit the background information—the rich life history that each unique individual brings to therapy—before proceeding to map out a detailed course of treatment. Once this information has been identified and discussed, logical links to community and family support can be prescribed.

Cultural Resiliency and Adaptability

According to Brave Heart (2003), historical trauma theory describes massive cumulative trauma across generations rather than the more limited diagnosis of posttraumatic stress disorder (PTSD). The Jewish Holocaust community, the descendents of the Japanese American World War II internment camps, African American descendants of slaves, and Latino survivors of colonization are some of those who share common features of all survivors of massive group trauma and have also endured a legacy of oppression, internment, genocidal practices, and racism. Native Americans are not unique in carrying this legacy. Sharing knowledge across massively traumatized groups can increase understanding and promote healing. The following is a process that the therapist and client may wish to explore, depending on the client's awareness of her own position in this historical context:

1. Become aware of trauma history within the tribe and its multigenerational impact on families, individuals, and community.
2. Grieve the losses and indignities the people have endured; acknowledge these losses and encourage a cathartic release.
3. Acknowledge and encourage the residual anger at the loss and the grief.
4. Finally, let go and move on with healing in an appropriate context.

Today, although many traditional values and beliefs are still taught, changes have taken a toll on Native families and communities. Our tribes and pueblos are not as united as they once were. Native people no longer look to each other for assistance and support when encountering trouble or difficult times. We are seeing increased problems with juvenile delinquency, gang activity, family violence, suicide, and substance abuse, which are claiming both young and old members of our communities. In many Native American communities, a wide array of services has emerged to address growing social problems. These services include community health care clinics, home visiting services, day care, community schools, and tribal substance abuse treatment and prevention programs, to name a few. One can usually obtain a community directory of services by contacting the tribal administrative offices, usually listed in the U.S. government listings in the local telephone directory.

Native people have withstood 500 years of change, grief, and loss and become stronger. They have emerged with their culture, language, and spiritual practices still largely intact. Native American women have been the organizers, the storytellers, and the keepers of the language, culture, and traditions. They keep native practices alive, in addition to taking care of the home and family. Today, life in a Native American community is rich and vibrant, full of laughter and humor. Humor is another attribute that has helped Native people through the worst of times. "Native humor" has been used historically through traditional icons, such as "clowns," to keep children in line or uphold community values and morals. Native humor is self-deprecating at times; the people tease each other and use laughter to make statements of fact about conditions of life or to build relationships between one another.

Native mothers are the teachers of the language. They speak to the child in the language right at birth. The Native language is the venue that leads to the heart of the culture and traditional practices. Without the ability to speak the language, one is unable to participate fully in the culture of the tribe. Songs, storytelling, and lessons about being part of the tribe are more meaningful in the Native language.

A celebration is about to take place in the small Pueblo village. When a birth, a death, a wedding, a baptism, or any other kind of celebration or gathering takes place in the Pueblo, the women swing into action at a moment's notice. The event about to take place in this community is the baptism of several new babies in the village. The women gather together to plan and organize. Relatives and friends are asked to come and help. Some are asked to prepare the food. The best bread makers are asked to make the bread, pies, and cookies; others are asked to cut meat, peel potatoes, clean the beans and/or make other foods, such as corn soup and chili stews. Amidst the fray is laughter and constant chatter in the Native language. Children are also playing about and vying for their mothers' attention. The children are part of a continuum that has been played out over several generations. They soon will be part of the fray, hustling and bustling, preparing a feast for their children's weddings and baptisms.

References

Brave Heart, M. Y. H. (1998). The return to the sacred path: Healing the historical trauma and historical unresolved grief response among the Lakota through a psychoeducational group intervention. *Smith College Studies in Social Work, 68*(3), 287–305.

Brave Heart, M. Y. H. (2003). The historical trauma response among Natives and its relationship with substance abuse: A Lakota illustration. *Journal of Psychoactive Drugs, 35*(1), 7–13.

Brave Heart, M. Y. H., & DeBruyn, L. M. (1998). The American Indian Holocaust: Healing historical unresolved grief. *American Indian and Alaska Native Mental Health Research, 8*(2), 56–78.

Duran, B., Sanders, M., Skipper, B., Waitzkin, H., Malcoe, L., Paine, S., & Yager, J. (2004). The prevalence and correlates of mental disorders among Native American women in primary care. *American Journal of Public Health, 94*(1), 71–77.

Geronimo, J. (2001, Summer). Mescalero Apache Scout. *Community Newsletter,* Mescalero, NM.

Niethammer, C. (1977). *Daughters of the Earth: The lives and legends of American Indian women.* New York: Collier Macmillan.

Tafoya, N., & Del Vecchio, A. (2005). Back to the future: An examination of the Native American Holocaust experience. In M. McGoldrick, J. Giordano, & N. Garcia-Preto (Eds.), *Ethnicity and family therapy* (3rd ed., pp. 55–63). New York: Guilford Press.

Underhill, R. M. (1989). *The Navajos.* Norman: University of Oklahoma Press.

CHAPTER 15

Healthy Living, Healthy Women

Barbara A. Stewart
Barbara F. Okun

Melissa, age 51, came for therapy because her anxieties were creating conflicts within her marriage and at work. She stated that she could not sleep more than 4 or 5 hours a night, was binge eating (she admitted to being 40 pounds overweight), and just "felt rotten." Melissa was a white middle-class Irish Catholic woman. An early couple's session (treatment consisted of primarily individual sessions with periodic couple sessions) revealed that these problems were not recently acquired, but that Melissa had been a lifelong "worrier" who could not tolerate well anyone's display of anger or conflict. Both husband and wife ascribed Melissa's current stressors to her adult children not "needing" her anymore and not choosing to be in as much contact with her as she (not they) desired. I (BFO) learned from her physician that he had found her healthy medically, but he did want her to become more physically active and to lose weight to alleviate her depression and to maintain her physical health. As she and I, in individual sessions, explored her resistance to these suggestions, it became clear that she believed that it was "selfish" to think about taking care of herself; her life script directed her to care for others because "that's what wives and mothers do." Our initial treatment goals were to start her on a daily 20-minute walk; teach her relaxation and make a tape with which she could practice; and plan and implement healthier nutrition. Once Melissa began to progress in these areas, she was able to focus on reconstructing her expectations and plan for the next phase of her life. Becoming aware of how she could help herself empowered her to take a more active part in decision making and problem solving.

This chapter focuses on women's experience in relation to both physical and mental health. Melissa exemplifies many of the major points that we want to emphasize throughout this chapter:

1. Health is not only the absence of disease but also the presence of vitality and is influenced by the reciprocal relationship of physical and mental health.

2. Women in the United States and throughout most of the world are socialized to be caretakers and find it hard to give attention to their own self-care; women exist within multiple contexts that affect their ability to attend to themselves.

3. It is important to facilitate collaboration between psychotherapist and physician.

4. To prevent disease and improve life for those with a disease, education for, and promotion of, healthy self-care and Western and alternative health care possibilities are essential components of psychotherapy.

In addition to exploring these points, we provide information on diseases that are prevalent for women, so that therapists can promote women's self-care.

We met as physician and patient 10 years ago. I (BFO) was referred to BAS by a previous male therapist (a psychiatrist interested in holistic medicine) after my male primary care physician told me that "my symptoms were in my head." Barbara was patient, thorough, listened to me, and took my symptoms, which were resulting in severe weight loss and weakness, seriously. Within a year, she had cured them with a 4-week dose of antibiotics; we believe I had some unknown gastrointestinal infection that did not show up in any of the diagnostic procedures. Over the years, we have collaborated on patient care and shared a commitment to the integration of physical and mental health issues. Both of us have in common the fact that we had children prior to attending graduate school. BAS grew up in a family that used homeopathic medicine; BFO grew up in a family that revered male physicians and where parental nurturing was available only during "sickness." We both entered male-dominated professions prior to the time when women practitioners and researchers developed notions of women's psychology and medicine. We both are invested in the promotion of healthy living in order to prevent physical and mental illness.

In this chapter we use a paradigm of health based on a biosociocultural model expounded by Johnson (2003). This model eschews psychological factors as equally primary as biological and sociocultural factors in determining health and illness. Furthermore, this model focuses both on wellness and prevention as well as diagnosis and treatment of disease. An important component of this model is psychoneuroimmunology (PNI), a "booming field within science" (DeAngelis, 2002). PNI examines the relationship between stress, the immune system, and health outcomes. Ray's (2004) review of research shows that as we change our minds (thoughts and beliefs), we change our brains and our physiology. Neurotransmitters, hormones, and cytokines act as messenger molecules carrying information between the nervous, endocrine, and immune systems.

Mental health workers need to consider the interrelationship of environment, mood, and physical health. Many diseases (e.g., cancer, multiple sclerosis) are typically accompanied by depression and anxiety; conversely, depression and anxiety can weaken the immune system, which, in turn, can lead to disease. Collaboration among psychotherapists, physicians, and other health care providers is more likely to lead to healthy outcomes than the isolated operation of each provider.

Women's health is also impacted by numerous additional factors: family, economics/class, race, ethnicity, religion, geographical region, generation, and sexual orientation. For example, the family history of an individual provides genetic, economic, and social information that may reveal the patient's ability to provide self-care and cope with illness. The economic circumstances in which a woman was raised contributes to her mindset regarding health and lifestyle, which may persist into adulthood. The socioeconomic situation in the family of origin, among extended family, and within the community also shapes her attitudes and expectations. Economics and class determine status and mobility, which affect access to quality education, preventive screening, and quality health care. For example, economics and class affect which foods are affordable; the need to cook quickly because of work and other responsibilities may also affect quality of nutrition. In addition, religion shapes attitudes toward self-care and seeking health care; some fundamentalist religions refuse medical intervention, believing solely in prayer and stoicism.

Race and ethnicity affect the likelihood of developing certain diseases as well as the likelihood of surviving these diseases. Class, race, ethnicity, and sexual orientation affect risk of diseases due to cultural attitudes about these differences. For example, minority and lower-class populations are less likely to get medical screening, less likely to have health insurance, and less likely to receive supportive follow-up. Throughout our discussion of the major health issues that affect women, we refer to these significant variables.

Health

"Health" refers to the absence of disease or incorrect bodily or mental functioning. More importantly, the state of health is characterized by a certain vitality, soundness, and vigor. Healthy people report feeling good, competent, energetic, alive, interested. These qualities are manifested in facial expressions, eyes, body language, posture, muscle tone and relaxation, eyes, and so on. Health is always precious, and, at the same time, it is precarious. It cannot be taken for granted but must be proactively maintained and nurtured— although many people ignore or deny this reality until they get sick. Sickness or disease can appear unpredictably, and many diseases (e.g., cancer, cardiovascular diseases) appear despite one's apparent health.

Adoption of certain behaviors associated with a reduction in disease incidence provides the best chance to achieve and maintain one's health for as long as possible. Mental health providers must understand that knowledge of, attention to, and support for healthy living relate significantly to the course and treatment of psychological difficulties. Lack of attention to, or ignoring, a patient's unhealthy behaviors can undermine and destroy health, sometimes irrevocably.

Healthy living results from our ability to pay attention to, and take responsibility for, our self-care. We cannot change our genetic predispositions toward certain diseases, but we can alter our behavior. Behaviors are estimated to contribute to 50% of an individual's health status (Institute for the Future, 2000). Unhealthy lifestyle behaviors include addictive activities such as smoking and drinking, workaholism, poor nutrition, over- or undereating, sedentary behaviors, not getting enough quality sleep, and lack of stress-management strategies. Healthy behaviors include managing and balancing individual, family, and work stressors, eating well (i.e., healthy nutrition with portion control), maintaining physical fitness, and good sleep habits. Obviously, women who take responsibility for self-care are likely to have healthier lifestyles than women who continuously put others' needs first, at the expense of their own. Likewise, women who are so self-involved that they are disconnected from relationships have problems as well.

Diseases Particularly Relevant to Women's Health

In this section we provide information about major diseases to which women are vulnerable. Our purpose is to educate clinicians about each disease and its symptoms so that they can encourage patients to seek medical evaluation early and to learn which behaviors can lessen risk for disease. Major diseases for women include cardiovascular disease; cancers; urogenital disturbances; issues related to aging, reproductive disorders, and sexually related issues (e.g., HIV); and obesity. As women achieve equity with men in the workforce and encounter an overload of stressors, they are beginning to experience the same rate of stress-related illnesses as men. For example, alcoholism is increasingly emerging as a major health issue for women (Kalb & Springen, 2004).

Cardiovascular Disease

Heart disease disables and kills far more women than does breast cancer today (but women worry more about breast cancer!); Hankinson, Speizer, Colditz, & Manson, 2002). Women need to pay attention to blood pressure and weight, exercise daily for ½–1 hour (Institute for the Future, 2000; Kalb & Springen, 2004), avoid smoking, and follow a low-cholesterol diet. Behavior modification can be life saving in heart disease and diabetes by lowering blood pressure and cholesterol. Additionally, medical checks can identify high-risk individuals, thus helping to reduce disability and death. Many drugs can reduce heart disease risk, but women need to carefully weigh the benefits and risks of these—or any—medication. In modern medicine, where discussion is sparse, the psychotherapist can work with the physician and/or patient to explore all aspects of treatment and prevention.

> As we were putting the final touches to this chapter, word came that a 53-year-old female psychologist colleague died of a heart attack on the way to the emergency room. She had several risk factors, she was overweight, had major allergies, and was asthmatic. She had casually mentioned to her physician that she felt chest sensations, and he had told her that he suspected it was the chest wall affected by the asthma. One night, when the chest sensations turned to pain, she phoned her cardiologist brother, and he urged her to go to the hospital. She never made it. As you read through this chapter, ask yourselves if this sudden death could have been prevented not just by her physician, but by a different attitude that would not allow her to ignore her body signals but to pursue help assertively.

Family history is a very significant predictor of cardiovascular disease, and socioeconomic class will influence access to health screening, intervention, and outcome. Anderson (2003) points out that smoking rates (related to cardiovascular and cancer diseases) are highest for those with less than a high school education, and that a high school education and socioeconomic class predict biological factors such as blood pressure and cholesterol. Anderson also reports studies showing that African American women are more likely to have high blood pressure than white women. High blood pressure may cause a thickening of the heart wall (a precursor of heart disease) more frequently in African American women than in white women who have high blood pressure. Many of the stress and mental health issues with which we deal are influenced by conditions such as hypertension; promoting women's self-care can help regulate blood pressure.

Men and women experience heart disease symptoms differently. Women may not feel chest sensation as do men and women's symptoms, such as fatigue, nausea, abdominal or back pain, may be vague and easy to attribute to exhaustion or "the flue." In women over age 70, heart symptoms are more likely to be vague (Charney, 1999).

A recent study from the National Institute of Mental Health (2002) found that people with heart disease are more likely to suffer from depression and anxiety disorders than people without heart disease. Conversely, the study found that people with depression are at greater risk for developing heart disease. This finding is in accord with the PNI model described previously.

Cancers

Lung cancer (largely related to cigarette smoking) is the number one cancer killer of women, with breast cancer next. In recent years early diagnosis and evolving treatments of breast cancer have heightened the survival rate. Continuous research has also resulted in new and emerging treatments that are improving outcomes for women with other kinds of cancer. Obviously, regular screening and early identification and intervention are critical for a positive prognosis. As psychotherapists, we must routinely ask our patients about their health status, using questions such as "When was your last physical exam?" and "How do you take care of yourself?" Here, as nowhere else, a woman who is depressed or who just doesn't feel right needs the support and encouragement of her therapist to fully explore the reason: Is it physical? Psychological? Both?

Socioeconomic class, race, sexual orientation, and ethnicity determine the availability of cancer screening, education about smoking, nutrition, and recognizing early symptoms, as well as attitudes about how, when, and where to access health care. Many of the community health centers located in poor neighborhoods are being forced by budget cuts to curtail outreach services. Likewise, there is a concentration of liquor and cigarette stores as well as hazardous waste and billboards in lower socioeconomic neighborhoods, along with higher depression rates and fewer social supports for healthy living. Furthermore, discriminatory mortgage lending practices strongly accompany discrimination in housing so that many are forced to live in conditions contributing to lead poisoning, rodents, or other toxins, which are being studied for a possible connection to cancer and other diseases (Anderson, 2003; Institute for the Future, 2000).

African American women have higher incidences of cancer (and obesity and diabetes) than do white women as well as African, Caribbean, Portugese, and Latina women of color. Anderson (2003) suggests that this data reflect healthier food processing and nutrition and safer environments in less-developed countries than in the United States. With time in the United States, immigrants' health becomes more like U.S.-born Americans' health. African American women are more likely to be diagnosed with late-stage cancer than are their white counterparts and thus are more likely to die of this disease. Physicians are less likely to order sophisticated tests for lower-class African American women than for lower-class white women, and this tendency certainly affects the early identification and treatment prognosis (*CA*, 2004). More specifically, the incidence of cancer of the uterine cervix, the stomach, and the liver are higher in minority groups than in whites.

Geographical location influences the type of screening and intervention that all women receive, particularly with regard to cancer diseases. Economic privilege enables some women to travel to major cancer centers or utilize public libraries or the Internet for research about experimental protocols. But a vast number of less privileged women in rural or regionalized nonmetropolitan locations may suffer long delays in screening and treatment. Travel may be impossible for these women, as they struggle to maintain their jobs and families.

Lesbians diagnosed with cancer may not receive support from their families or medical treatment that is sensitive to the unique needs of lesbian and bisexual women (Crary, 2004). Geographical location and local cultural norms also affect health care access for lesbians. Although there is a general misconception that lesbians are particularly prone to breast and ovarian cancers, there is no substantive data to document this view. There is some evidence, however, that lesbian women may struggle significantly to find health care providers who understand and appreciate their sexual orientation. Black lesbians, in particular, suffer from higher rates of obesity, diabetes, and cardiovascular diseases (Crary, 2004). They may be reluctant to seek help and feel uncomfortable discussing some of their health concerns with providers, which could lead to later diagnosis, affecting treatment and outcome.

Women with cancer are likely to experience anxiety and depression as they attempt to integrate lengthy treatments into their life schedules. Some may find it difficult to take time off from work (scheduling after-hours doctor appointments is always difficult); some may find the treatments arduous, exacerbating their anxiety and depression as well as their concerns about losing hair, sleeplessness, and lowered energy level. Cancer support groups, either online or in the community, can provide enormous education and support. Family support groups are also critical.

Urogenital Disturbances

Urogenital disturbances include urinary tract infections, incontinence with or without overactive bladder, and interstitial cystitis. All are frustrating and disturbing to women, because there is no clear understanding of the cause of these problems and the treatments vary from surgery to bladder training (using kegel exercises) and medication. Any of these disorders can affect a woman's sexual desire and sexual performance, and therapists need to be sensitive to this interaction.

New treatments for all of these disturbances are being developed, so presentation for evaluation by a physician should be encouraged.

> Recently, I (BFO) was asked to work with a woman who had just been released from the hospital after a 5-day stay in the ICU, fighting a life-threatening kidney infection. Dora, age 42, was a white working-class single parent of four children, ranging from 6 to 15 years. Her 6-year-old son had received one of her kidneys for a necessary transplant 1½ years ago. Dora lived hand-to-mouth; if a child needed her care, she earned no income for that day. She worked at the harbor, varnishing boats, which gave her some autonomy about her hours. Dora stated that she "did not have time or energy" to think about her health. However, she did take time to be with a series of boyfriends when her kids were in bed. She had endured lower abdominal pain for a month before she saw blood in her urine. Thinking the blood was from sexual intercourse, she did nothing until she passed out and was rushed to the emergency room by her (then) boyfriend. My work with Dora (scheduled in the evening to enable her attendance) focused on helping her to learn to value herself and take care of herself so that she never again had to struggle with the panic and shame of leaving her children untended. Fortunately, the boat community pitched in and provided for the children while she was in the hospital. Dora's physician and I arranged for some social service resources, which enabled her to heal before returning to her physically demanding work. During the 3 months of our weekly individual and family meetings, Dora learned to delegate some responsibilities to her teenagers and to take some time to tend to her own self-care. The stakes were high, given that she has only one kidney, and she was catapulted by this health crisis into being motivated to accept help. Her physician and I were successful in setting up monthly check-ins with the local community health center as well as her boating community, and after her treatment with me, Dora began to participate in a women's support group at the health center.

Aging Issues

While aging is not a health issue by itself, some aging-related symptoms may require medical attention. As women age, their energy levels, resilience after illness or injury, and overall health status change, and the necessary self-care for prevention and maintenance requires more time and energy. One's attitudes toward aging are shaped by family history, class, race, ethnicity, religion, and sexual orientation. And one's natural reaction to one's own genetic makeup differs by personality and temperament as well as by class, race, sexual orientation, ethnicity, and sociocultural variables.

All women may become more vulnerable to accidents and disease as they age, but planning and behavior modification may decrease this vulnerability. Depression and other mental health issues may become exacerbated as women deal with the onslaught of losses—loss of looks, of strength, of perceived value by others, of friends and family through death, and of familiar gratifying roles. As psychotherapists, we can help older women find sensitive health providers, develop optimistic attitudes, and discover gratifying activities and connections. These areas may be critical for enhancing and promoting life by strengthening the immune system.

In recent years older women's health has been affected by childbirth as health and technological advances enable conception and birth at older ages than previously possible. Far more women are reaching an age when their own medical issues start to demand greater attention at the same time as do those of their young children and their aging parents. In addition, across the spectrum of class, race, ethnicity, and religion, older women are assuming more caretaking responsibilities for their grandchildren and great-grandchildren. These additional responsibilities can create physical and emotional stressors that weaken the immune system, resulting in illness. These stressors can also prevent older women from seeking help early in the development of health issues.

Reproductive and Sexual Issues

Reproductive and sexual issues include infertility, premenstrual symptoms (PMS), menopause, sexually transmitted diseases, the inability to experience sexual pleasure, impact of the loss of ovaries, and so on. Although infertility is not a disease, it is an increasing phenomenon as women postpone childbearing until their late 30s and early 40s. Many of these women are shocked when they experience difficulty conceiving due to their age. Obviously, women with economic resources have more options, such as expensive *in vitro* fertilization procedures, use of donor eggs or sperm, or even freezing their eggs during their 20s or 30s. However, many women do not find these procedures successful and may suffer severe depression while coming to terms with their childlessness (which they may see as their bodies betraying them). Women who do come to terms with their inability to bear biological children can begin to consider alternative ways of parenting, a possibility that psychotherapists can help them explore. It is important to realize that all of the procedures available for insemination, parenting through nontraditional biological means, or parenting through non-biological means (e.g., adoption) not only take time, attention, money and energy, but may result in physiological side effects and/or psychological stressors related to the procedures.

Lesbian women who wish to have children typically consider a variety of methods that may involve much more thought and time than for heterosexual women, who assume they will bear children biologically conceived with their male partner's sperm. Sexual orientation, race, culture, and marital status may particularly affect parenting alternatives. For example, lesbian women, single women, and interracial couples, in particular, frequently experience discrimination if they want to adopt domestically or internationally.

PMS, as well as the long, developmentally normative process of menopause, may affect women's sense of well-being and their levels of energy and activity by altering physical functioning, mood states, and cognitive performance. For many years women were told that their PMS symptoms were psychological, but there is clear evidence that these symptoms are biologically based as well as psychologically and culturally influenced. It is helpful to ask patients about their experience of their first menstrual period: How were they prepared? By whom? How were they treated in their family? By their peers? How did they view it themselves? It is amazing how these questions produce such relevant data about the formation of a woman's attitudes, thoughts, and feelings toward womanhood, sex, and self-worth.

Many women who had negative experiences with menarche carry negative expectations into their adult experiences of their bodies, bodily functions, and sexuality, whereas those whose experiences were positive carry more positive attitudes and feelings. It is also helpful to ask women what they remember about their mother's experience with menopause and how this shaped some of their attitudes and expectations about this developmental milestone.

Women and their families often report that they (the woman) become a "bear" or are noticeably sad or depressed prior to their periods or when obviously going through a perimenopausal phase. Women may censor their communication less during these times, so that they are more reactive to the microaggressions than at other times, when they may allow subtle affronts to pass without comment because of their relational socialization. Given the multiple stressors in woman's lives today, PMS and menopausal symptoms may be exacerbated or may interact with sexist expectations in ways that are detrimental to women's health and good functioning. For example, in work settings, it is not unusual for colleagues to assume that women's moods are related more to "the time of month" or menopause than to the actual situation at hand. Although women may experience mood fluctuations related to their physiology, these fluctuations do not negate their relational perceptions of the frequency of unequal treatment in the workplace and elsewhere.

There are many treatments for menstrually related conditions. Increasingly, selective serotonin reuptake inhibitor antidepressants may be utilized to alleviate PMS and menopausal distress, as can sleep, exercise, and diet control. Many alternative health care strategies (discussed later) may also prove helpful. One of the major scientific controversies today concerns hormone replacement therapy for pre- and postmenopausal women. Findings of the Women's Health Initiative (2000) resulted in the cessation of millions of U.S. women's estrogen/progesterone therapy and the resurfacing of menopausal symptoms of hot flashes, mood swings, and skin and urogenital changes for many women. There have been varying reactions by the medical profession and by many women to the results of this study. Each woman needs to discuss her individual circumstances with her psychotherapist and physician to find a satisfactory treatment.

Heterosexual women have far higher rates of sexually transmitted diseases (STDs), including HIV, than lesbians. It is most important that therapists and physicians help patients strategize ways to prevent exposure to STDs. The most common STDs are human papilloma virus (the cause of most cervical cancer and most abnormal PAP smears), herpes, chlamydia, HIV, syphilis, gonorrhea, and hepatitis C (Cambrone, 2003). The risk of developing any one of these diseases is increased as the number of sexual partners increases, and with the use of IV drugs or excessive alcohol, which may reduce one's caution. There is a higher risk for the development of other STDs if one has contracted one type of STD.

Condom use and requiring a careful sexual history of the potential partner can reduce STD risk. STD testing before beginning a new sexual relationship is also advised. Condom use provides protection and is advised even for couples in a committed relationship, given each partner's previous sexual relationships. All STDs can be passed to sexual partners at an asymptomatic stage. The use of birth control pills by women, although an excellent contraceptive practice, may appear to obviate the need for condoms; in reality, STD exposure is still possible. Mental health providers can ask patients about the use of drugs or alcohol in relation to the use of contraception and condoms in order to educate them about the risk.

Psychotherapists help women clients become empowered to take the necessary steps for preventing exposure by educating them about boundaries, relationships, safe and risky sexual practices, treatment, and the risk of spreading STDs. Exploring with patients their underlying attitudes and anxieties about sex and relationships can be a surprisingly effective means of providing psychoeducation on STDs.

Obesity

Obesity has become a U.S. epidemic for all ages in recent years. Obesity is diagnosed when the body mass index, a measure of body fat based on height and weight, is over 30 (overweight is over 27); obesity is more severe than overweight, usually reflecting 25–30% overweight. Although there are certainly genetic, hormonal, and other biological variables, women who are overweight often delay visiting a physician due to their shame about getting on a scale. Obesity is a major health issue that increases the risk for diabetes, cardiovascular disease, and depression. Whereas some economically privileged women may seek a "quick fix," such as gastric bypass surgery or liposuction, many women respond to less drastic measures such as support group programs (e.g., Weight Watchers, Overeaters Anonymous). However, many women also find it difficult to maintain weight loss, and the resulting yo-yo effect may be hazardous to health as well. Hypnosis and acupuncture, two alternative health care methods, may be helpful for these women. It is critical that medical and psychological care be coordinated so that women do not merely lose weight but change their eating, exercise, and other behavioral patterns (e.g., rewarding oneself or celebrating in ways that do not involve food). Psychotherapists can help women create healthy attitudes and behaviors toward food that are ongoing, not just relevant to a maintenance phase (group or individual), in order to support permanent and different eating habits that allow them to maintain their weight loss.

Alcoholism

Alcoholism is increasingly a major issue for women, who are more likely than men to be secret drinkers and who can cunningly fool health care providers as well as family members about this condition for months at a time. Women tend to become addicted faster to alcohol, and are more in denial about having a drinking problem, than men. They require less alcohol to be affected than men, which may relate to gender differences in weight and the metabolizing of alcohol. Therapists and physicians may not learn about alcohol problems from the patient but, instead, from family members, called in to therapy or medical meetings to deal with a relationship crisis or anxiety or depression. Usually, interventions involving the family, psychotherapist, and physician are necessary. Women seem to respond well to women's recovery groups and residential programs. Group support is especially critical to recovery for women, because women are socialized to do better in relational contexts.

There is a tendency for women in minority groups to have a higher incidence of alcoholism (Anderson, 2003; Hankinson et al., 2002). One's perceptions and personal experiences of racism, ethnocentrism, homophobia and classism shape one's sense of self, of others, and the world and can result in interpersonal difficulties, higher levels of stress, and risk of physical and mental health symptoms. Environments where liquor is easily available contribute to women's (and men's) use of alcohol (which is cheaper and more readily available than medications) to allay symptoms related to these difficulties.

Allya, a 34-year-old immigrant from Santo Domingo, sought psychotherapy for anger management and help with relationships. A stunningly beautiful woman of dark color, Allya perceived that she was being discriminated against by both African Americans and European Americans at work and in her racially mixed neighborhood. Having been raised in an abusive, alcoholic single-parent family of color, Allya expected to feel "other" and had developed a hard protective veneer to cover her vulnerable feelings. She perceived alienation and discrimination even in situations where there was no clear evidence of these issues. After several sessions, Allya admitted that she drank at least one bottle of wine at night because that was the only way she could be sociable. She reported difficulties breathing and periodic episodes in which her heart raced as well as irregular, heavy periods. In spite of her physical symptoms, she had not seen a physician during the 7 years in which she had lived here. Allya believed that "doctors make you sicker and hospitals are to be avoided at all costs because they kill people." Allya's therapist explored with her the experiences that resulted in this belief prior to working to change her belief systems. After so doing, Allya's therapist worked with her to accept the necessity of a medical consult and located a neighborhood clinic where Allya could be seen by a Spanish-speaking nurse practitioner.

It was discovered that Allya suffered from some heart abnormalities as a result of untreated severe hypertension. The nurse practitioner and the psychotherapist collaborated to ensure Allya's compliance with a medication regimen and to correct her diet and other contributing lifestyle factors. Along with this focus, the therapist helped Allya to understand and manage her anger and her relationships more effectively. Through the 12 sessions she was allowed by her insurance, Allya became more trusting of other health care providers and better able to keep appointments and follow through with her nurse practitioner's recommendations.

This case example indicates how crucial health care education and information are, particularly for women who often are the major caretakers within their family systems. The active working alliance between the therapist and Allya was the medium through which Allya developed enough trust to make an appointment at the clinic. Allya was part of the collaboration and participated in the communications between physician and therapist; her participation was an essential point that enabled her to feel respected rather than marginalized. Allya's therapist referred her to a women's group for further education and support.

Self-Care and Healthy Living

Self-care exists on a continuum from positive to negative. On the negative or unhealthy side, there is a lack of attention to one's health, an avoidance of self-examination or of seeking a health care provider, as well as the perception and practice of known self-destructive behaviors. Positive or healthy self-care involves paying attention to one's health, which includes, as previously mentioned, seeking medical care early when one is not "feeling right" and scheduling regular checkups and screenings for disease. Screenings may include mammograms, colonoscopies, eye checkups, dental care, skin survey, breast exams, and blood pressure monitoring. Positive or healthy self-care also includes openness to education both by professionals and through self-education. The latter includes research, discussion with family, friends, and others, and keeping up with the "news" about current research findings—but without buying into the cultural myth of a "quick fix" promulgated by the media or pharmaceutical advertisements. Therapists can contribute to positive self-care by modeling, educating, and helping patients to plan strategies for achieving their goals.

Community health care centers and public health vans attempt to educate people and provide accessible screening in underprivileged neighborhoods. Nutrition programs attempt to teach willing consumers how to use food stamps healthfully. However, many people do not receive these services, due to lack of knowledge and curtailment of outreach services by budget cuts.

For a patient with a disease or a condition in the watching stage (e.g., prehypertension), healthy self-care involves a conscious collaboration between physician and patient and between physician, patient, and psychotherapist. A physician may refer a patient to a psychotherapist to address the patient's self-report or the physician's observations of symptoms of psychological distress. At this point, physical disease is ruled out for the time being. There are also many opportunities for psychotherapists to consider the possibility of an underlying disease or physical disorder to refer a patient to a physician. As Klonoff and Landrine (1996) elucidate, diseases such as temporal lobe epilepsy, multiple sclerosis, chronic fatigue syndrome, or fibromyalgia may manifest as affective disorders but are actually medical conditions.

Psychotherapist–Physician Collaboration

Psychotherapists may be skittish about contacting physicians whom they do not know. They may become frustrated with the physicians' response time lags and with a series of office personnel who put them "on hold." Often, I (BFO) ask the patient, who signs a release form at the first visit, to ask her physician to call me, because I am not sure whether the physician has a signed release. The physician is typically responsive to this request coming from the client, and I am able to join with him or her and establish a collaborative relationship in our first contact. Some physicians prefer to e-mail, although this is difficult with HIPPA, and sometimes voice-mail "tag" precedes any real contact. If there is information, such as a drinking problem or eating disorder, of which the physician is not aware, the therapist can either work with the patient to reveal these secrets or seek permission from the patient to tell the physician.

With patients' permission, psychotherapists might telephone patients' primary care physicians to introduce themselves and pave the way for collaboration. Some psychotherapists write a note and request whatever information the physician thinks might be helpful. It is difficult to always connect directly, given the pressures of time and paperwork. Neither physicians nor psychotherapists should personalize abrupt responses; many physicians and psychotherapists are not cognizant of the reciprocal relationship of mind and body and the benefits of collaborative treatment. There will be times when either the physician or the psychotherapist will be instrumental in locating an additional provider for the patient. It is likely that his or her selection will be someone with whom they have worked in the past, and this is a good foundation to develop.

> Johanna, a 48-year-old retail worker and daughter of an Armenian immigrant, came for therapy because of her growing fatigue, lack of energy, and unhappiness. Johanna was the primary caretaker for her mother; her brother was married and the family culture had prescribed this role for Johanna at her birth. Her mother was difficult, controlling, intrusive, and exceedingly demanding. The only life Johanna had for herself was at work.
>
> In the third session, Johanna reported that her mother had insisted that Johanna consult with her mother's primary care physician, who decided that Johanna needed a hysterectomy to alleviate her symptoms. The therapist suggested that Johanna seek an outside consultation with an independent specialist or ob-gyn physician. Johanna said that she did not have the strength to fight with her mother; it was much easier to do what her mother wanted than to risk upsetting her. Johanna had not seen a physician in 6 years; her insurance had

changed with her last job change, and she could no longer see her previous physician. Although the mother's physician, a general surgeon, was not on Johanna's plan, the mother had offered to pay all fees for this particular doctor and intervention.

The therapist had a dilemma: She was concerned about Johanna's health, and she also was aware that she did not have the time to make much inroad into the mother–daughter bind before the scheduled date of surgery. The therapist asked Johanna to bring in the most recent list of physicians on her health plan. As Johanna, who had received the therapist's name from a coworker, began to trust her and look forward to her sessions, the therapist was successful in obtaining Johanna's permission to schedule an appointment for her with one of two doctors she knew on the health plan's list. With Johanna in the office, the therapist phoned the doctors' offices, explained the urgency, and accepted the first appointment she could obtain. Johanna seemed relieved at this active support and wanted the therapist to talk to the doctor prior to Johanna's appointment. The therapist was able to talk to the consulting physician later that day.

When Johanna went to the doctor (without telling her mother), she discovered that not only were her life circumstances contributing to her depression, but that there was a strong indication that there was a thyroid imbalance. There was no evidence that surgery was necessary. Because of the timing, Johanna's new doctor got the results of the thyroid tests as quickly as possible and found that they confirmed the hypothesis. The therapist and the physician conferred after each session with Johanna—who did not have surgery. The focus of the therapy shifted to helping Johanna develop the ability to say "no" to her mother and her mother's physician. The active support of both the psychotherapist and the specialist enabled Johanna to work with them to achieve this goal. After this crisis, they were able to work with Johanna on developing self boundaries.

This case illustrates how physicians and psychotherapists need to collaborate in order to enable patients to consider different perspectives and utilize team support to actively participate in decision making and their own self-care. Therapists can help patients identify and specify their physical symptoms prior to visiting a physician. This effort applies to symptoms as benign as a common cold or as concerning as chest pain or dizziness. Helping the patient to understand why she may need medical attention is critical. For example, it is not normal to have a cold for 2 months. And all chest pain needs evaluation, because it is difficult to distinguish benign from life-threatening causes. If symptoms persist, therapists may have to push patients to get medical attention. Keep in mind that the symptoms of some diseases, such as ovarian cancer, can be vague but persistent.

Psychotherapists may need to help patients sort out their feelings about asking for and accessing help, including exploring patients' past experiences with seeking and receiving care. Look for clues about difficulties in seeking help, finding appropriate health care providers, and "working with the system." Learn how you can help your patients find physicians and work through the office staff system. Many patients, such as Johanna, develop inertia if their health plan changes and they no longer can see previous providers. For example, if a patient shows you a mole or you notice one that looks suspicious, and the doctor's office puts off an appointment for 2 months, coach your patient how to be more assertive or ask for her permission to phone the physician directly as a collateral health care provider.

It is also important to explain to your patient about today's health care system; doctors these days have only a short time to spend with each patient, so it is helpful if the patient is organized in presenting his or her concerns and asking questions. Suggest to your patient that she bring a medication list to the physician, including over-the-counter substances; also help her make a list of issues, questions, previous illnesses, and surgeries. Suggest she be accompanied by a partner or friend, when appropriate.

Often, the psychotherapist can function as a cultural broker between the physician and patient, explaining some of the significant cultural values. For example, when Johanna's therapist first talked to the consultant to explain the situation, she was able to explain the traditional Armenian view of the daughter's lifetime obligation to put her mother first.

When patients practice self-destructive behaviors or refuse to engage in self-care, the therapeutic relationship must focus on their assumptions and belief about self and self-care in order to progress. How well the therapist models healthy living and self-care is significant because it increases the therapist's credibility and authenticity. The point is that the focus of therapy must include attention to any destructive behaviors. Effective psychotherapeutic interventions include cognitive therapy, coping skills training, and positive reframing. These interventions may incorporate relaxation techniques, cognitive restructuring, and narrative therapy techniques.

Alternative Health Care

Today, medicine practitioners in the United States are more open to the possible benefits of alternative health care practices than ever before. Therapists should be aware of alternative health care for stress reduction, relaxation, and general attention to the state of body and mind. Some physicians recommend alternative health care as a supplement to Western-based medicine. Eastern medicine, the source from which many alternative formats are derived, has a different view of illness than does Western medicine. Eastern medicine is focused on mind/body/spiritual integration, achieving harmony and balance among all body systems and the soul and mind. In contrast, Western medicine is based more on a premise of mind–body duality and separation and locates the "disease" to eliminate it. Eastern medicine is more subjective, whereas Western medicine is, supposedly, more objective, based on "science." Currently, mind–body medicine is a discipline being integrated into Western medicine. This development is consistent with the PNI model described earlier in this chapter. Recent research (DeAngelis; 2002; Johnson, 2003; Ray, 2004; Weisman & Berman, 2004) confirms that the previously theorized connections between mind and body do exist and that interventions that address the mind and body as "out of balance" are effective.

The alternative health care interventions that are rated by patients and health care providers as helpful, on a continuum from little to great, include therapeutic massage, acupuncture, body work, meditation, relaxation, yoga, and tai chi (Kalb & Springen, 2004). Kalb and Springen (2004) also refer to research findings that support the significance of alternative health care pain management, which reduces reliance on medications with debilitating side effects. Some alternative health strategies, such as hypnosis and massage, are not derived from Eastern medicine but are included in alternative health care offerings.

Conclusions

Our intentions in this chapter were to (1) help mental health providers recognize the importance of both mental and physical health issues as critical reciprocally influencing elements of psychotherapy; (2) help mental health workers collaborate with other health care providers; (3) further the understanding of how race, class, gender, generation, and sexual orientation may inform how women understand and respond to health concerns; and (4) deepen our understanding of major health issues for women.

We emphasize that health care providers need to collaborate to foster responsible self-care and healthy living. More and more, we are learning that early screening, diagnosis, and treatment result in more favorable prognoses and that, although we cannot control our biological and genetic destinies, there is much we can do to lessen risk by developing healthy behaviors and extinguishing unhealthy behaviors. Obtaining satisfactory health care continues to be difficult, requiring self-advocacy and assertive persistence in today's changing health care system. Therefore, it is critical for us to empower our women patients to develop these necessary attitudes and skills.

References

Anderson, N. (2003, October 29). *Unraveling the mystery of racial and ethnic health disparities: Who, what, when, where, how and especially, why?* Paper presented at the Urban Health Research Symposium, Northeastern University, Boston.

CA: A Cancer Journal for Clinicians. (2004). *54*(1).

Cambrone, D. (2003). *Women's experiences with HIV/AIDS: Mending fractured selves.* New York: Haworth Press.

Charney, P. C. (1999). *Coronary artery disease in women.* Philadelphia: American College of Physicians.

Crary, D. (2004, June 21). Lesbian researchers examine their groups ignored health issues. *Boston Globe,* p. A3.

DeAngelis, T. (2002). If you do just one thing, make it exercise. *Monitor on Psychology, 33*(7), 48–68.

Hankinson, S. E., Speizer, B., Colditz, G. A., & Manson, J. (Eds.). (2002). *Healthy women, healthy lives: A guide to preventing disease from the landmark nurses health study.* New York: Simon & Schuster.

Institute for the Future. (2000). *Expanding meanings of health.* Menlo Park, CA: National Institute for Research Advancement.

Johnson, N. (2003). Psychology and health research, practice and policy. *American Psychologist, 58*(9), 670–677.

Kalb, C., & Springen, K. (2004, May 10). Health for life: Women's bodies. *Newsweek,* pp. 55–92.

Klonoff, E., & Landrine, H. (1996). *Preventing misdiagnosis of women: A guide to physical disorders that have psychiatric symptoms.* Thousand Oaks, CA: Sage.

National Institute of Mental Health. (2002). *Pathways to specialty mental healthy care.* Washington, DC: Author.

Ray, O. (2004). How the mind hurts and heals the body. *American Psychologist, 59*(1), 29–41.

Weisman, R., & Berman, B. (2003). *Own your health: Choosing the best from alternative and conventional medicine.* Deerfield Beach, FL: Health Communications.

Women's Health Initiative. (2000). *34*(2), 109–112.

PART V

Conclusions

CHAPTER 16

Connections and Future Directions

Barbara F. Okun
Karen L. Suyemoto
Marsha Pravder Mirkin

We began our summer retreat dialogue (after reading and editing all of the first drafts of the chapters) by asking the question "What do we want clinicians to learn from this volume?" Marsha replied that "context is always more complex and messy than we think. Learning about diversity is a lifelong process." Barbara added that "clinicians need to challenge previous assumptions from their earlier academic and clinical training in order to be open to new perspectives that are adaptive to our rapidly changing circumstances." Karen urged clinicians to "examine themselves and think about how they and others fit into social contexts—good therapy requires reflexivity." We agreed that we hope that exposure to the ecological/systemic perspective of our authors will enable clinicians to consider all the complex, complicated, interacting facets of the reciprocal influences of individual, cultural, and societal variables. This consideration will help us to avoid pathologizing that which we do not agree with or understand.

There were three major considerations we asked authors to consider as they wrote their chapters for this volume:

The first major consideration was that women experience multiple identities in reference to multiple systemic contexts. Identities and systemic contexts include, but are not limited to, race, class, gender, ethnicity, religion, sexual orientation, age, immigration status, and able-bodiedness. The meanings and implications of these identities and contexts change across the lifespan, across situational contexts, and as they interact with each other. We asked authors to consider not only a single context, identity, or status, but the interactions among them, and the ways in which they change in particular situational contexts. Thus, even if a chapter focused primarily on issues related to gender and race or a particular cultural group, we asked authors to engage questions of intersections with other statuses and systems, both marginalized and privileged. The experience of privilege in some systemic contexts and marginalization in others impact how a woman develops and how she understands and relates to herself and others. The intersections among these contexts help us understand women in complex, meaningful ways and challenge what we have learned from theories and research that exclude context. We need not be afraid of challenging the assumptions underlying major theoretical orientations and practice; what might have worked in one era may no longer be effective, as contexts change and new knowledge is disseminated.

A second major consideration was that one cannot talk about cultural groups without considering the diversity within each group. There is no monolithic phenomenon called "woman" or "Latina" or "lesbian." It is critical to explore diversity within a group, not just between groups. Part of this exploration involves looking at how a particular diversity intersects with others, for example, that a wealthy African American lesbian might have a different experience from a poor African American heterosexual woman. This point is, of course, related to the first consideration.

The third major consideration was that of self-reflection and awareness. We believe that the life experiences of an author or a clinician strongly affect the writing or therapy that is created. Thus we asked authors to situate themselves in relation to the topics within their chapters, so that readers would gain a sense of how the authors' own experiences may have shaped their thinking and presentation. We believe that it is impossible to separate the *person* of the author (or the therapist) from his or her writing, teaching, research, or clinical practice. All of us are shaped by our individual characteristics as well as by our sociocultural statuses. There is no reality to the concept of neutrality. However, with growing self-awareness and learning to ask ourselves hard questions about our internalized biases, we can learn to expose our students and patients to different perspectives without imposing our views on them.

In this final chapter, we would like to share with you some of the dilemmas that emerged for us, and our reflections on the outcome of our collaboration: the text you have just read. We do not intend to have "the final word." As our dialogue continues, we find that we have more questions than answers. Not only is learning a lifelong process, but our views of self, others, and the world are continuously evolving as we become more and more aware of the multiple, changing social contexts within which we live.

Dilemmas

What Is "Right"?

One of the first dilemmas with which we were confronted concerned the concept of "right" versus "wrong." Who decides and how? Who defines right and wrong, normal and abnormal, good and bad? What happens when the social construct is not in line with the individual's construct? What happens when the clinician believes that her way of thinking or living is the "right" or "best" way for others? These questions emerged repeatedly in our editing discussions. One of the challenges in discussing mental health in interaction with social contexts is that of engaging these questions. For example: Is it "right" (or healthy or adaptive) for women to advance in social class through education? How do we, as authors and clinicians, view people who choose not to "advance" or pursue education but instead choose to work to live rather than have work be a major part of their identity or reward? Is it "right" (or healthy or adaptive) for Asian immigrant women to become more "acculturated" and pursue careers for more personal gratification? Is it "right" (or healthy or adaptive) to encourage women to take time for self-care if it makes them "happier" to continually take care of others? Is it "right" to say that gender, race, sexual orientation, and so on, *do* create systems of marginalization and privilege? We all know women, and people of color, and gay or lesbian individuals who do not believe that sexism, racism, or heterosexism affects them or creates barriers.

Given the human proclivity to seek certainty as security, this variability can be troubling to many clinicians. If there is no clear "right" way or "truth," if we have to respect varying and differing perspectives, we must take responsibility for our own choices and actions as therapists, supervisors, authors, and editors. Thus we may have to rethink our notions about what is normal, what is pathological, what is healthy, and so on. We also grapple with whether there is a "bottom line" beyond which we do believe that our ideas are right/true, rather than just some of many possible right ideas. For example, we (the three editors) believe that genital mutilation is wrong, which could be seen as not respecting certain cultural values. We believe that depriving any person of integrity or possibilities because of race, class, gender, sexual orientation, religion, able-bodiedness, age, and so on, is wrong. But of course, the meaning of "integrity" and "possibilities" will vary considerably.

Individuals and Systems

A second dilemma that continually emerged for us was how to be true to our aims of focusing on interactive aspects of systemic and individual contexts and the heterogeneity of groups while still being able to say something useful about commonalities within and among groups. We continually found ourselves reading a chapter and thinking of the "exceptions to the rule." We pushed ourselves (and the authors) to continually articulate the assumptions underlying their statements. For example, when we talk to gay or lesbian couples about adopting or birthing children, we need to be open to discussing positive outcomes as well as risky and negative possibilities. In another example, when interracial couples insist that race is not the issue of their marital difficulties, we need to be respectful of their perspectives and hold the possibility that they are not experiencing an issue with race. When talking about women choosing to stay at home and to redefine career achievement, we need to acknowledge that economically challenged women would not likely have that option. When talking about women, religion, and spirituality, how do we acknowledge that religion has been a great source of strength for many women and also a great barrier for others? With all the convergences and divergences, all the intersections, how can a therapist ever be culturally aware or competent? How can we distinguish what is the norm for a particular community (e.g., middle class, lesbian Costa Rican) and what is idiosyncratic when we do not know enough people at that intersection and nothing seems to be written about it? How do we even know what to ask?

Clear Meanings

Although we can (and do) specifically describe our meanings of race, culture, class, sexual orientation, and religion, that does not always mean that we agree on the meanings of the boundaries implied in these concepts as they are reflected within lived experience. Some meanings of the social constructs themselves were less clear to us, reflecting the uncertainty about their meanings in colloquial discussions and, perhaps, our society's ambivalence about the categorizations themselves. The meaning of class seemed particularly variable to us, even as a social construct (i.e., we were not clear about whether there was an agreed-upon meaning of class): Is it just economic? Social status? Attitudes? Values? We believe that all of these variables comprise class and that shared attitudes, values, and customs are at least as important as finances in determining class. Some of the chapters discuss the complexities inherent in the concept of class, requiring us to reassess our own notions and recognize the complexities and multiple interpretations possible.

We seemed to have greater agreement, although certainly not without challenges, regarding race, ethnicity, and sexual orientation. However, these meanings also became more complicated when explored in interaction, as in many of the chapters. For example, although we understand and can discuss the differences between race and ethnicity, as we read the chapters, it was repeatedly clear that the confounding of these concepts reflects and interacts with lived experience—it is exceedingly difficult to clearly differentiate the influence of race and the influence of ethnicity when discussing an actual woman in context.

This dilemma of unclear meanings is related to the tension between individuals and systems; the meanings of an individual may not agree with the meaning of other individuals, of a group, or of a system. For example, as we explored our own class identities and backgrounds as part of situating ourselves and recognizing our potential biases (see below), we became aware that some of our self-assessments did not always jibe with how others saw us. Our self-reports about the class in which we were raised and in which we now live resulted in a great deal of questioning from each other and required each of us to reconsider our own constructs! We believe this reconsideration and awareness of the possible discrepancy between our self-views and how others see us have application to many of the chapters: Many of the clients discussed have problems stemming from the different meanings and understandings that are frequently related to systemic oppression and the intersection with adaptive living. For example, relational difficulties are frequently rooted in seeing ourselves or our situations differently from how others see us, and cultural "clashes" are clearly about different expectations based on different meanings.

Situating Ourselves

Another dilemma that confronted us was trying to acknowledge how our own backgrounds, values, and so on, affected the content and the process of creating this book. Our editorial and writing processes have been dependent on our ongoing dialogues. Like our authors, we have explored and discussed our own multiple identities, both in the chapters that we have contributed to this volume and among ourselves as part of our cooperative editing process. There are differences among us based on race, class, religion, ethnicity, and sexual orientation. What are the impacts of privilege on us as authors, as editors, and as colleagues and allies to each other? How do we recognize our own internalized racism, heterosexism, ethnocentrism, classism? What choices have we been given because of our privileges and how do we recognize that many people have limited, if any, choices? How do we avoid imposing our own views on each other and others (including our authors) while still holding ourselves and each other accountable to those of us who are marginalized? We have challenged each other and had long dialogues about the impact of privilege, judgment, and bias on our own thinking and clinical work. For example, as white Jewish editors, we (BFO and MPM) needed to confront whether we could see the marginalization experienced by an editor of color from our own place of racial privilege. Are we truly being allies with the editor of color? As a white, Jewish editor, I (MPM) recognized that there were moments when I was not the ally I hoped to be, and that Karen, rather than I, called attention to several of the racial dynamics related to our interactions as editors that a good white ally would have picked up on. We also questioned: Can the mixed bag of Jewish privilege and oppression be understood by someone who is not Jewish? As an Asian non-Jewish editor, I (KLS) had to weigh when to speak and when not to speak about race or about questioning racial privilege within the editing dynamics. From conversations we have had, I know that all three of us struggle with resisting a hierarchical mentality and a competition of oppressions, while also recognizing that some systems of oppression (such as race and gender) are more visible, some are more socially "accepted" (such as legal discriminations against gay and lesbian relationships), and some (such as race and class) seem to have greater social salience in terms of the scope and strength of their effect on access to power in multiple areas of living. I have needed to consider more the impact of religious marginalization and struggle. I have been challenged by my coeditors and by my own view of myself as an ally to better understand the history and current ramifications of religion as oppressed status and to find ways to integrate this understanding with my own commitments that focus more on race and ethnicity.

In addition to our differences, we also share roles and statuses as teachers, scholars, spouses, friends, daughters, clinicians. Two of us are mothers, one a grandmother. We share a work ethic, professional integrity and mutual respect, as well as a commitment to social justice. We also share an educational background and professional status. The social class implications of those shared statuses was the basis of some challenging conversations. One challenge related to recognizing our shared privilege with regard to education and career was questioning how much this intellectual engagement itself reflected privilege, and whether we could ever know how much our choices and values had been affected by our educational and career privileges.

As editors, we are committed to challenging ourselves, reflecting on ourselves and others, and holding ourselves accountable for our processes. Although we believe that all of us have multiple identities that change over the lifespan and across social contexts, we became aware throughout this process that we differ in which identity is salient for each of us at different times in our own lives: Gender? Race? Class? Religion? Sexual orientation? Ethnicity? Health status? Generation? Geographical region from where we came?

We began to wonder if our personal meaning of what is salient might be different from what others see about us. Obviously, our students and patients see us in a professional role; their images of what we are like personally may depend on their needs. Thus, as we consider closing here, we thought it would be important to take this opportunity to situate ourselves as editors, within this final reflective chapter:

I (MPM) assume that I am seen, as well as see myself, as a woman with race and class privilege. The fact of that privilege feels indisputable. The question is what I do with the privilege and how can I be an ally. For me, writing is the gift I feel I have been given to truly ally with those of less privilege. My religion and ethnicity are critical to me. I see being Jewish as not only my religion but also my ethnicity. I am aware that Jews of my generation and those who follow have privilege in this country that my parents would have never even imagined, and with that comes the responsibility to advocate for those who are marginalized. I am disturbed that many people whom I see as political allies do not recognize either the lack of privileges held by Jews in many other countries or the growing anti-Semitism in the United States. For me, an awareness of diversity and a commitment to social action are expressions of my religion and ethnicity as well as that of having white privilege.

As a multiracial Asian American woman, I (KLS) am continually uncertain about how others see me and whether my personal meanings are congruent with what is salient about me to others. I have had multiple experiences of exclusion from communities where I feel I should belong (such as Asian American communities) and of acceptance/belonging from communities with which I do not inherently identify (such as Native American communities, where I am frequently seen as belonging to the community because of my appearance). I believe that these experiences contribute to a way of seeing the world that simultaneously recognizes the social importance of boundaries and categorizations while also seeing those boundaries and categorizations as fluid, challengeable, contextual, and constantly interacting. The skills and understandings I have garnered through the earned and unearned privileges of education (related to my unearned class privilege) mean that I am in a position where my worldview can contribute to discussions that can foster resistance to oppression. I am committed to doing so, through my teaching, through my research, and through scholarship such as this that connects social systems with individual experiences and contributes to decreasing the potential negative effects of psychotherapy for marginalized clients.

I (BFO) have been privileged over my professional career to coordinate my roles as teacher, scholar, and practitioner in multiple contexts. Having been the first woman hired in my graduate department before the days of mentors and female colleagues, I have been sensitized to gendered abuse and oppression. I have realized that my privileged class and race have influenced my ability to cope with gender oppression, which in turn has strengthened my commitment to engaging with, and learning from, colleagues and friends of diverse cultures. I have only become attuned to my Jewish identity in the past decade, and being of an older generation, I am gaining perspective on generational differences.

One of the most gratifying aspects of these writing and editing experiences is how our differences have contributed to mutual respect and support. We have become a team wherein the responsibilities, time lines, and productivity are equally balanced, although not equivalent, as we each bring our own strengths and skills. We can agree to disagree and still remain respectful and even fond of each other. We can edit chapters that are stronger because the editing feedback has our multiple perspectives in it (all of the chapters in this book were edited by all of us). And we can write together, as we do in this chapter, in ways that simultaneously reflect our shared vision and our individual and sometimes divergent views.

Future Directions

In each section of this book, we have attempted to present material that considers intersections of contexts and experiences rather than singular categorizations. We are very pleased and excited about the results and feel that this book has much to offer clinicians who treat women. Of course, we could not cover everything in this one book, so at this stage in our process, we want to note the areas that we hope will receive further attention in the future.

A major contribution of the chapters in Part I is the authors' focus on the active incorporation of social justice issues into psychotherapy. Although this incorporation has been endorsed by feminist and multicultural psychotherapy theories and practice, the "hows" of application are just beginning to be explored (Goodman et al., 2004). Our authors discuss the links between the clinician's self-awareness and approach to sharing power, and the clinical work of helping people find their own voice, consciousness raising, focusing on strengths, and promoting coping and action strategies. The authors of Chapters 1 and 2 call our attention to dilemmas of complexity and emphasize reflectiveness and understanding of the impact of therapists' own contexts, privileges, and marginalized experiences on who they are as well as on the process of therapy. As pointed out in Chapter 3, how do we become allies? With our clients? Our professional colleagues? Our employers? Becoming an ally requires acknowledgment of power differentials and conscious commitment to confront power abuses. It requires following through on our commitments after the client leaves our office, perhaps with phone calls, e-mails, or social action.

We see it as a major contribution to have conceptual models that illustrate how clinicians may consider all of the convergences and divergences of multiple intersections. However, as we read these chapters we also see that this can be overwhelming! We wonder how a therapist can be culturally aware and competent, given this complexity. How does a therapist respect intragroup differences as well as intergroup differences? What is the best way to become culturally competent? Some clients from minority and/ or dominant groups may not see these differences as affecting them personally or in their therapy. However, we believe that even if a client does not consciously or immediately see the importance, therapists need to acknowledge and respect these differences in beliefs and value systems in a nonjudgmental manner.

We hope other authors will be inspired to consider how multiple contexts and intersecting identities and systems might affect other formats of psychotherapy, for example, group therapy. We also wonder if it might not be important to consider how individual and family therapy theories and specific orientations hinder or enhance multidiversity perspectives. How can the specific effective components of individual, group, and family therapy theoretical models be developed and expanded to a more ecological perspective?

A major contribution of the chapters in Part II is the focus on differences *within* relationships and the statuses of relationship partners, that is, differences in privilege, in culture/acculturation/generation, in class mobility and status. These chapters make us wonder about choices that affect mobility and connections/disconnections. For example, we wonder if it is ever preferable to remain situated in a working-class environment and identity and not seek upward mobility. Do wealthier or more educated women originally from a working-class background have trouble "fitting in" with people who have been economically privileged or educated for generations? How do race and ethnicity affect the consequences of upward mobility? Chapter 5, for example, brings up issues of whether it is better to love across differences or make active choices to love within homogeneous boundaries in order to maintain other important familial or community relationships.

In the future we would like to encourage that greater attention be given to women's friendships, which become ever so much more central to women as they get older. The vicissitudes and varieties of friendships— some endure, some fade and then reemerge, some are transient, some are work related, some are family related, some are intimate, others more casual—are an important component of women's feelings of connection. We would hope that future discussion about friendships would also include those of women with men as distinct from romantic relationships. Another area we would like to see developed are the strengths and challenges of relationships with people who are seemingly similar in one context, such as race or religion, but different because of another context, such as class or sexual orientation. Investigating these permutations of diversity would also be worthwhile in relation to the therapy relationship.

A strong contribution of all the chapters in Part III is their attention to the cultural aspects of career choice, development, and experience. These chapters also address class issues, disability, sexual orientation, and organizational contexts—issues that are relatively rarely addressed in relation to the experience and meaning of paid work.

In the coming years, we hope to see more scholarly work that focuses on diversity and leadership. How do consultants, for example, help a company to move toward recruiting people of color for management positions? Is the fact that so many women with privilege are opting out of the leadership track in professions and business likely to cause a backlash of deeply ingrained distrust of those women who choose to remain in leadership roles? Will graduate school admissions be affected by reemerging biases concerning women taking up precious slots in professional graduate schools and then leaving the field? Most of the career development theories and counseling models are based on the educated, dominant culture of the U.S. population. Although recent shifts in work practices have produced more flexible career paths, there is still a tendency to match an individual's interests and aptitudes with the "good fit" career or work organization. Do these models consider cultural differences and changing lifestyles? Are these models sensitive to men who enter traditional female positions, such as nursing or preschool teaching? Or to high-achieving and high-status men who wish to work "flexitime" to be more available to their families? Is it easier for a woman to become an engineer than for a man to teach nursery school? These are areas requiring further study.

With more space, time, and authors, we would love to have seen chapters addressing farming and rural work experiences for women, women in modern sweatshops, and women in blue-collar skilled trades. We look forward to seeing these chapters elsewhere.

A major strength of chapters in Part IV lies in their rarity. Chapters in this section address issues not commonly acknowledged as part of women's psychotherapy focus. The authors in these chapters connect our own and our clients' histories with current experiences and emphasize strengths and life balance as the salient psychotherapeutic focus. Because these chapters address uncommon topics, they are more general than chapters addressing topics with well-established foundations of understanding. We look forward to further development and study about women's play, spirituality, community connections, and self-care. For example, within the discussion of spirituality, we hope to see future scholarship develop considerations of non-Christian religions and religious communities as well as alternative healing approaches and their connection to spirituality and religious traditions. Within the discussion of play and self-care we hope to see future scholarship consider, more explicitly and in depth, how play and healthy living vary across class, race, gender, and so on. For example, how is an impoverished woman who works two jobs and also raises several children alone supposed to take time for physical fitness? How do different cultures, races, class, and ethnicities view play and playfulness? What are the rules for expression of feelings? Interpersonal space? Communication? Relationships? How can we avoid overgeneralizing about different groups with whom we have limited contact and experience?

Within the discussion of community, we hope future scholarship might consider how community (both present and historical) contributes to women's health and self-care in multiple racial and ethnic groups. What does community look like in the various racial and ethnic groups? How does social class affect the experience of community as a resource? How are lesbian communities different as resources for women's self-care? How does community help the women in these multiple and diverse groups to resist the negative effects of oppression (e.g., due to legacies of slavery, refugee trauma, colonization, or legalized discrimination)? Within the discussion of health, we hope to see future scholarship develop these ideas further, with greater explicit attention to, and deep development of, the influences of class, race, gender, sexual orientation, disability, and their intersections.

Overall, as editors and clinicians, we realize that the subject matter of this volume needs to be expanded with even more voices and perspectives. New populations emerge steadily, and their perspectives and needs must be incorporated into our theory and practice. For example, transgendered, disabled, Muslim American, and non-Western religious women have perspectives that need to be explored and published. Still other women in our society need broader and deeper consideration, for example, veterans, ex-prisoners, the elderly, and so on.

Furthermore, questions remain related to lifespan developmental issues. Perhaps we need a similar multidiverse intersection lens applied to human developmental issues. We also hope that, in the future, more attention will be paid to global issues, such as the effects of war, global warming, terrorism, and international relations on women's lives, because these issues affect all of our clients.

Finally, although we did not consider issues of training and training models in this volume, we believe strongly that these training models need to broaden their scope to include more diverse research topics and types of study. Our authors are all activists who empower not only their clients but are also involved in social justice advocacy. How can we integrate multidiverse perspectives into our graduate curricula, and how can we help trainees to experience diverse practica and internship placements? In other words, how do we inspire our colleagues and trainees to advocate for social justice as an integral part of professional psychology theory and practice?

Although this volume is a major step forward in exploring cultural and contextual sensitivity, we hope to see many more contributions aimed at expanding the fields of women's studies and women's psychotherapy in line with the always evolving sociocultural contexts. We hope that these readings inspire our colleagues and trainees to develop creative models of empowering psychotherapy that include social justice issues and all aspects of human functioning.

Reference

Goodman, L. A., Liang, B., Helms, J. E., Laira, R. E., Sparks, E., & Weintraub, S. R. (2004). Training counseling psychologists as social justice agents. *The Counseling Psychologist, 32*(6), 795–838.

Index